Emergency Care of the Abused

Emergency Care of the Abused is intended to assist the health care practitioner in managing the acute care of abused patients. Any general practitioner, pediatrician, or emergency physician will appreciate the easy-to-read, accessible information in this book. This book is not intended to be an exhaustive study of each topic, but rather a quick reference and practical guide for those in the clinical arena who see such patients. A wide range of abuse is covered here. Several topics not commonly included in textbooks, such as trafficking, torture, and cultural influences on managing and investigating abuse, are discussed. Each chapter has goals and objectives to maximize educational reading on the topic, photographs and tables to assist the clinician, legal aspects of the emergency situation, and quick reference pages to assist the practitioner who is dealing with an abused patient on an emergency basis.

Fiona E. Gallahue is Assistant Professor of Medicine in the Division of Emergency Medicine at the University of Washington School of Medicine and an emergency medicine physician at Harborview Medical Center in Seattle, Washington.

Laura D. Melville is Assistant Professor of Emergency Medicine at Weill Cornell Medical College and Director of Acute Care for Sexual Abuse, Child Abuse, and Domestic Violence, as well as an emergency medicine physician at New York Methodist Hospital, Brooklyn, New York.

Emergency Care of the Abused

Fiona E. Gallahue
The University of Washington School of Medicine

Laura D. Melville
Weill Cornell Medical College

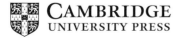

CAMBRIDGE UNIVERSITY PRESS
Cambridge, New York, Melbourne, Madrid, Cape Town, Singapore, São Paulo, Delhi

Cambridge University Press
32 Avenue of the Americas, New York, NY 10013-2473, USA

www.cambridge.org
Information on this title: www.cambridge.org/9780521867078

First published 2008

Printed in the United States of America

A catalog record for this publication is available from the British Library.

Library of Congress Cataloging in Publication Data

Emergency care of the abused / [edited by] Fiona E. Gallahue, Laura D. Melville.
   p.   cm.
Includes bibliographical references and index.
ISBN 978-0-521-86707-8 (hardback)
1. Medical emergencies.   2. Victims of crime – Medical care.   I. Gallahue, Fiona E.
II. Melville, Laura D.   III. Title.
[DNLM: 1. Emergency Medical Services – methods.   2. Crime Victims.
3. Domestic Violence.   4. Forensic Medicine.   5. Sex Offenses. WX 215 E515 2008]
RC86.7.E5628   2008
362.18–dc22   2008016977

ISBN   978-0-521-86707-8 hardback

Every effort has been made in preparing this publication to provide accurate and
up-to-date information that is in accord with accepted standards and practice at the time
of publication. Nevertheless, the authors, editors, and publisher can make no warranties
that the information contained herein is totally free from error, not least because clinical
standards are constantly changing through research and regulation. The authors, editors,
and publisher therefore disclaim all liability for direct or consequential damages
resulting from the use of material contained in this book. Readers are strongly advised to
pay careful attention to infromation provided by the manufacturer of any drugs or
equipment that they plan to use.

Contents

List of Contributors

Ann Botash, M.D., F.A.A.P.
Medical Director
McMahon/Ryan Child Advocacy
  Center

Neelofar K. Butt, M.D.
Instructor of Pediatrics
New York Medical College
Fellow, Child Abuse Pediatrics
Children's Advocacy Center at The
  Westchester Institute for Human
  Development

Jennifer Canter, M.D., M.P.H., F.A.A.P.
Director, Child Protection
Maria Fareri Children's Hospital at
  Westchester Medical Center

Stephanie Cooper, M.D.
Clinical Attending
Harborview Medical Center

Moira Davenport, M.D.
Clinical Attending
Allegheny General Hospital

Fiona Gallahue, M.D., F.A.C.E.P.
Assistant Professor
The University of Washington
  School of Medicine

Jonathan Glauser, M.D., M.B.A.
Assistant Professor
Case Western Reserve University

**Peggy E. Goodman, M.D., M.S.,
  F.A.C.E.P.**
Associate Professor
ECU Emergency Medicine

Laura Melville, M.D.
Assistant Professor
Weill Cornell Medical College
Director of Acute Care for Sexual Abuse,
  Child Abuse, and Domestic Violence
New York Methodist Hospital

**Jamie Hoffman Rosenfeld, M.D.,
  F.A.A.P.**
Medical Director
Queens Child Advocacy Center

Mary Ryan, M.D.
Assistant Professor
Weill Cornell Medical College
Assistant Residency Director
Lincoln Hospital

**Indrani Sheridan, M.D., F.A.C.E.P.,
  F.A.A.E.M.**
Assistant Professor
Director of International Emergency
  Medicine
Department of Emergency
  Medicine
University of Florida School of
  Medicine

United Nations Statement

Article 1

All human beings are born free and equal in dignity and rights. They are endowed with reason and conscience and should act towards one another in a spirit of brotherhood.

Article 2

Everyone is entitled to all . . . rights and freedoms . . . without distinction of any kind, such as race, color, sex, language, religion, political, or other opinion, national or social origin, property, birth, or other status.

Article 3

Everyone has the right to life, liberty, and security of person.

Article 4

No one shall be held in slavery or servitude; slavery and the slave trade shall be prohibited in all their forms.

Article 5

No one shall be subjected to torture or to cruel, inhuman, or degrading treatment or punishment.

Article 25

Motherhood and childhood are entitled to special care and assistance. All children . . . shall enjoy the same social protection.

Taken from the Universal Declaration of Human Rights adopted by the General Assembly of the United Nations on December 10, 1948.

Physical and sexual abuse of children

Jennifer Canter, M.D., M.P.H., F.A.A.P.; Jamie Hoffman Rosenfeld, M.D., F.A.A.P.; Neelofar K. Butt, M.D., and Ann Botash, M.D., F.A.A.P.

Goals and objectives

1. To understand the spectrum of child abuse that exists and may be seen by the clinician
2. To better identify, manage, and refer the child or adolescent who may have been neglected or physically abused
3. To better identify, manage, and refer the child or adolescent who may have been sexually abused

Introduction

Children and adolescent victims of physical abuse, sexual abuse, and/or neglect may initially present to an emergency department or primary care office. The patient–health care provider encounter may have significant emotional, legal, forensic, and medical implications for a child/adolescent and his/her family. In general, the emergency department setting is not ideal for the comprehensive, multidisciplinary assessment of the child/adolescent who may have been abused. Whenever and wherever possible, a coordinated, protocol-based collaboration between an emergency department and the nearest child advocacy center or program is recommended. Nonetheless, the emergency department provider should have a thorough understanding of the detection, triage, management, documentation, and treatment of the maltreated child or adolescent.

Epidemiology

The U.S. Department of Health and Human Services reports that approximately 872,000 children were victims of child maltreatment in 2004.[1] Their report is based on national data collected from child protective services (CPS) agencies in the United States, which were analyzed by the National Child Abuse and Neglect Data

System, the Children's Bureau, Administration on Children, Youth, and Families in the Administration for Children and Families, and the U.S. Department of Health and Human Services. The majority of these children, 62.4 percent, were victims of neglect, 17.5 percent were victims of physical abuse, 9.7 percent suffered sexual abuse, and 7 percent were emotionally abused.[1] Children under three years of age had the highest rate of overall victimization (16.1 per 1,000 children); 72.9 percent of these cases were cases of neglect.[1] Females comprised 51.7 percent of the victims overall.[1] This gender difference in victimization is even more pervasive when looking specifically at sexual abuse, with some reports concluding that females are sexually abused three times more than males.[3] Abused males, however, seemed to be at increased risk for serious harm or injury when compared with females.[3]

In addition to gender differences, racial disparities also exist among child victims. African-American (19.9 per 1,000 children), Pacific Islander (17.6 per 1,000 children), and American Indian or Alaskan Native children (15.5 per 1,000 children) have rates of victimization out of proportion to their percentage within the general population.[1] Asian children had the lowest rate of victimization, 2.9 per 1,000 children, whereas White and Hispanic children had rates of 10.7 and 10.4 per 1,000 children, respectively.[1]

By definition, child abuse is committed by a person legally responsible for the child, such as a parent, caretaker, or guardian; therefore, in the majority of instances, the perpetrator is known to the child. The majority of perpetrators of neglect are mothers, and because neglect is the most common type of child abuse, mothers are the most common perpetrators of maltreatment.[1] Ninety percent of sexual abuse is committed by males and by individuals known to the child, with family members representing one-third to one-half of the perpetrators against girls and 10 to 20 percent of the perpetrators against boys.[2]

In 2004, a total of 1,490 children died as a result of abuse or neglect, with more than one-third of these deaths being ascribed to neglect.[1] Of these child fatalities, more than 80 percent of the children were under four years of age.[1] The aforementioned data do not take into account victimization of children by persons not legally responsible, including child-on-child abuse, "stranger" abuse, and certain authority figures that are not recognized as legally responsible under state law. Thus, as staggering as these statistics are, these numbers are derived solely from reported cases to CPS agencies and, therefore, may be a significant underestimation of the true scope of the problem.

Reporting child maltreatment

Although the role and right of families to raise children as they see fit is honored in the United States, the state has the right to intervene if a child is not protected from preventable harm. The federal government demonstrated its commitment to issues of child protection with the establishment of the Children's Bureau in 1912. The Child Abuse Prevention and Treatment Act (CAPTA), a key federal law established in 1974, ensures that victimized children are identified and reported to appropriate authorities.

All states have the responsibility, under CAPTA, to comply with child maltreatment guidelines and have enacted child maltreatment laws that define the parent–child relationship, the role of mandated reporters, and the specific tasks of the Child Protection Agency, the Civil Court, and the Criminal Court. Because each individual state has some autonomy in the design of the specific regulations for reporting and response to maltreatment, it is important for professionals to be familiar with the child protection structure in their own states. A summary of state reporting laws is available at the State Statutes section of the National Clearinghouse on Child Abuse and Neglect website (www.calib.com/nccanch/statutes).

Although there are some differences among states, most reporting laws define and identify which professionals are recognized as mandated reporters; enumerate the criteria and the threshold for reporting; and describe the reporting process, the response to a report of child maltreatment, and penalties for failure to report. The following are general principles of the Child Protection Process:

1. Identification

The first step in the process is the identification of children who have been subjected to maltreatment or who are at significant risk of maltreatment. Medical providers, particularly those whose jobs place them on the front line, must be familiar with the definitions of sexual abuse, physical abuse, and neglect. A recent study by Flaherty and Sege[4] revealed that physicians under-identify and under-report child abuse, leaving children at risk for victimization and harm. The authors of this study conclude that identification and reporting of child abuse can be improved by a program of continuing education that covers not only identification but also information about child protective interventions and outcomes.

2. Reporting

State laws generally define what conditions are reportable; how, when, and by whom a report should be made; the duty to share information; as well as the boundaries of information sharing. In most states, reports are made orally, generally via telephone, although many states require that a written report follow. Reports must be made promptly and based on suspicion because a delay in reporting for confirmation or "proof" may be placing a child at imminent risk.

3. Mandatory reporters

Those individuals who are mandated reporters risk civil and criminal liability for failure to report. Any person may make a report of child abuse or neglect to the agency that is authorized to receive such reports. In 18 states, any person who suspects child abuse is required to make a report. In the majority of states, however, mandated reporters are those individuals who suspect child abuse from an interaction in their professional capacity. Physicians and other health care professionals are always included among the list of mandated reporters. Although the specific language may differ from state to state, a report must be made when the reporter has reasonable cause to know, suspect, or believe that a child has been abused or neglected.

The response to a report of suspected maltreatment

In most states, the Child Protection Agency is authorized to receive reports of suspected child abuse. Some states require that certain types of abuse, such as sexual abuse and severe physical abuse, are reported to both Child Protection and law enforcement. In most states, when the Child Protection Agency receives a report there is a system in place for information to be shared with law enforcement and the prosecutor's office when appropriate. After a report is made, there is an initial screening procedure that determines whether the information meets the state's statutory and agency definitions of maltreatment as well as the urgency of the investigation.

Penalties for failing to make a report and immunity provisions for reporters

To encourage reporting and eliminate perceived barriers to reporting, state statutes provide protection for reporters by conferring immunity from civil lawsuits, if a report is made in "good faith". On the other hand, most states impose penalties for mandated reporters who knowingly or willfully fail to report suspected abuse. In general, failure to report is a misdemeanor. Information sharing is generally protected by statute such that medical providers who make a report are not only permitted to share relevant medical information but are also required to cooperate with the investigation.

Child protection teams and child advocacy centers

One of the most significant changes in the field of Child Maltreatment over the past two decades has come about with the recognition that child abuse is not an issue that falls exclusively within the purview of the medical, social service, or legal fields. National, State, and local efforts to create integrated and collaborative models to address this complex issue have emerged. Concomitant with the development of collaborative programs was the emergence of Child Abuse Pediatrics as a subspecialty within Pediatric Medicine. In June 2005, the American Board of Pediatrics (ABP) accepted a petition to begin a new subspecialty within pediatrics certified by the ABP. Child Abuse Pediatricians, or forensic pediatricians, provide children, families, and communities with expertise in the recognition and management of child abuse, provide consultation to child protection and law enforcement professionals, participate on multidisciplinary teams, engage in child abuse research, and serve as medical directors of child advocacy centers.

Multidisciplinary teams are the result of community cooperation in an effort to provide a coordinated response to suspected child maltreatment. Through interagency agreements and established guidelines, teams work together to investigate and prosecute child abuse as well as protect children from ongoing harm. The objective of this collaborative model is to lessen the trauma to the child/adolescent victim and their families by reducing the number of times that a child is interviewed, minimizing duplicative services as well as enhancing communication and information sharing among involved agencies. The core membership of multidisciplinary teams includes professionals from child protective services, law enforcement agencies, local prosecutor's offices, victim advocacy groups, and medical experts. Broader membership might include participation by Departments of Education, domestic violence agencies, and disability agencies.

Hospital-based child protection teams are essential to the proper detection, reporting, coordination, and management of abuse cases. These may include a pediatrician or child abuse pediatrician, social work services specifically trained in the field of child abuse, an administrative unit (particularly for a children's hospital), and other health professionals, such as psychologists.

Child advocacy centers provide a centralized, child-friendly venue for the work of the multidisciplinary team. Although models differ throughout the country, child advocacy centers generally provide a single site for investigation, provision of victim support, and other mental health services, as well as expert medical evaluation. The National Children's Alliance website (www.nca-online.org) provides information on advocacy centers as well as listings of those certified through the organization across the United States.

Although acute care settings such as emergency departments will often be the point of initial recognition of child maltreatment, they are not appropriate locations for the conduction of an investigation including forensic interviews of children. In addition, expert medical services are not necessarily available in those acute care facilities. Every primary care practice/program and emergency department must have a triage algorithm that includes clear guidelines for how to respond to suspected maltreatment. The decision tree outlines which cases must be evaluated at the time of presentation and which cases can be referred for evaluation to a child protection team or child advocacy center. Specific information about effective and appropriate triage is included in sections on physical and sexual abuse elsewhere in this chapter.

General history taking

Taking a history and effective triage in child or adolescent abuse
Effective triage
> *Adapted from www.childabusemd.com*
>
> Once a child or adolescent presents for an evaluation due to a concerning physical sign or symptom, worrisome behavioral sign or symptom, or because they have made a statement that suggests that they have been abused, the medical provider must proceed with caution to avoid the "runaway train" scenario that may develop if a report to child protective services or law enforcement agency is triggered inappropriately or prematurely. Effective triage requires that the provider do the following:

- Gather and document pertinent information
- Determine the safety and welfare of the child/adolescent
- Determine who should examine the child/adolescent and when
- Determine whether you are mandated to report this situation

Gather and document pertinent information
> The importance of a careful and detailed history cannot be emphasized enough. In a stepwise fashion, the reason for the abuse concern must be understood. The presenting caregiver must provide the answers to the following questions:

1. Who are you and what is your relationship to the child/adolescent?
2. What is your reason for concern regarding abuse?
   - Is this a referral from a child abuse investigative agency?
   - Have you witnessed the abuse?
   - Did the child/adolescent disclose abuse? If so, to whom was the disclosure made? What are the exact words the child/adolescent used?
3. Who is the suspected perpetrator and what is that person's relationship to the child/adolescent?
4. Does the child/adolescent live with the suspected abuser or have regular contact with that person? Is the child/adolescent safe from the suspected perpetrator now?
5. Are you safe? Do you think your present situation is dangerous?
6. Is there a medical concern such as pain, bruising, bleeding, alteration in mental status, acute change in behavior, or possible pregnancy?
7. When was the last time that the child/adolescent had contact with the suspected perpetrator?

Determine the safety and welfare of the child or adolescent

As the responses to the above questions are being gathered, the provider must have the safety of the child or adolescent foremost in his or her mind. If there is any indication that the suspect has accompanied the child for the medical visit, he/she must be separated from the patient. This might be done by bringing the patient into the exam room while asking the adults to remain in the waiting area. If there is any chance of a dangerous situation developing, the facility's security should be called or local law enforcement contacted by dialing 911 if necessary. If the decision is made that the patient needs to be sent to another facility, for example, a child advocacy center, for evaluation, utmost care must be taken to arrange for and assure safe transport. If the child is being referred to another facility, the transfer of accurate and complete information is as important as the safe transport of the child. If the accepting institution does not understand the referral source's concern about abuse, effective evaluation and treatment will be jeopardized.

Determine the most appropriate location for evaluation and the most appropriate provider to conduct the evaluation

It goes without saying that the very first step is to determine whether the child or adolescent is medically stable. Any and all investigatory steps may need to be delayed if the child requires emergency medical treatment.

If the child/adolescent has any of the following and has presented to a primary care office setting, a local emergency response team should be notified with appropriate referral to an emergency department.

- Unstable vital signs
- Symptoms of head trauma: vomiting, headache, syncope, lethargy, visual disturbance
- Symptoms of abdominal injury: vomiting, abdominal pain, bruising to the abdomen/flank/back, hematuria
- Symptoms or history of recent traumatic sexual contact: bleeding from the vagina or rectum, genital pain, or other signs of injury

If a sexual abuse incident has occurred within 96 hours and the child/adolescent is medically stable, refer to the appropriate local resource, emergency department, or specialized center for forensic evidence collection.

The nature of sexual abuse is such that most exams are not an emergency. There are powerful disincentives for children to disclose, therefore sexual abuse of children often comes to medical attention after a delay. If the child/adolescent is safe, the examination can usually be deferred until the next working day. Making a report to CPS and/or an appropriate law enforcement agency cannot be deferred. In areas where there is an effective multidisciplinary response to child maltreatment or a child advocacy center, the coordinated investigation and medical exam may be deferred in some cases once there has been an assessment of immediate risk. If there is a local child abuse expert, refer the child/adolescent to that medical provider. If this is not an option, proper photo documentation and clear medical record documentation of the examination are essential so that a forensic pediatrician can interpret the findings. If your facility does not offer the appropriate services for medical care, determine which facility offers the best services for this child/adolescent and family.

Determine whether you are mandated to make a report

A discussion of mandated reporting is located elsewhere in this chapter.

Physical abuse

Cutaneous manifestations of abuse

Cutaneous manifestations of child physical abuse include abrasions, bruises, lacerations, burns, oral injuries, and bite marks. Labbe and colleagues evaluated 1,467 children and adolescents aged 0 to 17 from the general population and noted that over 75 percent of nonabused children had at least one recent skin injury and 17 percent of the total sample had at least five injuries.[5] This same study demonstrated that children under eight months of age rarely had skin injuries, a finding echoed by Sugar and colleagues who found bruising extremely rare in infants younger than six months.[6] This study led to the commonly voiced axiom, "Those who don't cruise, rarely bruise." In other words, the assessment of any injury must take into account the developmental stage of the infant or child. In pre-ambulatory infants, the opportunities to bruise are few. Although the clinician must always consider non-visible signs of trauma, up to 90 percent of physical abuse victims present with discernible skin manifestations.[7]

To distinguish physical abuse from accidental or medical conditions, the clinician must consider location, number, and patterns of injury as well as underlying medical conditions, presenting history, and developmental capabilities of the child or adolescent.

Contusions, lacerations, and abrasions

A contusion represents hemorrhage into the skin secondary to blunt trauma. Contusions that are diffuse are referred to as bruises, and those that are focal, as hematomas. A laceration represents tearing of the skin secondary to crushing, cutting, or shearing forces. An abrasion, or "scrape," is removal of superficial skin layers secondary to friction.

Bruises are the most common type of injury seen in children greater than eight months of age; in infants less than eight months of age, scratches are the predominant type of injury.[5] The most common location for accidental bruising in mobile children is the anterior tibia or knee, followed by the forehead, scalp, and upper leg, with accidental bruising in all age groups most commonly found over bony prominences.[6]

Bruising in protected areas of the body, such as hands, ears, neck, buttocks, medial and posterior thighs, and upper arms, should raise concern for physical abuse. Although forehead bruising is commonly, seen bruises located primarily on the facial soft tissues, such as, cheeks, should raise concern because the bony facial structures project making them the most likely points of impact. As mentioned previously, bruising in babies and children who are not independently mobile is rare and should also raise concern.

There are clearly identifiable patterns of injury that may be evident while examining a child. Emergency department clinicians should be familiar with pattern injuries and the objects used to produce them.

The appearance of a bruise depends on site of injury, depth of tissue, skin complexion, age, and characteristics of each individual's inherent healing capabilities. Therefore, visual dating of bruises has been demonstrated to be inexact,[8,9] although an assessment of acute or fresh vs. old may be made by the experienced examiner. In contrast to bruises that are in the advanced stage of resolution, fresh bruises may be accompanied by tenderness, swelling, and palpable induration. The presence of bruises at multiple stages of healing should raise concern because this suggests multiple episodes of inflicted injury.

Bite marks

The presence of abrasions, ecchymoses, or lacerations in an elliptical or ovoid pattern should raise concern for abuse as they may be indicative of bite marks. The positive pressure created by the closing of teeth, or the negative pressure created by suction, often creates a central area of contusion. As opposed to animal bites, which tear flesh, human bites compress flesh. Human bites rarely lead to avulsion of tissue. The general medical provider is cautioned about attempting to make a determination of whether a bite is from an adult or child though they may feel pressured to do so. The intercanine distance is the linear distance between the central point of the cuspid tip and will measure more than 3.0 cm in an adult and less than 2.5 in a child; this measurement should only be made by a professional who has been trained to do so.[10] Bite marks should be evaluated by a forensic odontologist (or a forensic pathologist if an odontologist is not available).

These specially trained professionals may be of assistance in evaluating the pattern, size, contour, and color of the bite mark. If none is available, a physician or dentist with experience in child abuse should photographically document the bite mark with an identification tag and scale marker. The photograph should be taken so that the camera lens is over the bite and perpendicular to the plane of the bite. The American Board of Forensic Odontology (ABFO) created a special photographic scale for this purpose, which is available at www.abfo.org. A polyvinyl siloxane impression of the bite mark should be made only after, in acute cases, the mark is swabbed for DNA through proper forensic techniques (see below). Some authors suggest daily photographs for at least three days to document the evolution of the bite.

As mentioned, DNA evidence may be obtained from fresh bites. Also, blood-group substances can be secreted in saliva. Even if saliva and cells have dried, they should be collected by using the double-swab technique as follows:

1. A sterile cotton swab moistened with distilled water is used to wipe the area in question, dried, and placed in a specimen tube.
2. A second sterile, dry cotton swab cleans the same area and then is dried and placed in a specimen tube.
3. A third control sample should be obtained from an uninvolved area of the child's skin. All samples should be sent to a certified forensic laboratory for prompt analysis.[11]

Burns

Epidemiology

Inflicted burns are mostly seen in younger children with the majority being less than two years of age.[12] Burns comprise approximately 10 percent of all cases of child abuse.[13] Moreover, 10 percent of children with burns requiring admission to an inpatient burn unit have inflicted injuries. Compared with children who present with accidental burn injuries, children with inflicted burns tend to be significantly younger and have higher mortality rates.[12]

The hallmark of a first-degree burn result is erythema of the epidermis; medical conditions such as cellulitis, erysipelas, sunburns, contact dermatitis, rash from a drug reaction, and diaper rash may mimic the appearance of first-degree burns. Second-degree burns extend into the dermal layer and cause erythema and blister formation; medical conditions that involve blistering may mimic second-degree burns, such as bullous impetigo, Staphylococcal scalded skin syndrome, toxic epidermal necrolysis, Epidermolysis bullosa, phytophotodermatitis, and varicella.

Third-degree burns involve the entire dermis with destruction of all the dermal appendages, including nerves, and are typically insensate.

Thermal injuries and imitators

Scald burns comprise the most common type of inflicted burn in children.[14,15] If a scald burn results from forcible immersion of a child, there may be a bilateral or symmetric distribution that is typically circumferential, described as a "stocking-glove" distribution; the entire burn is generally uniform in depth due to the dunking of the affected body part in a standing body of liquid. Typically, immersion burns will have minimal or no splash marks which would be expected if the mechanism was one of a splash or spill.[14,15] Burns of the perineum and buttocks may occur with sparing of the skin in the intertriginous folds and other areas where the skin is in close opposition because of the child's flexed position. An area of central sparing of the buttocks may reflect that the child was forcibly held down against the cooler surface of a tub or sink which had a protective effect.[14,15] Accidental splash burn injuries do occur in ambulatory children, but because the hot liquid cools as it runs down the surface of the body, these types of burns tend to be non-uniform in shape and depth, with irregular borders that are more superficial.[14] Studies of temperature vs. duration of exposure have demonstrated that, at sufficiently high temperatures, significant burns can occur in a matter of seconds. As a result of these studies, the American Academy of Pediatrics recommends that home hot water heaters be set at a maximal temperature of 120 degrees Fahrenheit. People who live in apartments, however, may not have the ability to regulate their own hot water temperatures, and children may fall victim to water temperature that has changed abruptly due to someone else in the building flushing a toilet. Providers should ask about the hot water realities in the home.

Contact injuries and imitators

When a hot object is brought into contact with skin, a contact burn results. Often the appliance or object used is suggested by the pattern or imprint of the burn injury, such as an iron, curling iron, or hair dryer. Cigarette burns are typically well-demarcated, circular, full thickness burns which acutely develop a black eschar that subsequently granulates inwards, resulting in the healed appearance of a crater-like or punched-out lesion. Accidental cigarette burns are typically ovoid "brushed lesions" and are more superficial.[14,15] There are some traditional folk medicine practices that may mimic abusive contact burn injuries. Moxibustion is an Asian practice that involves burning incense, yarn, or herbs on the skin's surface.[14] Cao-Gio or coin-rubbing is a Vietnamese practice that involves the placement of hot coins on the skin. Cupping is a practice that involves placing a cup on the skin after the rim is brushed with alcohol and ignited, which may create circular burns with ecchymotic central areas.[14]

Other burns and imitators

Inflicted chemical burns usually result from forced ingestion or splashing of caustic substances, such as sulfuric acid and hydrochloric acid, or alkalis, such as lye and calcium chloride. Electrical burns result from the combination of heat with the

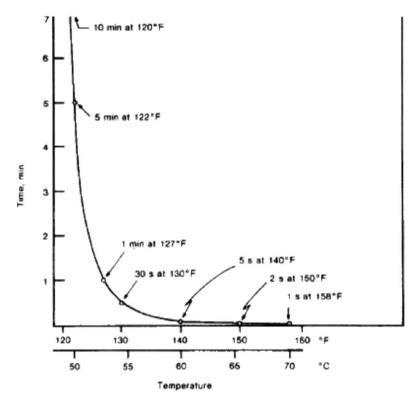

Figure 1.1   Relationship of water temperature and time of exposure to burn depth. This graph
demonstrates the duration of exposure required at different water temperatures to cause
superficial partial thickness burns of adults. (Derived from original data from Moritz and
Henriques[26], and reproduced from Katcher ML. Scald burns from hot tap water. *JAMA.*
1981; 246: 219–22, with permission.)

direct effect of polarization of molecules in the tissue. Cutaneous burns from stun
guns usually consist of a pair of small superficial circular marks.

Oral injuries

Injuries to the face, head, and neck occur in over half of child abuse cases.[16,17]
Therefore, a thorough intraoral and perioral examination is necessary in all cases
of suspected abuse and neglect.

Oral injuries may be inflicted with instruments, and therefore, the examiner
should pay careful attention to patterns. Documentation of oral injuries is often
challenging; a dentist or otolaryngologist may be a valuable asset in collaborating
with optimal documentation.

The lips were the most common location for non-accidental oral injuries (54%) in one study see color inserts.[18] The presence of discolored teeth indicates necrosis of the pulp and may be secondary to previous trauma.[19,20] Bruises or scarring at the mouth corners may represent gagging.[21]

Visible injuries to the oral cavity are rare in sexual abuse, even though oral–genital contact is a common form.[19] When oral–genital contact is suspected, children should, whenever possible, be referred to specialized clinical settings, such as child advocacy centers, that are equipped to conduct comprehensive examinations.

Fractures

Non-accidental fractures represent a serious form of physical abuse and are the second most common presentation of inflicted childhood injury.[22] Up to 55 percent of seriously abused children will have fractures identified on evaluation.[23–25] Most of the fractures occur in children less than three years of age and approximately 80 percent in the 18 months and younger age group.[26] Much of what we understand about abusive skeletal injury is extrapolated from the literature on accidental fractures and the mechanisms and forces required to produce those fractures.

Forty to eighty percent of extremity fractures in children less than 12 months of age result from non-accidental trauma.[27] It is critical to have a basic understanding of the biomechanics of extremity fractures in children in order to assess the consistency between the type of injury and the explanation for the fracture provided in the history.[27] Whether a given force results in a fracture, and the particular "fracture morphology"[27] that results, depends not only on the strength and vector of the force and the rate at which it is applied, but also on the characteristics of the bone impacted.[27] Bone mass and density, which are affected by the extent of bone mineralization, are directly related to the strength of bone. Bones of children differ from those of adults in that they are less mineralized and the periosteal membrane is more loosely attached and more vascular than adult bones.[27] Furthermore, the areas of transition between the metaphyseal and cortical areas of bone are especially vulnerable to compression injury, which usually manifest as the typical "bucket handle" fracture.[27]

Mechanism and developmental level play a critical role in discerning accidental from abusive injury.

Certain types of skeletal injury, such as metaphyseal fractures and rib fractures, are highly associated with non-accidental trauma.[28] According to one study, rib fractures had a 95 percent positive predictive value as an indicator for non-accidental trauma.[28] In this same study, rib fractures were the only manifestation of physical abuse in 29 percent of cases.[28] In abused infants, CPR may be proposed as a potential explanation for rib fractures that have been discovered on skeletal survey. In several studies, CPR has not been implicated as a cause of rib fractures in infants and should not be accepted as a plausible explanation, particularly when the history does not reveal that CPR was ever performed.[29–32] The absence of rib fractures from CPR is most likely related to the elasticity of the infantile rib cage. When determining the consistency between the historical account and the injury, it is important to remember that certain types of fractures are generally associated with greater magnitudes of force; these include displaced, transverse, and comminuted long bone fractures, as well as fractures of the femoral neck.[27] Whereas a fall on an outstretched arm in a mobile child may result in a buckle fracture to the arm, buckle fractures in children less than nine months of age are uncommonly accidental because of the fact that infants are non-ambulatory.[27] Bucket handle and corner fractures are descriptions of radiographic patterns of metaphyseal injury that are considered "pathognomonic" for abuse or non-accidental trauma. These characteristic inflicted fractures result from a transmetaphyseal disruption of the bony trabeculae[33] at the ends of long bones. These types of lesions usually result from shearing forces that occur when a child is violently pulled or shaken while being held by the trunk or extremities.[27,33] Mild injury may produce either subtle or absent radiological changes, whereas moderately severe force frequently results in the characteristic corner fractures and bucket handle appearance.[33] Fraying of the metaphyseal region may result from repeated injury.[33] The direction of the forces required to produce the classic metaphyseal lesion are such that these types of fractures are not seen as the result of appropriate handling of infants or from accidental means.

Spiral fractures result when a bone is rotated along its longitudinal axis. This type of injury has also traditionally been thought to be highly associated with non-accidental trauma. However, the finding of a spiral fracture is not necessarily diagnostic of physical abuse as this injury may occur in accidental settings, such as when a child trips while running or from a stair fall.[27,34] Integral in the determination of whether a spiral fracture is the result of an accident or from abuse is the required element of twisting or torque around the long axis of the extremity. In the running child, there is often a history that the foot is planted or entrapped and the fall occurs with a twisting motion around the fulcrum that is created by the foot. Stair falls can result in femur fractures in children, especially if the caregiver falls with the child.[34] Spiral fractures of the femur usually only occur as a result of a stair fall in ambulatory children associated with a history of their leg twisting beneath them as they fell.[34] Complex fracture morphologies, such as comminuted fractures and classic metaphyseal lesions, with an accompanying history of a stair fall should always be cause for a high index of suspicion of non-accidental trauma.[34] It is also important to note that a significant amount of energy is needed to result in transverse and oblique fractures; therefore, their presence within the historical context of an uncomplicated stair fall should also prompt an assessment for possible non-accidental trauma.[34]

A transverse fracture occurs when the fracture line is perpendicular to the long axis of the bone.[27] This type of fracture is frequently associated with non-accidental trauma[27] and may be the result of the extremity having been directly impacted with an object. Transverse fractures may also occur when a child falls from a significant height or if the caretaker falls down steps with the child in their arms.[27] In one study of childhood femur fractures, transverse fractures were more common in the abuse group, yet spiral fractures were more commonly reported as suspicious for non-accidental injury.[35] The authors concluded that, by having a higher index of suspicion for abuse when faced with spiral femur fractures, abusive transverse fractures may be missed.[35]

In summary, one must consider presenting history and developmental capabilities when evaluating fractures, particularly in small children. The skeletal survey is a valuable tool in these situations and should be routine in children under three years of age if abuse is being considered. Further, one must always consider bone mineralization defects before concluding that a fracture is secondary to abuse; a child abuse pediatrician and an evaluation outside of the emergency department setting are recommended in these circumstances.

Medical Conditions that Predispose a Child to Fractures:

Osteogenesis Imperfecta
Menkes' Kinky Hair Syndrome
Congenital Syphilis
Congenital Indifference to Pain
Drug Therapy (Prostaglandin therapy, MTX therapy, Phenobarbital, and
   Phenytoin)

Shaken Baby Syndrome (SBS)

Child abuse is the leading cause of serious head injury in infants,[36] and head injury is the most common cause of child abuse deaths.[37] Each year, a total of 1,400 American children require medical attention for shaking injuries; 21 percent die, and 43 percent suffer serious sequelae.[38] Many new parents lack experience and coping skills to deal with crying babies, and some react with a physical response that can have permanent and tragic consequences. Recent literature suggests that

Table 1.1 Common types of fractures seen in childhood

The specificity of radiological findings and abuse

High specificity
- Classic metaphyseal lesions
- Rib fractures, especially posterior
- Scapular fractures
- Spinous process fractures
- Sternal fractures
- Any infant with an unexplained fracture

Moderate specificity
- Multiple fractures, especially bilateral
- Fractures of different ages
- Epiphyseal separations
- Vertebral body fractures and subluxations
- Digital fractures
- Complex skull fractures

Common but low specificity
- Subperiosteal new bone formation
- Clavicular fractures
- Long bone shaft fractures
- Linear skull fractures

up to 6 percent of parents of six-month-old infants have smothered, slapped, or shaken their baby at least once because of its crying.[39]

Pediatric radiologist John Caffey first described "whiplash shaken baby syndrome" in 1972, referring to a spectrum of clinical findings in young babies, including subdural and/or subarachnoid hemorrhage and retinal hemorrhages, often with little or no signs of external cranial or other trauma.[40] In 1971, Guthkelch[41] postulated that acceleration–deceleration, or whiplash forces, resulted in subdural hematomas due to the tearing of cortical bridging veins.

Shaken baby syndrome most often involves children younger than two years, but may be seen in children up to five years of age or older.[42–45] There is a spectrum of clinical severity, and symptoms may go unrecognized when they are less serious and when caretakers, who are not responsible for the injuries, are unaware of the traumatic forces that the infant was subjected to. For these reasons, SBS must feature prominently on the differential when an infant or young child presents with symptoms such as lethargy, irritability, and vomiting. Most often, there is a lack of external evidence of trauma, thereby making thorough radiological and clinical assessment critical.

Table 1.2 Criteria for determining biomechanical and fracture type compatibility (biomechanical match)[34]

Biomechanical conditions[15]	Fracture types	Biodynamic history examples
Torsional loading	Spiral/long oblique	Twisting or rotation of leg as child slips and leg folds underneath body
Bending load	Transverse/short oblique	Perpendicular impact of leg such as leg caught between stair and caretaker
Compressive loading	Buckle/impaction	Knee impacts along longitudinal axis of femur as child falls down stairs
Tension and/or shear loading	CML	Pulling or yanking of leg
High-energy event (any loading condition)	Open and/or comminuted	Pedestrian leg impacted by fast-moving vehicle

Shaking of an infant resulting in this syndrome is violent, and the reasonable observer would recognize this as dangerous. Routine childcare activities, such as bouncing a baby on the knee, do not result in SBS. Similarly, there is no peer-reviewed scientific literature that demonstrates short falls, seizures, or vaccinations as a cause for SBS. Shaking alone, or shaking with impact, have both been proven to result in the injuries seen in SBS.[46–48]

Caretakers who are experiencing stress as a result of sleep deprivation or environmental, social, biological, or financial hardships are more at risk for the loss of control that may result in shaking. Children living in homes with domestic violence and/or substance abuse may also be at higher risk of SBS.

Shaken baby syndrome is uncommonly an isolated incident as up to 40 percent of all cases have evidence of prior intracranial injury from shaking.[49,50] Males are more frequently the perpetrators in SBS, which is the case with other forms of physical abuse as well.[42,51]

The shaken infant may present with nonspecific symptoms, such as vomiting and irritability, or more severe symptoms, such as seizures. The SBS victim may have a several-day history of vomiting; change in behavior, such as lethargy or irritability; and/or poor feeding. Establishing the time of symptom onset is the most accurate way to establish the time frame for when an injury occurred. The emergency department clinician's history and documentation thereof may play a critical role in understanding the timeline of the child's condition. A carefully recorded timeline obtained through collaborative efforts of medical and investigative professionals is paramount. Ideally, the sooner a multidisciplinary approach is elicited, the better the investigative and protective outcomes. In rural or medically underserved areas in which one or more of these specialists is not available, a regional consultation network for child abuse cases should be developed. With prompt notification, law enforcement and child protective investigators may be able to explore the scene of the injury and elicit a detailed history from the caretakers.

The medical evaluation of the shaken infant includes meticulous and thorough assessment for other traumatic injuries, such as rib or long bone fractures, bruises, and abdominal injuries. Any external signs of trauma should be properly photographed. All children with possible inflicted head trauma should have a dilated retinal examination by a pediatric ophthalmologist, pediatric neurologist, pediatric neurosurgeon, or other experienced physician who is familiar with such hemorrhages and has the proper equipment.[44,45,52] Retinal hemorrhages that are multilayered and extensive have a high diagnostic specificity for SBS and the number, character, location, and size should be recorded.

Xanthochromic cerebral spinal fluid from an atraumatic spinal tap for the evaluation of meningitis should raise suspicion of cerebral trauma. Clotting abnormalities associated with cerebral trauma should be fully evaluated at the time of presentation and thereafter to assure resolution or diagnose a potential underlying disorder.

Although a CT scan may fail to uncover details of intracranial injury,[53] it remains the first-line imaging study for the child with suspected intracranial hemorrhage. The non-contrast CT scan should be completed with bone and soft-tissue windows as an integral part of the assessment. The use of MRI as an adjunct to CT is now routine in the evaluation of SBS.[54] MRI can be of great value in evaluating potential repeated or old injuries due to variations in the presentation of hemoglobin on the scan.[53]

A skeletal survey including skull films should be obtained once the child is medically stable. Skull films are an important adjunct to CT bone windows as they may add greatly to the ability to detect skull fractures.[55] Although simple linear skull fractures may occur with minor household trauma, when skull fractures are multiple, bilateral, diastatic, or so extensive that they cross suture lines, they are more likely to be abusive in nature.[55] A repeat skeletal survey two weeks after the first study has also been demonstrated to be of great value as some acute fractures may not be detectable on the initial study.[54]

Children who survive severe braininjury may have cortical blindness, seizure disorders, and other severe neurologic outcomes.[53]

A child abuse pediatrician may be a helpful adjunct to the evaluation of a child with potential SBS, specifically in excluding medical conditions that may mimic elements of SBS. For example, one must exclude the possibilities of perinatal trauma and coagulation disorders before attributing a subdural hematoma exclusively to abuse.

Abdominal injuries

Abdominal trauma is the second most common cause of death in cases of child physical abuse. The overall mortality rate of inflicted abdominal injuries in child physical abuse is reportedly between 40 and 50 percent[56]; this is likely due to the fact that even extensive visceral injury may have little or no immediate external signs or symptoms, often resulting in delayed identification.[56] Although perforation of a hollow viscus, such as the stomach, small intestine, or colon, rarely occurs in accidental trauma, it has been reported as a result of inflicted abdominal injury in children. The liver is frequently affected in cases of both abusive and severe accidental blunt abdominal trauma, such as a motor vehicle accident.[57] Coant[56] studied 49 children who had no evidence of abdominal trauma, but were suspected of being abused; four children had elevated liver enzymes, three of whom had evidence of liver lacerations when a CT scan was done. This study illustrated the value of liver transaminases as a screen for occult liver injury. The pancreas may also be injured from inflicted abdominal trauma and may result in pancreatitis, as well as some of the known complications associated with pancreatitis, such as traumatic pancreatic pseudocyst.

Possible signs and symptoms of abdominal injury include: abdominal tenderness or distension, bruising of the abdomen, absent or decreased bowel sounds, occult bleeding as evidenced by hypotension, low hematocrit, hematuria, or the presence of blood in the stool or nasogastric aspirate. Because even extensive abdominal injury may be clinically silent, it is important to have a low threshold for completing a comprehensive laboratory and imaging evaluation in order to detect occult abdominal injuries; laboratory studies should include a complete blood count with platelets, AST, ALT, alkaline phosphatase, amylase, lipase, urinalysis, and stool guaiac. Abdominal radiographs may detect free air from injury that resulted in the perforation of hollow viscera, and therefore if ordered, must include at least two views of the abdomen with an upright, cross-table lateral, or left lateral decubitus view in addition to the supine view. Plain films alone, however, are not adequate to determine the presence or absence of intra-abdominal injury. Computed tomography of the abdomen with and without contrast is necessary as this imaging study can identify occult solid organ injury, such as liver and splenic lacerations.

Once abdominal injury is identified in a child, it is critical to ascertain whether the mechanism of injury was accidental or intentional. Whereas the history and the consistency of the historical account with the type and severity of injury are still paramount in making this determination, some studies have identified some additional features that may be helpful; Ledbetter and colleagues[58] reported that inflicted visceral injury was more common in younger children with injuries to hollow viscera, who presented with vague histories and had delayed medical care. In this same study, children with abusive abdominal injuries were also noted to have a higher mortality rate (53%) compared with those who sustained accidental abdominal trauma (21%). Price and colleagues, however, reported that liver lacerations were the most common injury (52%) in their review of 33 fatal cases of inflicted blunt visceral trauma.[59] Thirty-three percent of cases had mesenteric injury, 30 percent showed small bowel injury, 15 percent had injury to the pancreas, and 6 percent had evidence of adrenal injury.[59]

Diagnostic imaging

Skeletal survey

Appropriate diagnostic imaging is essential in the evaluation of infants and children who present to the emergency room with physical injury. In cases of suspected child abuse, diagnostic imaging not only defines the extent of physical injury in the acute setting, but can also provide evidence of occult or previous injury, thereby increasing the clinical suspicion of non-accidental trauma. The assessment of skeletal trauma is especially important as the detection of occult or multiple fractures is a strong indicator of abuse.[60,61] Furthermore, certain types of skeletal injury, such as rib fractures and metaphyseal lesions, are highly associated with non-accidental trauma.[60,62,63]

The skeletal survey is used as a screening tool in cases of suspected child abuse for the detection of occult or prior injury. The standard skeletal survey recommended by the American Academy of Pediatrics consists of bilateral anteroposterior (AP) views of the humeri, forearms, femurs, lower legs, and feet; an oblique posteroanterior (PA) view of the hands; AP and lateral views of the thorax; an AP view of the pelvis, including the mid and lower lumbar spine; lateral views of the cervical and lumbar spines; and two views, frontal and lateral, of the skull.[60] The addition of two oblique views of the thorax increases the detection of rib fractures, and is routinely being included as part of the standard skeletal survey at many institutions.[60,63,64]

A complete skeletal survey is indicated in all cases of suspected non-accidental injury in children younger than two, and in some instances younger than three years of age, as these children are more likely to have occult injuries detected than older children.[25,61,65] Although the majority of children in whom occult injuries are identified are less than one year of age,[61] occult skeletal injury has been detected in older and disabled children[25,61,63]; therefore, it is still important to consider

Table 1.3 Disorders that mimic abuse (see color inserts)

Normal Bruising

Mongolian Spots/Slate Grey Nevus

Disorders of Blood Vessels and Collagen
- Capillary Hemangiomas
- E. multiforme
- Henoch-Schonlein Purpura
- Ehlers-Danlos

Dermatitis
- Phytodermatitis
- Reaction to Millipedes
- Contact Dermatitis

Coagulation Disorders
- Hemophilia
- Von Willebrand's Disease
- Vitamin K Deficiency

Acquired Conditions
- Idiopathic Thrombocytopenic Purpura
- Leukemias

Folk/Alternative Medicine
- Cupping
- Cao-Gao
- Moxibustion

radiographic investigations in these children if there is a high clinical suspicion of physical abuse.[25,61,63]

Some fractures may not be apparent on an initial skeletal survey.[25,64–67] Therefore, bone scintigraphy and repeat skeletal surveys are indicated in certain situations.[63,64,67] Bone scintigraphy has higher sensitivity than plain radiographs in detecting rib fractures and acute skeletal fractures as it can identify early periosteal elevation within several hours of injury, whereas skeletal survey may initially be negative in the acute setting.[60,65,66] The skeletal survey may also provide additional information that bone scintigraphy cannot, such as the stage of healing or age of the injury.[65] Follow-up skeletal survey and bone scintigraphy studies are indicated in some instances and are best evaluated in conjunction with a child advocacy team and pediatric radiologist.

Accidents and abuse: How to distinguish

One of the challenges in emergent evaluation of children is discerning what is reported as accidental injury from what may be inflicted injury. The emergency

Research Regarding Histories of Falls:

AUTHOR	INCLUSION	NUMBER OF CHILDREN	TYPES OF INJURIES/ CONCLUSION/ COMMENTS
Helfer et al.,[68] 1977 (Pediatrics)	Falls from beds	161	• 3 clavicle fractures • 2 skull fractures • 1 humeral fracture • None of the children suffered serious life-threatening injury
Nimityongskul & Anderson,[69] 1987 (J Pediatr Orthop)	Falls from upper and lower bunk beds and cots	76 (78% were younger than 6 years)	• 25 fractures • 27 minor head injuries • 12 lacerations requiring repair • 21 soft tissue injuries of limbs • 14 requiring inpatient admission
Barlow,[70] 1977 (Nurs Mirror Midwives J)	Falls	61 (50% were younger than 4 years)	• Less than 3 stories: 100% survival • 5–6 stories: 14 (50%) died, 11 sustained "severe brain injury"
Williams,[71] 1991 (J Trauma)	Falls from varying heights	106	• 15 had no injuries, 7 of these fell >10 feet • 77 had minor bruises, abrasions, or simple fractures, 43 of these fell >10 feet • 14 required intensive care • One fatality of a child who fell >70 feet
Musemeche et al.,[72] 1991 (J Trauma)	Falls >10 feet	70 (50% were 3 years old or younger)	• No fatalities • 39 suffered head trauma, with 2 subdural hematomas, and 3 eqidural hematomas

AUTHOR	INCLUSION	NUMBER OF CHILDREN	TYPES OF INJURIES/ CONCLUSION/ COMMENTS
Smith et al.,[73] 1975 (*J Trauma*)	Falls from varying heights, 50% were 12 feet or less	66 (50% were younger than 5 years)	• 2 subdural hematomas • 10 skull fractures • 26 upper extremity fractures • 10 lower extremity fractures • No rib or cervical spine fractures and no retinal hemorrhages
Chadwick et al.,[74] 1991 (*J Trauma*)	Falls from varying heights	317	• 100 had histories of falls <10 feet • 7 of these 100 children died from head injuries, 2 fell from a standing position, 2 from a bed/table, 2 from the arms of an adult, and 1 fell down stairs • In one of the seven fatalities there were clear indicators of abuse • In the other 6 fatalities, there were either multiple injuries or the histories were so discrepant for the degree of head injury sustained that child abuse was obvious
Selbst et al.,[75] 1990 (*Am J Dis Child*)	Falls from bunk beds	68	• None suffered internal injuries or fatalities • 52% suffered injuries to the head, 13% to the lower extremity, 12% to the face, 10% to the upper extremity, 4% or less to the mouth/teeth, eye, buttocks, or trunk

(continued)

(continued)

AUTHOR	INCLUSION	NUMBER OF CHILDREN	TYPES OF INJURIES/ CONCLUSION/ COMMENTS
Mayr et al.,[76] 2000 *(Eur J Pediatr)*	Falls from bunk beds	218	• 42% suffered major trauma • 58% suffered minor trauma • No cases of intracranial bleeding or fatalities
Joffe & Ludwig,[77] 1988 *(Pediatrics)*	Falls down stairs	363 (median age of 38 months)	• 90% had no major injury (10% with no injury, 80% with minor injury) • No life-threatening injuries or multiple injuries • In the younger age group, most of the injuries were sustained to the head
Mayr et al.,[78] 1999 *(Acta Pediatr)*	Falls from high chairs	103	• 100% sustained head injuries • 16% had skull fractures, 14% had concussions, 2% had limb fractures, and 69% had either simple contusions of the head or scalp/facial lacerations • There were no instances of intracranial bleeding or fatalities

Research Regarding Straddle Injuries:

AUTHOR	INCLUSION	NUMBER OF CHILDREN	TYPES OF INJURIES/ CONCLUSION/ COMMENTS
Waltzman et al.,[79] 1999 *(Pediatrics)*	Injuries from playing on monkey bars	204	• 59% sustained long bone fractures, most to the upper extremity • 10 children had closed head injuries without any evidence of intracranial bleeding
Dowd,[80] 1994 *(J Pediatr Surg)*	Straddle injuries	100	• 72% occurred in girls • The girls mostly complained of bleeding while the boys mostly complained of pain • 25% incurred injury from a bicycle bar, 23% from furniture, 10% from playground equipment • Of the girls, 79% had minor lacerations or bruises of the labia, 16% had injuries to the posterior fourchette, and 9% had vulvar hematomas • 7 incurred vaginal injury, and 2 sustained hymenal injury; 3 of these children had penetrating injuries • 5 of the children were ultimately diagnosed with sexual abuse

Research Regarding Walker Injuries:

AUTHOR	INCLUSION	NUMBER OF CHILDREN	TYPES OF INJURIES/ CONCLUSION/COMMENTS
US Consumer Product Safety Commission,[81] 1994 (Federal Register)	Walker injuries	25,000 children seen in US Emergency Departments in 1993 due to walker/jumper injuries	• 75 percent received injuries classified as "less severe" which includes lacerations, contusions, abrasions, hematomas, dental injuries, punctures, and strains or sprains. • 23% sustained "more severe" injuries such as concussions, burns, fractures, and injuries to internal organs • From 1989–1993 there were 11 deaths due to walkers, 4 drowned, 4 suffocated, 2 fell down stairs, and one fell out of the walker and suffered a fatal head injury

Research Regarding Strangulation, Suffocation, and Asphyxia:

AUTHOR	INCLUSION	NUMBER OF CHILDREN	TYPES OF INJURIES/ CONCLUSION/COMMENTS
Drago et al.,[82] 1997 (Arch Pediatr Adolesc Med)	Injuries from clothing drawstrings and window cords	230	• Of the 47 children who suffered injuries from being entangled by drawstrings on clothing, 8 died • There were 183 cases of fatal accidental window-cord asphyxiations, 93% of whom were younger than 3 years of age
Drago & Dannenberg,[83] 1999 (Pediatrics)	Deaths from infant mechanical suffocation	2,178 cases of infant suffocation in the US in 1995	• 14.4% were younger than 2 months of age • 879 resulted from wedging, 512 were from oronasal obstruction, 180 from overlaying, 145 from entrapment by suspension, and 142 from hanging

Research Regarding Falling Objects:

AUTHOR	INCLUSION	NUMBER OF CHILDREN	TYPES OF INJURIES/ CONCLUSION/ COMMENTS
Bernard et al.,[84] 1998 (*Pediatrics*)	Injuries from toppled television sets	101	• 73 injuries • 28 fatalities
DiScala et al.,[85] 2001 (*Arch Pediatr Adolesc Med*)	Injuries from toppled television sets	183 children who incurred injury	• 68% had head injuries • 44% had injury to multiple areas of the body • 5 fatalities were reported • 25% developed functional limitations

Research Regarding Drowning:

AUTHOR	INCLUSION	NUMBER OF CHILDREN	TYPES OF INJURIES/ CONCLUSION/ COMMENTS
Kemp et al.,[86] 1994 (*Arch Dis Child*)	Bathtub submersion	44 children involved in drowning or near-drowning incidents	• 64% were 8–15 months of age who were unsupervised • There were 25 fatalities • 10 had histories considered to be consistent with abuse or homicide
Lavelle et al.,[87] 1995 (*Ann Emerg Med*)	Bathtub near drownings	21 children involved in bathtub submersions	• 75% were younger than 2 years of age • There were 8 fatalities • Two-thirds of the children had circumstances consistent with neglect or abuse
Byard & Lipsett,[88] 1999 (*Am J Forensic Med Pathol*)	Drowning deaths	32 cases of children less than 2 years old involved in drowning	• Abuse was suspected in 2 cases

Research Regarding Toppled Television Sets:

AUTHOR	INCLUSION	NUMBER OF CHILDREN	TYPES OF INJURIES/ CONCLUSION/ COMMENTS
DiScala et al.,[89] 2001 (*Arch Pediatr Adolesc Med*)	Retrospective review of medical charts hospitalized for injuries documented in the National Pediatric Trauma Registry (1988–1999) caused by falling television sets.	183 children, 7 years of age and younger	• 57.4% of the children were male • 68.3% of the children sustained head injuries • 43.7% of the children sustained multiple injuries to various regions of the body • 28.4% of the children had injuries classified as moderate to critical severity • 31.1% of the children required admission to and intensive care unit • There were 5 fatalities (2.7%) • 26.2% of the children developed functional limitations
Bernard et al.,[90] 1998 (*Pediatrics*)	Retrospective analysis of incident cases reported to the US Consumer Products Safety Commission (CPSC) from January 1990–June 1997	73	• The mean age of the children was 36 months • Of the 73 cases reported, there were 28 fatalities • The most common site of injury was the head, accounting for 72% of the injuries overall • Injuries to the head accounted for 13 of the 14 fatalities that were further investigated by the US CPSC

department clinical evaluation should take into account the type of injury, developmental capability of the child, setting of the event, and future risk to the child, as well as a wide body of literature regarding plausibility of certain injuries with provided histories.

Motor vehicle crashes

Children and adolescent victims of motor vehicle crashes often present in the emergency department, and the treating clinician must assure any issues of potential abuse or neglect are adequately handled. There are certain circumstances where abuse should be considered, such as when a car seat was not used, when the driver was under the influence of alcohol or other drugs, or when reckless behavior contributed to the crash. Emergency medical services is a valuable asset in obtaining these historical elements.

Sexual abuse

Portions adapted with permission from Botash AS. Child Abuse Evaluation and Treatment for Medical Providers. http://www.ChildAbuseMD.com

Presentation

Appropriate handling of child and adolescent sexual abuse requires that the practitioner understands something about the dynamics of this complex topic, including the ways that children disclose abuse and the behavioral and physical indicators of possible sexual abuse.

Overview

Evaluation of possible sexual abuse of a child or adolescent requires that the medical provider understand the myriad ways that this form of abuse may present to medical attention. Because of the hidden and intra-familial nature of the problem, cases of possible sexual abuse may present with worrisome behavioral symptoms, such as depression, anxiety, aggression, or sexually acting-out behavior. Child sexual abuse may present with signs or symptoms of genital injury or sexually transmitted infections, such as dysuria, discharge, genital pain, or bleeding. Children may make statements or disclosures about sexual abuse, although those statements may be partial or incomplete as the child hints at the abuse to "test the waters" for the reaction that such a statement might generate.

Physical signs and symptoms

The following list represents some physical signs or symptoms that should trigger the consideration of sexual abuse. None of these are diagnostic of sexual abuse;

however, if abuse is not in the differential diagnosis, then sexual abuse will be missed.

- Dysuria
- Vaginal discharge which might indicate the presence of a sexually transmitted infection
- Genital lesions which might indicate the presence of a sexually transmitted infection
- Genital pain; may cause difficulty walking or sitting
- Genital bleeding
- Visible signs of trauma, such as bruising of mons pubis, labia, penis, scrotum, or perianal region
- Pregnancy in an adolescent; no assumptions can be made about the relationship of the teen female and the person who impregnated her

It is equally problematic for sexual abuse to be assumed when a child presents with any of the above signs or symptoms. Providers need to be aware of the full spectrum of possibilities when faced with any of the above. For example, vaginal discharge can be caused by a number of non-sexually transmitted organisms in the pre-pubertal child. A common scenario is when a child presents with a purulent discharge and a beefy red vulvo-vaginitis. Routine bacteriologic cultures may reveal Group A beta-hemolytic Streptococcus. Careful history often uncovers a concomitant or preceding sore throat and fever. There is an extensive differential diagnosis for genital bleeding and although abuse should be on the differential, there are certainly medical conditions that cause a female to bleed. Similarly, there are common medical conditions that present in the emergency setting and may be confused with abuse. These include:

Genital Bleeding – Sexual abuse should be considered with a history of new onset genital bleeding. However, other medical or traumatic causes of genital bleeding exist. These include menstruation, irritant vaginitis, foreign body, urinary tract infection, newborn estrogen effects, urethral prolapse, or accidental trauma such as a straddle injury.

Vaginitis – Vaginitis refers to inflammation of the vulvar structures. It may present with symptoms of burning, pain, bleeding, itching, or discharge. An infection of the urinary tract must be excluded. It is rarely a presenting sign of sexual abuse; however, it is commonly mistaken as such. Vaginitis may be secondary to infectious, allergic, or irritant triggers, therefore warranting a through history and review of precipitant factors such as use of bubble baths, or presence of signs of infection such as lymphadenopathy or fever. Vaginitis, if infectious, is best treated with topical and systemic antibiotics; if allergic or irritant, with removal of the identified trigger.

Sitz baths, use of loose cotton underwear, and hypoallergenic soap are recommended.

Urethral Prolapse – This is a condition more common in African-American females and associated with constipation, cough, or other increased intra-abdominal pressure-related conditions. The urethra outpouches create visible red–purple mucosa at the urethral site. Children may experience pain with urination, general pain in the urethral area, and commonly present with bleeding. In its minor form, the condition is best treated with Sitz baths and Bacitracin. Estrogen cream has also been demonstrated to be an effective treatment. Severe cases may require surgical intervention and should be referred to a pediatric urologist.

Labial Adhesions – This is a common condition that children may be born with or develop over time as a result of chronic irritation. The labiae are fused together at varying degrees and may create symptoms such as vaginal odor, discharge, or bleeding as the adhesions lyse. If asymptomatic, this condition may spontaneously resolve and does not require treatment. If symptoms are present, treatment may include Estrogen cream or, in its most severe forms, surgical intervention.

Evaluation of the physical findings

Because of the importance of medical confirmation of sexual abuse, the members of the multidisciplinary team often wait anxiously for the results of the medical exam to decide how to proceed with the investigation. The many factors that affect the likelihood of finding signs of traumatic injury or sexually transmitted infection have been already touched on in this chapter. Because there is a tremendous amount of variability in the ano-genital anatomy, the examination for sexual abuse should be done by the most experienced provider available. Care should be taken not to over-interpret normal variation as abnormal. Even when there are abnormalities noted on exam (for example, signs of inflammation), the findings may have a broad differential of which sexual abuse might be one possible etiology. In one study of Pediatric Emergency Physicians' interpretation of physical findings in pre-pubertal girls who alleged abuse, 79 percent of the "worrisome" findings were judged to be normal or nonspecific by trained child abuse physicians.[91]

There have been multiple attempts to classify the historical and behavioral elements, the examination findings, and the results of testing for sexually transmitted infection into levels of certainty for a diagnosis of sexual abuse. Some findings are considered normal variants or nonspecific findings, whereas others have a greater level of diagnostic significance, particularly when there is an associated history. Some findings, which were considered suggestive of abuse in the early stages of this field, have been better elucidated through empirical research and are now considered within the full range of normal. For example, vaginal opening size has largely been abandoned as an indicator of prior penetrating trauma; it is a measurement that is technically difficult to do and will vary with, amongst other things, the degree of patient relaxation and the amount of traction applied to the labia. The following are generally considered to be normal variants[92]:

- Labial adhesions particularly in a diaper-wearing girl
- Erythema of the vestibule (often intense vascularity is confused with abrasion or contusion)
- Perianal erythema, pigmentation, and venous engorgement
- Urethral dilatation with traction
- Midline avascular area of the fossa navicularis or posterior fourchette
- Concavities that are shallow and smooth, particularly when found in the anterior 180 degrees of the hymen
- Visible intravaginal ridges behind a qualitatively normal hymen and are not fully exposed
- Perianal smooth areas or skin tags in the midline
- Brief anal dilatation to less than 2 cm

The following are generally felt to be highly suggestive of sexual abuse[92–95]; these must be assessed in light of the history. Accidental injury and medical conditions that may be "mimics" of trauma must be considered:

- Acute trauma to the external genitalia and/or anal tissues, including lacerations and bruising in the absence of a credible accidental explanation
- Scar of the perianal area, posterior fourchette, or fossa navicularis
- Acute trauma to the hymen and perianal region, including tears and ecchymosis
- Healed hymenal transection or missing segment of hymen; multiple techniques are employed by expert examiners to confirm this finding
- Presence of a sexually transmitted infection that indicates contact with infective secretions. These are considered elsewhere in this chapter.
- Pregnancy, once voluntary sexual activity has been assessed
- The presence of DNA evidence when retrieved as part of a forensic sexual assault evaluation is considered a diagnostic indicator of sexual abuse/assault

Once again, the medical provider is reminded that the history is the foundation of all medical diagnosis.

Behavioral signs and symptoms

As with physical signs and symptoms, there is no behavior which is diagnostic of sexual abuse, that is, there is no behavior that when demonstrated leads to a certain conclusion that sexual abuse has occurred. The converse is also true, that is, not all children and adolescents who have been abused will demonstrate behavioral or emotional sequelae, so the absence of these does not indicate that abuse did not occur. Referrals are frequently made to child abuse evaluation programs when children behave in a manner that is considered sexualized. First, it is important to realize that all children engage in sexual behaviors that are normative. It is important for pediatric health care professionals to be familiar with the behaviors that are displayed at certain developmental stages so that they can provide reassurance and guidance to family members and educators who may be uncomfortable after having witnessed some of these behaviors. Even when a child demonstrates behaviors that fall outside of what is considered normal, this does not mean that the child has been sexually abused, although any evaluation would not be complete unless it included an assessment for sexual abuse.

The following list represents some behaviors that might be seen in children and adolescents who have been victims of sexual abuse. In evaluating these cases, sexual abuse must be included in the differential diagnosis.

- Externalizing behaviors, such as tantrums, aggression or fighting, and arguing
- Internalizing behaviors, such as depression and anxiety
- Sleep disturbance
- Appetite disturbance
- Declining school performance
- Truancy
- Sexualized or sexually acting-out behaviors

Younger children may display a knowledge of sexual matters which is inappropriate for their age and development. Families and educational staff may be upset by a child's masturbation, a behavior that is nearly universal in children. It is useful for medical providers to familiarize themselves with the literature on normative sexual behavior in children so that education and reassurance can be provided. In very general terms, masturbation is abnormal when it has a compulsive quality to it and when the child does not respond to redirection or the suggestion that self-touching should be done in private.

Statements or disclosures of sexual abuse

Studies of adults who admit to past histories of child sexual abuse demonstrate that many children do not report the fact that they are being or have been abused. More than half of the children who have been victims of sexual abuse do not report the abuse to anyone, and only a small minority of cases ever come to the attention of professionals, such as law enforcement or child protective services.[96] The reasons are complex but include the fact that very young children may not understand that they are being abused, and older children may be pressured or even overtly threatened not to tell. Sexual abuse disclosure for many children is a process. Sorenson and Snow[97] note that disclosure may be accidental and that initial disclosures may be followed by recantation. Other factors that interfere with a child's ability to successfully report his/her abuse include the closeness of the victim to the perpetrator and the absence of support from a non-offending caretaker.

When a medical provider is faced with a case where a child has reported abuse, their role is very clear. A history must be taken from the accompanying adult and from the victim to obtain sufficient information to decide what steps need to be taken next. Foremost in the provider's mind should be these questions:

1. What questions do I need to ask to ensure the safety of this child/adolescent?
2. What information do I need to decide whether I must report this to child protective services and law enforcement?
3. What information do I need to perform appropriate tests and render appropriate treatment?

It is important for medical providers to understand that they are not conducting a forensic interview, rather they are taking a history. The questions that should be asked make up what is referred to as a "minimal facts" history. It is inappropriate for a medical provider to overstep their role and enter the investigatory domain. A forensic interview must be done by someone who has had specialized training and only after the appropriate professionals have been assembled to listen to and/or participate in the interview.

Sexual abuse disclosure

The process of disclosure, when a child/adolescent reports their sexual abuse, may be hampered by many things, including fear, guilt, and embarrassment. The youngest of victims may not even understand that what has happened to them is abusive. The sexually abusing adult may start off by buying presents or paying special attention to the child, a process referred to as "grooming." The perpetrator may employ overt threats, such as "I'll kill you or you mother," "nobody will believe you," or "you will be taken away from your mother." Early statements made by a child may be partial disclosures, an attempt by the child to test the waters and to observe the consequences of telling. For example, one 7-year-old female initially disclosed digital/vaginal contact by an adult male; during her initial CAC evaluation, she disclosed that the adult male "touched my private part (pointing to her vagina) with a hand. My pants and underpants were off. He didn't touch me with any other part of his body." The child was subsequently brought back to the CAC three weeks later for another medical examination after she disclosed penile/vaginal penetration by the same adult male. If a child sees that the disclosure has elicited negative reactions from the person to whom they have confided or has caused distress to family members, the initial disclosure may be quickly followed by a recantation.

When a child discloses, the medical provider should:

- Control the natural response of shock, disgust, or horror
- Support the child or adolescent for telling
- Use age-appropriate language and make the child comfortable in using their own words to describe the abuse, including their own labels for their private parts
- Ask only those questions that are necessary to determine whether a report must be made to CPS and to assess for imminent risk. This "minimal facts interview" includes determining the most basic information of who, what, when, and where
- Do not ask leading questions
- Do not make promises that you cannot keep, such as "everything will be alright"
- Explain what will happen next, including the fact that the child will most likely need to repeat what they have told you to someone else

TRIAGE: Appropriate level of care

The following are guidelines for deciding where and when the sexual abuse evaluation should take place. For ease of understanding the issues related to the urgency of the evaluation, three levels have been devised: emergent, urgent, and to be scheduled for a later time.

Emergent evaluation

An emergent evaluation is one that should occur on the same day as the initial contact with the child or adolescent. If there is a local child abuse expert, refer the child/adolescent to that medical provider for an immediate consultation. In many places, this immediate consultation is not available, and the child/adolescent must go to the local emergency department. In that case, proper photo documentation and clear medical record documentation of the examination is essential so that a forensic pediatrician can interpret the findings. In some cases, the child may be medically unstable due to physical trauma and the emergency department is the most appropriate resource for evaluation and treatment. Indications for an emergent evaluation:

- Imminent danger
- Loss of consciousness
- Bleeding or history of bleeding
- Pain (genital or other)
- Extensive bruising or bruises that may resolve quickly

- Possible fractures
- Abdominal trauma or other medical emergency concerns
- Pregnancy possibility
- Need for STD prophylaxis
- Psychiatric emergency
- Forensic evidence collection

Imminent danger

Imminent danger refers to the risk of further abuse to the child/adolescent. When imminent danger is suspected, evaluate the child/adolescent as soon as possible. The provider must ascertain the possibility of injury and begin to access the social services system in order to protect the child/adolescent from further harm.

Medical need

Immediately evaluate a child/adolescent who has severe pain, loss of consciousness, bleeding, possible fracture, possible abdominal trauma, extensive bruising, signs of suffocation, or other emergent medical concern. Following is a more complete list of symptoms which indicate the need for an emergent medical evaluation in a facility that is equipped to handle the evaluation:

- Symptoms of head trauma: vomiting, headache, syncope, lethargy, visual disturbance, change in mental status
- Symptoms of abdominal injury: vomiting, abdominal pain, bruising to the abdomen/flank/back, hematuria
- Symptoms or history of recent traumatic sexual contact: bleeding from the vagina or rectum, genital pain, or other signs of injury

Evaluate immediately if the possibility exists that the child/adolescent may benefit from prophylactic treatment for sexually transmitted diseases or pregnancy. Post-pubertal females with a history of exposure to semen are at risk for pregnancy and may receive prophylaxis up to 120 hours after the incident. All children/adolescents with history of exposure to bodily fluids may be at risk for a sexually transmitted disease. These situations should be considered on a case-by-case basis by collaborating with a professional trained in the forensic examination of abused children and a pediatric infectious disease specialist where appropriate.

Psychiatric emergency

Certain situations, such as a suicide attempt, parental or child emotional instability, acute psychotic crisis, or other significant mental health concern, warrant an immediate evaluation.

Medical/legal issues

An immediate evaluation is appropriate when there is a possibility of forensic evidence collection or documentation of an injury that may resolve quickly. Because of the advent of emerging DNA technology, the time period during which forensic evidence may be collected has been extended to 96 hours. Collect evidence when there is a suspicion of sexual abuse within the previous 96 hours that includes the potential for exposure to bodily fluids:

- Penile/vaginal contact
- Penile/anal contact
- Oral/penile contact
- Oral/vaginal contact

Forensic evidence kits were developed for use in situations of acute sexual assault of teens and adults. In most cases of child sexual abuse, the collection of forensic evidence will not be appropriate either because of the time delay between abuse and discovery or because the reported contact does not carry the potential for recovery of bodily fluids. In a study of child sexual abuse and the sensitivity of the forensic evidence kit, there were very few positives in children when the kits were performed beyond 24 hours after the abuse. In those instances where DNA was discovered, it was more likely to be found on clothing or bedding than on the child. For this reason, it is important to ask about clothing and bedding.[98]

Urgent evaluation

Urgent evaluations should take place within 24 hours of the referral. Consider these situations carefully, as sometimes it is more appropriate to have the child/adolescent seen emergently.

Indications for an urgent evaluation:

- Bruises or need for documentation of minor injuries that may resolve quickly
- Vaginal discharge
- Supportive evidence for a legal case

Documentation of an injury that may resolve

Genital injuries may resolve rapidly.[99] Document them by using proper photographic equipment and chart sketches. Evaluation and interpretation by a professional trained in the forensic evaluation of children is valuable and should be arranged whenever possible.

Non-genital injuries and bruises are variable in their resolution and should be considered on a case-by-case basis. It is sometimes advisable to perform an immediate medical evaluation if injury resolution will occur before an urgent examination can be scheduled.

Medical concerns

Evaluate urgently if the child/adolescent complains of genital pain even though the incident of abuse may have occurred more than 96 hours ago. Genital injuries are often accompanied by a history of pain or bleeding.

If there has been an otherwise asymptomatic vaginal discharge that has been present for some time, the child/adolescent needs to be seen as soon as possible. In general, the evaluation is not an emergency.

Most situations of medical neglect require an urgent or emergency evaluation. Children suffering from injuries due to physical abuse and who do not fit the criteria for an emergency evaluation should be evaluated within 24 hours.

Supportive evidence

Occasionally, in order to move forward with an arrest in a case, legal professionals are awaiting physical examination results on a child/adolescent who may have healed findings. Consider on a case-by-case basis if these situations warrant an urgent examination.

Evaluation scheduled for a later date

All children/adolescents with a suspicion of child abuse and/or neglect are entitled to a medical evaluation. An examination can be scheduled for a later date when there is no urgency for documentation of injury, forensic evidence collection, treatment, or prophylactic treatment.

Indications for an evaluation scheduled for a later date:

- Abuse was not within the week
- Nature of the abuse is not likely to result in findings
- Family or child/adolescent needs reassurance
- Concern is limited to a behavioral problem
- Custody issues

Unlikely need for treatment or evidence collection

Activities such as genital fondling over the clothes may not result in injury or need prophylactic treatment. However, children and adolescents often disclose abuse in a piecemeal fashion. The possibility of additional activity and possible healed physical findings must be considered.

Need for reassurance

In some circumstances the nature of the evaluation may be for the psychological reassurance of wellness. Some children/adolescents without contact types of abuse may still benefit from an evaluation, including:

- Siblings of abused children/adolescents
- Children/adolescents with histories of exposure to pornography

Behavioral concerns

In many cases, the only concern regarding abuse is due to "sexual acting out" or an acute behavioral change. These children should be examined with careful attention to the history of the problem and social concerns.[100]

Family issues

Some of the most challenging evaluations involve allegations by one parent against another concerning child abuse. These allegations should be taken seriously. In all cases, the child is being victimized either as a pawn in a parental dispute or as a victim of emotional, sexual, or physical abuse or neglect. These children usually benefit from referral for evaluation by a medical professional with expertise in evaluating abused children.

Domestic violence impacts the entire family. A child/adolescent exposed to parents or caregivers who engage in domestic violence is a child/adolescent at risk. States vary with regard to whether or not children being exposed or witnessing domestic violence constitutes a mandatory report to the agency designated to receive such reports, often referred to as the Child Abuse Hotline. Although the literature is quite clear that children who grow up in households where there is violence are at risk for developing a host of long-term sequelae, this is not inevitable. Because there may not be immediate risk to children in households where there is violence, some states have not made exposure a reportable event in the absence of direct harm to a child. Providers need to familiarize themselves with their own state reporting laws.

The physical examination

The physical examination consists of the preparation for the examination, a complete and thorough physical examination, collection of forensic specimens, testing for sexually transmitted infections when appropriate, and "wrapping up" with the child and accompanying adult, if present.

Preparation for the examination

The purpose of the physical examination should be explained to the child and accompanying adult, including a demonstration of any special equipment that will be used, such as a colposcope. The colposcope is an instrument that was initially developed for cervical evaluation during the gynecologic exam. It has been adopted by the child abuse medical community as a device that enables viewing of the genitalia and anal regions with magnification and an enhanced light source. This instrument allows for photo documentation of the exam with 35-mm, digital, or video image capture. Photo documentation of the examination findings allows for teaching, second opinion, case conferencing, and important evidence at trial. In cases where the evaluation is inconclusive, the images may serve as important "baseline" documentation. Many colposcope systems allow for the child or adolescent to view the exam in "real time." The patient's anxiety may be lessened if they are able to see what is happening "down there" while the medical provider is doing the exam. After the exam is complete, the medical provider can use the photos or video to teach the patient about their own anatomy and, most of the time, can reassure the child/adolescent that they are healthy and undamaged. Even when the colposcopic exam has revealed traumatic injury, emphasizing that the injuries are so small as to require the colposcopic magnification to fully appreciate them is crucial. The victim should be reassured that injuries heal completely in the majority of cases and residual traumatic injury does not have any physiologic importance and cannot be detected by a future sexual partner.

The physical examination must not be traumatic. If the child or adolescent is not able to cooperate with the exam, more time should be spent preparing the patient and helping him or her to relax. The patient should never be forced or restrained. It is far better to reschedule the exam for a later date when the child or adolescent has had time to prepare for the exam. In instances where there is a medical imperative to the exam, such as acute hemorrhage, consideration should be given to using sedation or anesthesia.

The child or adolescent should be accompanied into the exam by a supportive adult. Adolescents may choose to be examined alone, and this request should be honored. This enables the medical provider the private venue for asking teens about confidential issues, such as voluntary sexual activity and cigarette, alcohol, or other drug use.

Although a non-offending parent or guardian is generally the most appropriate person to accompany a child during a sexual abuse examination, instances where it might be detrimental include:

- The parent is distraught or disbelieving, and this behavior may have a negative effect on the child/adolescent
- When a parent is acting to censor information the child/adolescent may provide

• When a history of sexual abuse in the parent may trigger emotions in the parent that may affect the child/adolescent's behavior

In general, it is not appropriate for non-medical members of the multidisciplinary team, such as child protective workers or law enforcement personnel, to be in the exam room during a sexual abuse exam. There are some unique circumstances where a child might be accompanied by a non-family member, such as a foster agency caseworker, and if the child requests, this person may serve, in the absence of a parent, as the supportive person during the exam.

Conduct a complete and thorough physical examination

It is never appropriate to begin a physical examination by examining the genitalia first. The physical exam should be conducted in the manner that children and adolescents are accustomed to. Additionally, there are potentially, many other physical exam indicators of sexual victimizations, such as suction marks or "hickeys" on the skin or bruises from being restrained during a sexual assault.

Special consideration for the examination of the female patient

The female genitalia are an area which engenders a lot of misconception and misinformation. Of utmost significance is the myth of the "intact hymen." It is commonly accepted within the general population as well as the larger medical community that the hymen is a membrane, which in its natural state covers the opening of the vagina and therefore must be "popped" or broken for vaginal penetration to occur. A far better description of the hymen is that of a "cuff" of tissue that surrounds the natural opening of the vagina. In instances where the entirety of the vaginal opening is covered, the diagnosis of imperforate hymen may be made. This is a condition which might require surgery prior to menarche since the absence of a patent orifice for the outflow of menstrual blood would create a primary amenorrhea and ongoing symptoms, such as abdominal pain.

The examination of the pre-pubertal girl often requires employing several positions. Most providers start with the girl supine with the bottoms of the feet pressed together and the knees abducted toward the exam table. In this position, known as the supine frog-leg position, the examiner should first look at the skin of the inner thighs and the labia majora before even touching. The labia must be spread gently to visualize the labia minora, clitoris and clitoral hood, hymen, vaginal opening, fossa navicularis, and posterior fourchette. This technique is called Labial Separation.

The next step is to use the Labial Traction technique, which entails grasping each labia majora between the examiner's thumb and forefinger and gently abducting laterally while also pulling downward and outward toward the examiner. This technique enables enhanced visualization of the genital structures and is often required to adequately see the hymeneal rim, particularly the posterior aspect. The

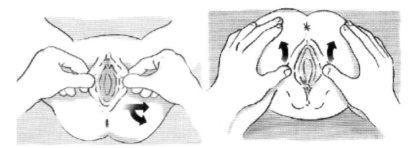

Figure 1.2   Figure A: Labial traction in the supine frog-leg position. Figure B: Labial traction in the prone knee–chest position. Reprinted from the New York State Department of Health *Child and Adolescent Sexual Offense Medical Protocol.*

hymeneal tissue may be folded and flop inward into the vaginal canal or outward to lie flat against the fossa navcularis. The hymen may temporarily adhere to the surrounding tissues due to secretions. The medical provider may need to gently manipulate the hymen with a small swab, such as a wire Dacron or Calgi-tipped swab, to adequately examine its architecture. Another tool is the use of water, gently squirted with a syringe, to cause the agglutinating secretions to wash away or to cause the hymeneal tissue to float, allowing it to be examined optimally. Another position is the prone knee–chest position. In this position, the patient lies with the chest pressed down toward the table, the buttocks raised in the air, and the legs spread. This position may allow for better visualization of the posterior hymen, which may flop down or unroll with the help of gravity. This position may also allow for viewing deeper into the vaginal canal to look for foreign bodies.

The medical provider must carefully describe what they see on the examination. Using the word "intact" to describe the hymen's appearance is discouraged since it is not descriptive and has no universally understood meaning. In fact, it fuels the erroneous notion that the hymen's presence or absence is a legitimate diagnostic test for sexual abuse or assault. Medical providers who conduct sexual abuse or assault exams should be familiar with the variety of hymeneal configurations as well as the nomenclature that was standardized by the American Professional Society of the Abuse of Children (APSAC).[101]

The hymen may be annular or crescent-shaped and its appearance can change over time. The annular hymen is the most common shaped in infancy, whereas the crescent-shaped hymen is more common in school-age pre-pubertal girls. This is most likely a developmental phenomenon[102] and may be due, at least in part, to the hormonal milieu.

The hymen's appearance changes again as a girl approaches puberty, such that the estrogenized mucosa has greater redundancy as well as resilience.

The examiner must be on the lookout for signs of inflammation and acute injury as well as old or chronic injury. The position of noted findings should be described using position on a clock face (with the exam position also noted). When a patient is supine, anterior is at 12 o'clock and posterior is at 6 o'clock.

Category	Examine and document presence or absence of
Labia majora and minora	Skin lesions, unusual pigmentations, or other skin changes
Clitoris	Unusual size or changes of the clitoris or hood
Urethral meatus	Inflammation, edema, or other lesions of the periurethral tissue
Perihymenal tissue (vestibule)	Vascularity, abrasions, lacerations, scarring, or lesions which might be an indication of a sexually transmitted infection
Hymen	Configuration (annular, redundant/fimbriated, crescentic, dorsal/anterior), transections (depth), hemorrhages, abrasions, bruises, ecchymotic areas, healed scars or adhesions, rounded or thickened edges, and abnormal vascular patterns, areas of scant or absent hymenal tissue and whether this absence represents a shallow notch, a deep notch, or a complete transection[1]
Posterior fourchette and fossa navicularis	Lacerations or scars, bruises, healing abraded areas, lesions which might be consistent with a sexually transmitted infection, or an unusual vascular pattern that might indicate neovascularization
Vagina	Bleeding, discharge, lesions, foreign bodies, abnormal vascular pattern, petechiae, or other lesions on the walls of the vagina
Cervix	Bleeding, discharge, STD lesions, cervicitis, tears, or other signs of trauma

In the extreme circumstance where the inside of the vagina must be visualized, sedation or anesthesia must be considered.[2]

Category	Examine and document presence or absence of
Penis	Tanner stage, circumcised, lesions that might indicate a sexually transmitted infection, bite marks, edema, hematomas, lacerations, abrasions, or dried secretions
Urethral meatus	Scars, lesions, discharge, or bleeding
Scrotum	Erythema, ecchymoses, abrasions, bite marks
Testes	Tanner Stage, descent of testes, any signs of atrophy or differential in firmness of the tissue, testicle size, scrotum, and phallus development

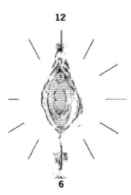

Figure 1.3   Figure C: Clock face superimposed on female genital area. Reprinted from the New York State Department of Health *Child and Adolescent Sexual Offense Medical Protocol.*

Important key concepts

(1) The terms "intact, broken, virginal, marital, or missing" are not sufficient to describe hymenal findings and may be inaccurate and misleading.
(2) Examiners should never use a speculum or perform an internal examination in a pre-pubertal girl or in the post-pubertal female without a medical indication to perform such an examination.

The examiner must also carefully visualize the anus and perianal tissues, taking into account scars, bruises, tears, abnormalities of tone, and remarkable dilatation in the absence of stool in the rectal vault.

Following is a more detailed listing of the specific findings that should be looked for and carefully catalogued during an examination for sexual abuse/assault.

The following should be assessed and documented in the examination of the sexually abused child.

Anal/rectal examination

With either the supine or prone knee–chest position, the examiner should use both hands to separate the buttocks for viewing of the anal area in males or females. In general, traction techniques are not necessary when these positions are used. Note in the medical record the exam position that is used and the degree of relaxation.

The anus is readily visualized in the prone knee–chest position. Because this position may cause some victims unusual embarrassment or recall memories of prior abuse, other positions that may be more acceptable are the lateral decubitus (knee–chest) position, supine knee–chest (hugging the knees to the chest), and standing while bending forward over the exam table. In the lateral decubitus position, the child should be curled so that the knees are as close to the chest as possible, usually with one leg flexed more than the other. The examiner can separate the buttocks with one hand on each gluteal area, using the thumb and fingers for leverage.

Examination of the Anus

Category	Examine and document presence or absence of
Buttocks	Fresh/healed lesions, wet/dry secretions, ecchymoses, rashes, potentially infectious lesions, bruises (indicate shape, size, location, and photograph), scars
Perianal skin	Inflammation, wet/dry secretions, bruising, lacerations, fissures, tears located on the external surface, internal to the sphincter, or that extend across the pectinate line
Anal verge/folds/rugae	Prominent, normal, or flattened verge or anal sphincter skin folds when child is in a relaxed state
Tone	Increased or decreased anal tone. Avoid a digital rectal examination in children unless there is suspicion of internal trauma. On visual exam, note the presence of anal spasm
Anal laxity	An anus that greatly dilates with gentle buttocks traction when there is no stool in the vault should be documented. Always record the presence or absence of stool in the rectal ampulla
Rectal examination	A rectal examination is rarely necessary in the evaluation of sexual abuse. If intra-abdominal/rectal trauma or a foreign body is suspected, a digital examination is justified. Consider further evaluation using anoscopy and possible sedation. In situations following an acute assault involving trauma to the rectum, perform a guaiac exam

Once the examiner has completed the exam, they will be called on to render an opinion about the significance of any examination findings. Members of the multidisciplinary team often wait anxiously for the exam results, expecting that their decisions, both protective and grounds for arrest, will be predicated on the medical evidence. Providers should realize and be able to explain to their non-medical colleagues that a normal physical exam is common even when sexual abuse has occurred. In studies that assessed for presence of abnormal findings in sexually abused children and adolescents, normal exams were reported in 26 percent to 73 percent (mean 50%) of girls and in 17 percent to 82 percent (mean 53%) of boys.[103] Even when the exam was not normal, most findings were nonspecific, meaning that they were not diagnostic findings of sexual abuse.[103]

There are many reasons why the exam for sexual abuse is frequently normal:

- Delayed disclosure/discovery of abuse so that trauma may have completely healed
- Some types of sexual abuse (including fondling and oral–genital contact) would not be expected to cause visible signs of trauma

- The hymeneal tissue is elastic and can stretch to allow for some degree of penetration without injury; epecially once a female enters puberty
- Perceived "penetration" by a female may actually be penetration into the vulvar space rather than past the hymen into the vaginal canal ("Vulvar coitus")
- The anal sphincter has remarkable capacity to stretch to allow for passage of large caliber stools
- Lubricants may be used
- Because of the delay in time between the sexual abusive event and medical assessment, it is frequently too late to attempt to collect forensic specimens. In a study of pre-pubertal children, forensic evidence was rarely found beyond 24 hours from the abuse, and when it was retrieved, it was more likely to be on bedding or clothing than on the children.

Sexually transmitted disease

The following table is from the www.childabusemd.com website as adapted from the Cincinnati Children's Hospital, Mayerson Center Child Abuse Team, and internet information on sexually transmitted disease. www.cincinnatichildrens.org/svc/alpha/c/child-abuse/sexual/disease/

Home Appendices

APPENDIX E: Evaluation of Sexually Transmitted Diseases

Infections with very high likelihood of sexual transmission			
Infection and sites of infection	Incubation period and symptoms	Transmission	Diagnostic tests
Gonorrhea (GC) *Neisseria gonorrheae* • Vagina • Cervix • Urethra • Rectum • Throat • Pelvis (PID) • Systemic	Vaginal infection (vaginitis) in pre-pubertal girls usually causes discharge within 2–7 days. Rectal and throat infections in all ages, as well as cervical infections (cervicitis) in adolescents, are often asymptomatic.	During delivery, an infant may be infected. Eye infections are most common and result in eye discharge within a few days of life. Vaginal and rectal infections are also possible. Vaginal infections beyond the newborn period should be presumed to be from sexual abuse. There is little known about the persistence of asymptomatic rectal and pharyngeal infections.	The **only** acceptable testing method for diagnosis is bacterial culture using a modified Thayer-Martin Medium in a CO_2-rich environment. A positive culture must be confirmed by two other identification tests before the diagnosis is made. Misidentification will occur if these methods are not followed. Note: NAAT tests are suitable for screening but not diagnosis.

Infections with very high likelihood of sexual transmission			
Infection and sites of infection	Incubation period and symptoms	Transmission	Diagnostic tests
Chlamydia *Chlamydia trachomatis* • Vagina • Cervix • Urethra • Rectum	Most chlamydia infections do not cause symptoms. Tissue culture tests should be positive 5–7 days after contact. Identification earlier than this is very unlikely.	Perinatal infection may be unrecognized for years. Asymptomatic vaginal and rectal perinatal infections have been documented for up to 3 years. Chlamydia pharyngitis has not been reported and pharyngeal chlamydia tests are not recommended. A chlamydia infection should be presumed to be from sexual abuse if perinatal infection has been excluded.	The **only** acceptable method for diagnosis is positive bacterial tissue culture. Misidentification will occur if other methods are used. Institutions have specific requirements for the obtaining, transport, and/or storage of the particular type of medium used. Note: NAAT tests are suitable for screening but not diagnosis.
Syphilis *Treponema pallidum* • Primary infection causes a painless ulcer at the site of contact.	Primary infection usually occurs about 3 weeks after exposure (range from 10–90 days). Secondary syphilis causes rash, fever, and other symptoms 1–2 months later. Condyloma latum, a wart- like rash, may be seen around the anus and vagina.	Perinatal infection often occurs. It is routine practice to screen for maternal syphilis. Infection is almost always spread by direct sexual contact. Non-sexual transmission, other than perinatal infection, would be extremely unusual. Infection should be presumed to be through sexual abuse unless acquired by perinatal (congenital) infection.	Although definitive diagnosis can be made by microscopic identification, adequate specimens are usually not available for this type of testing. Most cases of syphilis are diagnosed through serologic blood tests. A presumptive diagnosis of syphilis can be made if there is a positive non-treponemal test (RPR, VDRL, or ART) and a positive treponemal test (FTA-ABS or MHA-TP).

(continued)

(*continued*)

	Infections with very high likelihood of sexual transmission		
Infection and sites of infection	Incubation period and symptoms	Transmission	Diagnostic tests
HIV/AIDS Human immunodeficiency virus • Causes systemic illness	Signs of illness are delayed for up to 6 or more years. Symptoms include swollen lymph nodes, failure to thrive, or fungal and other infections.	Infection is spread by contact with infected semen, blood, cervical secretions, or human milk. The incidence of developing HIV infection from a single episode of abuse is very low. Other methods of infection in children include contaminated blood or blood products during transfusion, IV drug abuse, or sexual abuse.	Finding HIV antibodies in the blood makes a presumptive diagnosis. Other tests confirm the diagnosis. In infants under 18 months old, other tests are needed if the infant's mother is HIV positive. Tests are often positive within 6–12 weeks after exposure, but may take as long as 6 months to become positive.
Trichomonas *Trichomonas vaginalis* • Vagina • Urethra	Many infections are asymptomatic. Male urethral infection is often asymptomatic. Vaginal discharge may develop between 4–28 days after contact.	Perinatal vaginal infection may persist for many months following birth. Infection is usually by sexual contact. Non-sexual transmission is very unlikely, although possible.	Microscopic identification or bacterial culture of vaginal secretions. Must be differentiated from other types of trichomonas if identified in analysis of urine or stool.

Infections with possible likelihood of sexual transmission			
Infection and sites of infection	Incubation period and symptoms	Transmission	Diagnostic tests
Herpes Herpes simplex virus, types I and II • Vagina • Penis • Anus • Mouth	Painful ulcers occur within 2 weeks following contact. Reactivation of the infection often occurs and results in ulcers at or near the site of primary infection.	The most common infection in children is gingivostomatitis, an infection of the mouth. It is not transmitted sexually. Infection of the genitalia or infection around the anus may be due to sexual contact. Non-sexual transmission is also possible.	The diagnosis can be made based upon the appearance of the ulcers. The virus can be cultured if the diagnosis is in question. Type I and type II both cause genital and perianal ulcers. Identification of the virus type does not differentiate sexual from non-sexual transmission.
Condyloma acuminata (venereal warts) Human papillomavirus (HPV) • Vagina • Penis • Anus • Hands	Infection may cause skin-colored growths that vary in size from a few millimeters to many centimeters. Infections may cause no visible warts. The incubation period may be 2 years or longer.	Infection may be transmitted prenatally, perinatally, through sexual contact, or by non-sexual contact.[104] Sexual abuse should be considered in any child with anal or genital warts. Evaluation for other STDs should be considered. In a child younger than age 3 with a diagnosis of venereal warts, detailed history of mother's past gynecologic problems may suggest perinatal transmission.	The diagnosis is usually made by their appearance on physical examination. In some centers, the virus type can be determined. It is unclear if determination of the wart type is of any value when evaluating for sexual abuse.
Pubic lice (crabs) *Pediculus pthirus* • Eyelashes • Eyebrows • Genital hair • Perianal hair • Beard • Arm pits • Scalp (rarely)	The most common site of infection in young children is the eyelash. Nits (eggs) can be seen as well as the movement of lice.	In adolescents, transmission is usually sexual. Non-sexual transmission through contaminated towels is possible. Sexual abuse should always be considered in children infected with pubic lice.	The diagnosis is made by the clinical appearance of the lice. Head lice do not infect eyelashes. Lice infestations of the eyelashes are pubic lice. Microscopic examination of the louse can be done if there is any doubt about the type of louse causing the infestation.

(continued)

(*continued*)

| Hepatitis B virus (HBV) • Causes systemic illness Hepatitis C, E may also be sexually transmitted. | Some children will have no symptoms. Others will have loss of appetite, stomach pain, and jaundice. Infection can cause death. The incubation period is 45–160 days after contact. | Perinatal transmission occurs. Both sexual and non-sexual transmission occurs. Children living with HBV carriers and in institutions for the developmentally disabled are at risk. Infection is transmitted through infected blood, wound secretions, semen, cervical secretions, and saliva. | The diagnosis is made from serologic blood tests (HepBsAg and Ab). Vaccination is recommended for all children. It is 90–95% effective in preventing infection. |

Infections with low likelihood of sexual transmission			
Infection and sites of infection	Incubation period and symptoms	Transmission	Diagnostic tests
Bacterial vaginosis (BV) *Gardnerella vaginalis* and other bacteria • Vagina	May cause vaginal discharge. Some infections are asymptomatic.	This organism is most often seen in sexually active women but has been found in girls and women who have had no sexual contact and have not been sexually abused.	Identification is made by microscopic analysis and other methods.
Molluscum contagiosum poxvirus • May occur anywhere on the body	Small bumps with a central depression. The incubation period is 2 weeks to 6 months.	This virus is spread by direct contact. It is most often transmitted by non-sexual contact.	Diagnosis is made by the clinical appearance of the rash.
Candida *Candida albicans* • Muco-cutaneous infection (thrush, vulvovaginitis), gluteal or other skin folds, paronychia and onychia • May be disseminated in immunocom-promised patients	May cause itching, discharge, or vaginal pain. Incubation period is unknown.	Most infections are due to endogenous organisms. Person to person transmission can occur, including perinatal transmission.	Diagnosis is generally based on physical examination findings. Identification can be made of yeast and pseudohyphal forms by microscopic examination of swabs/scrapings suspended in 10% potassium hydroxide (KOH).

Infections with low likelihood of sexual transmission			
Infection and sites of infection	Incubation period and symptoms	Transmission	Diagnostic tests
Scabies *Sarcoptes scabiei*, subspecies *hominus* Sites of predilection in older children and adults: • Interdigital folds • Flexor aspects of writs • Extensor surfaces of the elbows • Abdomen • Folds of skin • Other areas In children younger than 2 years: • Head • Neck • Palms • Soles	Intense, pruritis of a papular rash. May see burrows in the skin. Incubation is usually 4–6 weeks.	Transmission occurs by close personal contact.	Diagnosis is clinical or based on identification of the mites' eggs or scybaia (feces) from the skin scrapings of unexcoreated lesions.
Streptococcal perianal cellulitis[105] or vaginitis *Streptococcus pyogenes* or Group A beta-hemolytic streptococci • Causes pharyngitis, pyoderma, or impetigo most commonly. • May cause vaginitis, pericarditis, pneumonia, sepsis, otitis media, cervical adenitis, or perianal cellulites.	Painful defecation, beefy red perianal area, sometimes peeling. May be chronically infected with exacerbations over several months. Incubation period for pharyngitis is 2–5 days and for impetigo is 7–10 days. For vaginitis and perianal cellulitis, the incubation period is not known but likely within one week.	Person to person contact. Streptococci are endogenous to the perianal area.	Diagnosis by swab of the vagina or rectum and plating on sheep blood agar with use of bacitracin sensitivity discs. The use of rapid strep antigen tests for genital or perianal infections has not been well studied.

Evidence collection

Many states in the United States have forensic evidence kits that include all of the necessary materials for collection of forensic specimens, for example, swabs, slides, labeled envelopes, and so on, and comprehensive and detailed instructions for doing the "rape kit." Most sexual offense medical protocols recommend performing a rape kit if the abuse or assault has occurred within the past 72 to 96 hours. Every facility must establish a protocol so that all collected specimens and the sealed kit are handled with careful documentation of every person who participated in the process; this is referred to as an "unbroken chain of evidence." It must be remembered that, in the setting of child sexual abuse, because of the frequent delay in reporting abuse, the last abusive event may not have occurred within this 96-hour window. Additionally, the type of abusive contact may be such that performing evidence collection would not be appropriate. The health care provider must always consider the risk–benefit ratio when performing any procedure; it might be appropriate to collect some specimens but not all of them. Some of the procedures, such as pubic hair combing, might be particularly offensive to the patient and should therefore be skipped. At no time and under no circumstance should a victim of abuse or assault be forced to undergo a forensic examination.

Consent for collection of forensic specimens is separate from the general consent for evaluation and treatment. Providers should be familiar with their state laws that deal with a minor's right to consent to confidential treatment for issues involving reproduction, sexuality, and sexual assault. A minor who understands the implications of the evaluation and treatment may have the right to access this type of care without the knowledge and/or consent of their parent or guardian. The converse is also true; no minor can be forced to undergo such an exam. By the same token, parents do not have the right to force a teen to submit to a "virginity check," which has no medical basis or purpose.

Detailed instructions about forensic evidence collection is beyond the scope of this chapter. Every facility should check to see if their State Departments of Health have published guidelines. For example, New York State has a comprehensive manual that can be downloaded from the Internet at http://www.health.state.ny.us/ professionals/protocols_and_guidelines/sexual_assault/index.htm.

Consideration must also be given to the possibility that drugs or alcohol were used to facilitate the sexual assault. Symptoms such as memory loss or lapse, dizziness or disorientation, and other evidence of intoxication should prompt collection of blood and urine for toxicology. Some states have collection kits, similar to the "rape kit," that include blood tubes for serum and a urine specimen container.

Photography

Many State laws allow for photographic documentation of injuries in child abuse evaluations even without consent of the parent or guardian. Guidelines for photo documentation include the following recommendations:

1. Include a full body photo including the patient's face for identification purposes.
2. Document a finding by taking several shots from multiple angles and include a recognizable body part in at least one photo to enable the viewer to orient to the location of the injury.
3. Include a card with the patient's name and the date in the photo.
4. Develop a system for labeling the photo with the child/adolescent's name, medical record number, date, and the name of the person taking the photo.

Every facility must have a written protocol that carefully outlines who is authorized to take photos within the facility and under what circumstances. The protocol must also describe how photographs should be stored and to whom they may be given.

Diagnostic testing

Transmission of sexually transmitted infections (STI) can take place during sexual abuse of children and adolescents. The symptom of infection may be what brings the child or adolescent to medical care, and the detection of an STI may be the only evidence that sexual abuse occurred. The various STIs have differing significance with regard to the likelihood that sexual abuse took place. For example, Neisseria gonorrhea and Chlamydia trachomatis, which are primarily sexually transmitted in adults, may be the result of perinatal acquisition in infants. Long asymptomatic latency periods of Human Papilloma Virus infections make it difficult, if not impossible, to pinpoint if and when sexual abuse or assault may have taken place. Herpes simplex may be shed asymptomatically and can be auto-inoculated from one anatomic site to another. A considered approach to diagnostic testing requires that the provider take into consideration mode of transmission, transmissibility, and the organism's incubation period. Selective testing has been recommended to avoid the discomfort and cost of unnecessary testing.[106–108] Testing should be considered in the following circumstances:

- The patient has genital or anal symptoms, such as discharge, pain, or dysuria
- The alleged perpetrator is known or believed to be in a high-risk group (e.g. intravenous drug use, incarcerated, high-risk sexual behavior)

- A disclosure or history of oral, anal, or genital contact
- Contact history includes pain, bleeding, or contact with blood or semen of perpetrator
- STI prevalence in the community is high
- Physical examination reveals abnormal findings, such as indications of infection and/or trauma
- The child is too young to give a clear history, or the family (or child) are anxious about the possibility of infection
- Adolescent victims, because they are in an epidemiologically high-risk group

The following table provides information "at a glance" to assist with deciding whether or not testing is appropriate in the setting of sexual assault. The reluctance to avoid testing of sexually active adolescents because of the concern that identifying the teen's sexual activity may discredit the teen's testimony in the legal arena is probably unfounded. The use of a victim's previous sexual history, including any preexisting STIs to undermine the adolescent's testimony is strictly limited by law in most if not all states.

Child and adolescent sexual offense post-assault testing and treatment

Providers need to be familiar with the testing methods that are available at their own facilities. More detailed coverage of this topic is available at the website of the Centers for Disease Control and Prevention; the 2006 treatment guidelines are available at http://www.cdc.gov/std/treatment/ and can be downloaded.

It should be noted that, at the time of this publication, the use of nucleic acid amplification tests for Neisseria gonorrhea and Chlamydia trachomatis in the setting of sexual abuse and sexual assault is controversial and still being evaluated. These tests offer an attractive alternative to traditional culture tests because they do not have difficult transport and storage requirements; a single swab can be used for both GC and CT, and urine can be tested rather than vaginal or cervical swabs. In addition, the NAAT sensitivity for Chlamydia may be higher than tissue cell culture, the current "gold standard." The problem with these tests remains the Positive Predictive Value (PPV) or ability to detect a true positive, which may be unacceptably low given the potential consequences of a false positive. If the presence of a STI is going to be "proof" of sexual abuse or assault, identifying true infections is of utmost importance. At this time, these tests have been studied more extensively in the adult or pubertal population than the pre-pubertal group. Once again, facilities are advised to be familiar with the available testing and discuss the advisability of using NAAT or cultures with local experts.

The following chart from the New York State Department of Health Guideline for Child and Adolescent Sexual Assault nicely summarizes current recommendations for post-assault treatment and testing:

Medical Care	Hours 24	48	96	120	Weeks 1	2	Months 1	2	3	4	6	12
❶ Acute & Follow-up Examinations					Follow-up Exam 1 to 2 weeks		Exams for physical and emotional well-being may be done at any time.					
❷ Forensic Specimen Collection												
❸ HIV Post-Exposure Prophylaxis & Testing	36 hours						Re-test 4-6 weeks		Re-test 3 months		Re-test 6 months	
❹ Pregnancy Testing & Prevention	72 hours				Follow-up Serum ßhCG 1 to 2 weeks							
❺ STI Testing					Follow-up cultures 1-2 weeks		RPR, HBV 4-6 weeks		RPR, HBV, HCV 3 months		HCV 6 months	
❻ STI Treatment					Treatment may be offered in the acute post-assault setting. Treatment decisions are guided by results of diagnostic testing.							
❼ Drug Facilitated Sexual Assault Testing												

Treatment

The decision to provide prophylactic treatment for STIs must be made on a case-by-case basis. Many providers feel more inclined to treat adolescents who present for medical care after an acute sexual assault. The greater concern in adolescents is predicated on many factors, including the following:

1. Follow-up may be more difficult in this age group
2. The prevalence of some STIs is high in sexually active women, and the visit for medical care after a sexual assault may represent an opportunity that should not be "missed"
3. There is a risk of complications from untreated ascending infections from Chlamydia and Gonorrhea

As a general concept, prophylactic treatment is not generally indicated in pre-pubertal children who have been sexually abused. Treatment in these instances will be guided by the results of the microbiologic testing.

Consult the Centers for Disease Control website for the most up-to-date recommendations regarding STD prophylaxis. At the time of this publication:

Prophylaxis	Order
Gonorrhea Children less than 45 kg:	☐ **Ceftriaxone** 125 mg intramuscularly in a single dose. ☐ **Spectinomycin** [40 mg/kg (max. 2 gm)]_____mg IM in a single dose. (not recommended for treatment of gonococcal pharyngitis).
Children greater than or equal to 45 kg:	☐ **Cefixime (Suprax®)** 400 mg by mouth in a single dose. (Suspension of 200-mg/5-mL formulation of cefixime oral suspension) ☐ **Ceftriaxone (Rocephin®)** 125 to 250 mg intramuscularly in a single dose. ☐ **Ciprofloxacin (Cipro®)** 500 mg by mouth in a single dose. ☐ **Levofloxacin (Levaquin®)** 250 mg by mouth in a single dose.

Chlamydia
Children less than or equal to 45 kg:
 	
Children greater than or equal to 45 kg and less than 8 years old:
Children greater than or equal to 8 years old:
	☐ **Erythromycin base or ethylsuccinate** 50 mg/kg/day by mouth divided into four doses daily for 14 days.
	      Erythromycin _____ _____mg four times daily for 14 days.
	            (Specify base or ethylsuccinate) (Dose)
	☐ **Azithromycin (Zithromax®)** (20 mg/kg) _____mg by mouth in a single dose.

	☐ **Azithromycin (Zithromax®)** 1 gm by mouth in a single dose.
	☐ **Azithromycin (Zithromax®)** 1 gm by mouth in a single dose.
	☐ **Doxycycline (Vibramycin®)** 100 mg twice daily for 7 days.
Bacterial Vaginosis & **Trichomoniasis**	☐ **Metronidazole** 2 gm by mouth in a single dose
Hepatitis B	☐ **Hepatitis B virus vaccine** 1 mL intramuscularly (deltoid) at 0, 1, and 6 months. **and/or** ☐ **Hepatitis B immune globulin** 0.06 mL/kg intramuscularly in a single dose; within 14 days of exposure.
Human Immunodeficiency Virus **Zidovudine (Retrovir®)** + **Lamivudine (Epivir®)** + / − **Lopinavir/ritonavir (Kaletra®) for 4 weeks.**	**Zidovudine** ☐ 12 years of age: 160 mg/m²/dose, 3 times a day, by mouth or 180–240 mg /m²/dose, by mouth twice daily (max. 200 mg/dose three daily or 300 mg /dose, twice daily. Zidovudine _____mg by mouth _____times daily for 4 weeks. ☐ Greater than or equal to 13 years: 200 mg/dose by mouth 3 times daily, or 300 mg /dose by mouth twice daily. Zidovudine _____mg by mouth _____times daily for 4 weeks.

	Lamivudine
	☐ Less than one month of age: 2 mg/kg/dose by mouth twice daily.
	   Lamivudine _____mg by mouth twice daily for 4 weeks.
	☐ Less than 37.5 kg in body weight: 4 mg/kg/dose by mouth twice daily.
	   Lamivudine _____mg by mouth twice daily for 4 weeks.
	☐ Greater than or equal to 37.5 kg in body weight: 150 mg/dose by mouth twice daily.
	   Lamivudine _____mg by mouth twice daily for 4 weeks.
	
	Lopinavir/ritonavir (Kaletra®) available as 400mg/100mg/5 mL solution
	☐ Children 7 kg to 14 kg and 6 month to 12 years:
	   Kaletra® (12 mg/3 mg per kg per dose) _____mg by mouth twice daily for 4 weeks.
	☐ Children 15 kg to 40 kg and 6 month to 12 years:
	   Kaletra® (10 mg/2.5 mg per kg per dose) _____mg by mouth twice daily for 4 weeks.
	☐ Children over 40 kg:
	   Kaletra® (400 mg/100 mg per dose) _____mg by mouth twice daily for 4 weeks.

Alternative for children 13 years and older and 40 kg or more.	☐ **Lamivudine/Zidovudine (Combivir®)** 1 tablet by mouth twice daily and Tenofovir (**Viread®**) 300 mg by mouth daily.
Emergency Contraception	☐ **Levonorgestrel (Plan B®)** 2 tablets of 0.75 mg. One tablet (0.75 mg) should be taken by mouth within 72 hours after unprotected intercourse. The second tablet (0.75 mg) should be taken 12 hours after the first dose.

The decision to provide prophylaxis against HIV is a complicated one. Although the risk of HIV acquisition through sexual abuse or assault is most likely low, infection has been reported in people where abuse and assault was the only identifiable risk factor. Sexual assault may be a particularly risky contact because of the possibility of traumatic vaginal, anal, or oral penetration. Because studies of post-exposure prophylaxis have demonstrated benefit in occupation exposure of health care providers, it has been extrapolated that benefit might exist in other types of exposure, including after sexual assault. Medical providers should consult HIV experts in their institutions for recommendations about treatment in each case of sexual assault. Another very valuable resource is the National Clinician's Post-Exposure Prophylaxis Hotline (PEPLine), telephone: 888-448-4911.

Recommendations for PEP assessment of adolescent survivors within 72 hours of sexual assault[109]

- Assess risk for HIV infection in the assailant
- Evaluate characteristics of the assault event that might increase the risk of transmission
- Consult with specialist in HIV treatment if PEP is being considered
- If the survivor appears to be at risk for HIV transmission from the assault, discuss antiretroviral prophylaxis, including toxicity and lack of proven benefit
- If the survivor chooses to start antiretroviral PEP, provide enough medication to last until the next return visit; re-evaluate the survivor in three to seven days after the initial assessment and assess tolerance of medication
- If PEP is started, perform baseline CBC and serum chemistries; initiation of medication should not be delayed pending results
- Perform HIV antibody test at original assessment; repeat at six weeks, three months, and six months

Other diagnostic and treatment considerations

In adolescents, a pregnancy test is always indicated. Once it has been determined that the teen is not pregnant, emergency contraception should be offered if the sexual assault was within the prior 72 hours. Because the high dose of hormonal therapy, particularly when coupled with the prophylactic antibiotics and antiretrovirals, can cause nausea, an antiemetic may be prescribed.

Concluding the visit

At the end of the visit, the medical provider must ensure that the child is safe. This means that, if the medical provider is not comfortable with the immediate discharge plans, the child should not be allowed to leave the emergency department or other facility. Although the local child protective agency has the authority to make the decision about whether the child will return to his or her home or be removed and placed into protective custody, there is always someone at a more supervisory level who can be reached in an emergency. The medical provider may need to enlist the assistance of their social worker, risk management, or legal department if there is genuine concern about a child's well being.

The medical provider should answer any questions that the child and non-offending parent or other guardian have about the medical evaluation. A written discharge document should include the name and doses of any medications that were given or prescribed. The dates and times of follow-up visits or referrals (e.g.

to a child advocacy center or program) should be written down. This becomes particularly important in cases when a child will be removed from their home and placed with a substitute caregiver.

Although the medical provider may feel compelled to reassure the child with statements such as, "Everything will be alright," such promises should not be made. In fact, for some time to come, things may not be "alright." Sexual abuse or assault is devastating to children and their families, and in the aftermath of disclosure, families are frequently in turmoil. A child should be told that there are people who are working very hard to help them and their families. Children should be thanked for their cooperation and bravery and reassured that they are not to blame.

Medical providers should make sure that the child and supportive family members have had the opportunity to meet with a counselor or victim advocate. At the least, a referral should be made to a victim advocacy program or agency; these professionals can often be accessed through a local child advocacy center.

Sexual abuse: case examples

Abuse in children with disabilities

It is important for medical providers to be cognizant of the fact that children with disabilities are at greater risk of maltreatment of all kinds than their peers without disabilities. A large epidemiological study by Sullivan and Knutson[110] revealed that the relative risk of maltreatment in children with disabilities is about 3.5. Although the issue is multifactorial, some of the reasons that children with disabilities are at greater risk include the following[111]:

- Children with disabilities may have developmental or communication difficulties that make disclosure of abuse difficult or impossible
- Children with disabilities may lack correct information or education about abuse prevention, sexuality, and self-protection strategies (e.g. the right to say "no")
- Children with disabilities may not understand the difference between a hygienic touch, an affectionate touch, or an abusive touch
- Children with disabilities may have physical disabilities that prevent a child from defending themselves or getting away
- Children with disabilities may depend on others to meet even their most basic needs (bathing, toileting, feeding), which creates an extreme imbalance of power
- Children with disabilities may have a desire to please or may have cognitive difficulties that make them overly trusting and easier to trick
- Children with disabilities may place higher emotional, physical, economical, and social demands on their families. There are limited specialized childcare facilities to provide families with respite

The medical provider in the acute care setting may be influenced by the myth that nobody would hurt a child with a disability and therefore may be blind to the red flags of child abuse. The approach to the evaluation of possible child abuse in children with disabilities is similar to that in children without disabilities; however, providers should be prepared for each stage of the evaluation to take longer. It is just as important for providers to understand a child's communicative limitations and to take steps to maximize the child's ability to recount their abuse as it is to provide an interpreter for a child who communicates best in a language other than English. It behooves providers in acute care settings to locate professionals with disability expertise to assist in the evaluation of a child with a disability. The health care provider is also in a unique position to assist the other members of the multidisciplinary team with their investigations by helping them to understand the child's strengths and limitations.

Failure to thrive

Failure to thrive (FTT) is identified either when a child weighs below the fifth percentile for age or when their weight is less than 80 percent of the ideal weight for their age, when plotted on the standard pediatric growth charts from the National Center for Health Statistics (NCHS).[112] FTT is also identified when a child demonstrates an inadequate rate of weight gain that results in the crossing of two percentiles on a standard pediatric growth chart.[112] Many children with nutritional FTT are managed in an outpatient clinical setting with close follow-up. However, those children who have FTT due to neglect may not be followed regularly by a pediatrician, if at all, and may first present to the emergency room.

There are many medical conditions that may result in a lack of useful nutrition which subsequently lead to FTT. However, the traditional distinction between organic and inorganic FTT is no longer considered diagnostically helpful since children with "organic" conditions that cause FTT may also have psychosocial or environmental factors that contribute as well.[112] The underlying cause(s) of FTT can usually be identified by completing a thorough history and physical examination and by reviewing prior growth parameters as well as the state newborn screening program results. Some laboratory studies may be indicated, based on the history and physical exam; these include: CBC and differential, to identify chronic or occult bleeding, iron deficiency anemia, lead toxicity, malignancy, and infection; urinalysis or urine culture, to identify kidney or bladder infection or renal disease; serum electrolytes, to identify renal tubular acidosis or other causes of acidosis; T4 and TSH, to identify hyperthyroidism or hypothyroidism; PPD; serum albumin, calcium, phosphorus, or liver function tests, in order to identify rickets or liver disease; erythrocyte sedimentation rate; stool guaiac, culture, ova and parasites, and fecal fat, to identify GI causes of malnutrition; and HIV testing. Further management decisions, such as inpatient admission or further testing, may be based on the results of these studies. A chest radiograph or a skeletal survey may also be indicated in certain cases.

Medico–legal issues

Documentation

The professional, accurate medical record should contain information pertinent to medical diagnosis and treatment. The records should be professional, precise, legible, dated, and signed.

Protective custody

Consider taking protective custody of a child or adolescent if there is a reasonable cause to believe that the child/adolescent may be in imminent danger if in the care of the presenting guardian. Specific laws vary from state to state; refer to your institution's legal counsel or hospital administrator for specific guidance. In most states, if a hospital-based medical provider believes a child/adolescent would be in imminent danger if returned to the care and custody of the parent or guardian, that provider can have the child/adolescent placed in protective custody at that hospital. This action requires immediate notification of the local CPS and notification of the child/adolescent's parent or caretaker. CPS must, in turn, begin an investigation and, if warranted, appropriate legal proceedings.

It is important to distinguish hospital-based protective custody from inpatient medical diagnosis and treatment. If a child/adolescent does not require inpatient or emergent hospital care, CPS should make arrangements for the transfer of the child/adolescent to a community-based facility, respite care, or foster care.

Confidential and privileged communication

Typically, medical providers cannot reveal confidential patient information without specific consent. When a medical provider suspects child abuse and is mandated to report, certain exceptions to physician–patient confidentiality may apply.

When a case involves child abuse, it is safe to assume that medical records will become available for release in a criminal or civil legal matter. However, do not assume that any police, attorneys, or others are privy to this information without determining whether authorization exists. When contacted by an attorney, determine whether you are authorized to talk to the attorney by seeking guidance from your institution's legal counsel or administrator.

Consent by mature or emancipated minors

In general, any person who is 18 or older, who is or has been the parent of a child, or who is or has been married, may give effective consent for medical, dental, health, and hospital services for him/herself. Any pregnant female may give effective consent to medical, dental, health, and hospital services relating to prenatal care. When in a medical provider's judgment, there is an emergency requiring immediate need of medical treatment, and the delay of time in an attempt to secure consent would increase the risk to the person's life or health, medical, dental, health, and medical care may be rendered without parent or guardian consent.

There may be specific laws regarding consent to an HIV test, testing and treatment of sexually transmitted diseases, contraception, termination of a pregnancy, and drug/alcohol abuse treatment. The Center for Adolescent Health & the Law has produced a monograph that summarizes the minor consent laws for all 50 states and the District of Columbia; this is downloadable for free at http://www.cahl.org.

Releasing information

HIPAA, or the Health Insurance Portability and Accountability Act, pertains to the security and privacy of patient health information. The text of the HIPAA regulations can be found at http://www.hhs.gov/ocr/hipaa/. The American Bar Association publication "The Impact of HIPAA on Child Abuse and Neglect Cases" is available at http://www.pcsao.org/HIPAA/HIPAAChildAbuse.pdf. In general, when medical information is critical to the protection of the child, sharing of that information is recommended and ethically responsible.

The judicial system

Child abuse cases may be addressed in civil court, criminal court, or both. Courts are established on federal, state, and local levels. Jurisdiction and procedure vary at each level. Specific court structures may vary from state to state, and in different areas within states. Refer to your own institution's legal counsel or administrator for guidance should you be called on for a legal proceeding related to child abuse.

Hearsay and medical documentation

Hearsay is most often not allowable testimony in court proceedings because it is seen as less reliable evidence, and because the individual who made the statement is not testifying to it and cannot be cross-examined. There are several exceptions to the hearsay rule, and the law regarding admission of hearsay varies from state to state. In some states, medical records indicating disclosures of abuse and medical testimony regarding patient information given as part of routine care may be allowed in court as exceptions to hearsay rules. This is why accurate documentation is critical in cases of child abuse; the child's or the caretaker's precise words may become admissible to a court proceeding in these situations. In these instances, assure and document that the child/adolescent understood that he/she was seeing you for medical diagnosis and treatment. In some states, statements made in response to an unusual and startling event may be admissible in court proceedings. In child abuse cases, document the specific words the child/adolescent used and that the child/adolescent was in an excited state, if that was the case.

Testifying as a fact witness

A fact witness testifies regarding observations, findings, and diagnoses. For example, a physician treating a child for bruises, abrasions, fractures, or other injuries may be asked to give an opinion as to whether such injuries were inflicted or accidental.

Testifying as an expert

It is the responsibility of the attorney to provide the court with expert testimony. The medical provider who happens to treat a child/adolescent with potential abuse need not offer him/herself as an expert. However, in particular circumstances, the medical provider may either be called to testify about cases in which he/she has played no prior role, or be asked to render an expert opinion about a case he/she provided treatment for.

A qualified expert is allowed to testify regarding matters that would be outside the normal scope of knowledge and experience of the judge or jury. The purpose of expert testimony is typically to provide education for the court about a specific medical issue. Before being "qualified" as an expert, the judge will determine whether the individual possesses the appropriate knowledge, skill, experience, training, or education to assist the jury. If qualified, the expert must resist testifying beyond the limits of his/her expertise, especially if an attorney asks questions on topics about which that person is not an expert—it is better to answer "I don't know" or "That is beyond my area of expertise." An expert is most effective when the information is presented in a knowledgeable, unbiased manner without a personal agenda or advocacy position. Expert testimony should be reliable and based on sound scientific principles.

Provider qualifications

The role of medical providers in the recognition, treatment, and follow-up of children and adolescents who may have been abused varies between states, and according to the availability of child abuse pediatricians.

In general:

> Child abuse pediatricians/forensic pediatricians are medical specialists who are certified or eligible to be certified by the American Board of Pediatrics, which designated the field as a formal subspecialty in 2006. These child abuse specialists are identified nationally through the Helfer Society: http://www.helfersociety.org.

Nurse Practitioners, general pediatricians, family practitioners, or physicians' assistants may have training and expertise in the area of child abuse and be considered experts within certain regions.

Emergency medicine physicians should have knowledge about the developmental and emotional needs of child and adolescent abuse victims, be able to recognize behavioral indicators and clinical signs of abuse, know when it is appropriate to obtain laboratory tests, radiographs, and photographs, know how to collect forensic evidence, and how to determine an appropriate treatment plan. Further, it is essential that they are familiar with local CPS and other services available to abused children/adolescents and their families. However, the emergency medical provider need not consider him/herself an expert in child abuse and may defer a formal opinion on a child abuse matter if he/she is not qualified to do so.

Registered nurses are mandatory reporters, and therefore, should be aware of the indicators of child abuse.

Forensically trained nurses are registered nurses who have successfully completed either a Sexual Assault Nurse Examiner (SANE) course or a Sexual Assault Forensic Examiner (SAFE) course and corresponding mentorship. These nurses have been primarily used to evaluate adult sexual assault victims in order to assist treating physicians or physician extenders in the acquisition of forensic evidence as well as to contribute to the assurance of well being of the adult sexual assault victim. There are significant differences in the forensic examination of a child versus an adult. In some geographical regions, these nurses may be part of collaborative teams that evaluate children or adolescent victims of sexual abuse. These examinations must be performed in conjunction with a physician or qualified physician extender.

The importance of peer review and supervision in child and adolescent sexual abuse evaluations

The field of child abuse pediatrics has rapidly developed over the past 20 years. Some findings that examiners may have interpreted as abnormal at one time have since been determined through research to be normal variants. Thus, the examiner must be familiar with the most up-to-date research and literature, as over-interpretation of findings in sexual abuse may result in severe consequences, including incarceration of an innocent person. In the current state of child and adolescent sexual abuse, examiners should be engaged in regular, quality peer-review and, if not fully trained, be mentored by a child abuse specialist. This will ensure optimal medical care and the most specific and evidence-based findings to be used in legal proceedings.

References

1. U.S. Department of Health and Human Services and the Administration on Children, Youth and Families. Child Maltreatment 2004 [online]. (Washington, DC: U.S. Government Printing Office, 2006.) Retrieved February 3, 2007, from http://www.acf.hhs.gov/programs/cblpubs/cm04/chapterthree.htm.

2. Finkelhor D. Current information on the scope and nature of child sexual abuse. *Future Child*. 1994; 4: 31–53.

3. The Federal Interagency Forum on Child and Family Statistics. (1997). America's Children: Key Indicators of Well-Being. Retrieved November 16, 2006, from www.cdc.gov/nchs/data/misc/amchild.pdf.

4. Schulman ST. Child abuse. *Pediatr Ann*. 2005; 34(5): 338.

5. Labbe J, Caouette G. Recent skin injuries in normal children. *Pediatrics*. 2001; 108(2): 271–6.

6. Sugar NF, Taylor JA, Feldman KW. Bruises in infants and toddlers: those who don't cruise rarely bruise. *Arch Pediatr Adolesc Med*. 1999; 153: 399–403.

7. Stephenson T. Bruising in children. *Curr Paediatr*. 1995; 5: 225–9.

8. Langlois NEI, Gresham GA. The aging of bruises: a review and study of the colour changes with time. *Forensic Sci Int*. 1991; 50: 227–38.

9. Bariciak ED, Plint AC, Gaboury I, Bennett S. Dating of bruises in children: an assessment of physician accuracy. *Pediatrics*. 2003; 112: 804–7.

10. Wagner GN. Bitemark identification in child abuse cases. *Pediatr Dent*. 1986; 8: 96–100.

11. National Research Council, Committee on DNA Technology in Forensic Science, Board of Biology, Commission on Life Sciences. *DNA Technology in Forensic Science*. Washington, DC: National Academy Press, 1992.

12. U.S. Department of Justice. Burn injuries in child abuse. June 2001. Retrieved from http://www.ncjrs.gov/pdffiles/91190-6.pdf.

13. Chester DL, Jose RM, Aldlyami E, King H, Moiemen NS. Non-accidental burns in childrens are we neglecting neglect? *Burns*. 2006; 32: 222–8.

14. Reece RM, Ludwig S (eds). *Child Abuse: Medical Diagnosis and Management*, Second Edition. Philadelphia, PA: Lippincott, Williams & Wilkins, 2001.

15. Zitelli B, Davis H (eds.) *Atlas of Pediatric Physical Diagnosis*, Third Edition. Singapore: Mosby-Year Book, Inc., 1997.

16. Tate RJ. Facial injuries associated with the battered child syndrome. *Br J Oral Surg*. 1971; 9: 41–5.

17. Naidoo S. A profile of the oro-facial injuries in child physical abuse at a children's hospital. *Child Abuse Negl*. 2000; 24: 521–34.

18. O'Neill JA Jr, Meacham WF, Griffin JP, Sawyers JL. Patterns of injury in the battered child syndrome. *J Trauma*. 1973; 13: 332–9.

19. Kittle PE, Richardson DS, Parker JW. Two child abuse/child neglect examinations for the dentist. *ASDC J Dent Child*. 1981; 48: 175–80.

20. Blain SM, Winegarden T, Barber TK, Sognnaes FR. Child abuse and neglect. II. Role of dentistry [abstract]. *J Dent Res*. 1979; 58 (spec issue A): 367.

21. Vadiakas G, Roberts MW, Dilley DC. Child abuse and neglect: ethical issues for dentistry. *J Mass Dent Soc*. 1991; 40: 13–15.

22. Scherl SA. Orthopedic injuries in child abuse. *Curr. Pediatr*. 2006; 16: 199–204.

23. Galleno H, Oppenheim WL. The battered child syndrome revisited. *Clin Orthop*. 1982; 162: 11–19.

24. Herndon WA. Child abuse in a military population. *J Pediatr Orthop*. 1983; 3: 73–6.

25. Merten DF, Radkowski MA, Leonidas JC. The abused child. A radiological reappraisal. *Radiology*. 1983; 146: 377–81.

26. Worlock P, Stowen M, Barbor P. Patterns of fractures in accidental and nonaccidental injury in children: a comprehensive study. *Br J Med*. 1986; 293: 100–2.

27. Pierce MC, Bertocci GE, Vogeley E, et al. Evaluating long bone fractures in children: a biomechanical approach with illustrative cases. *Child Abuse Neglect*. 2004; 28: 505–24.

28. Barsness KA, Cha ES, Bensard DD, et al. The positive predictive value of rib fractures as an indicator of non-accidental trauma in children. *J Trauma*. 2003; 54: 1107–10.

29. Bush CM, Jones JS, Cohle SD, Johnson H. Pediatric injuries from cardiopulmonary resuscitation. *Ann Emerg Med*. 1996; 28: 40–4.

30. Spevak MR, Kleinman PK, Belanger PL, Primack C, Richmond JM. Cardiopulmonary resuscitation and rib fractures in infants. *JAMA*. 1994; 272: 617–18.

31. Feldman KW, Brewer DK. Child abuse, cardiopulmonary resuscitation, and rib fractures. *Pediatrics*. 1984; 73: 339–42.

32. Bulloch B, Schubert CJ, Brophy PD, Johnson N, Reed MH, Shapiro RA. Cause and clinical characteristics of rib fractures in infants. *Pediatrics*. 2000; 105; e48.

33. Kleinman PK, Marks SC, Blackbourne B. The metaphyseal lesion in abused infants: a radiologic-histopathologic study. *AJR*. 1986; 146: 895–905.

34. Pierce MC, Bertocci GE, Janosky JE, et al. Femur fractures resulting from stair falls among children: an injury plausibility model. *Pediatrics*. 2005; 115: 1712–22.

35. Scherl SA, Miller L, Lovely N, Russinoff S, Sullivan CM, Tornetta P III. Accidental and nonaccidental femur fractures in children. *Clin Orthop Relat Res*. 2000; 376: 96–105.

36. Alexander R, Levitt C, Smith W. Abusive head trauma. In: Reece RM, Ludwig S, eds. *Child Abuse: Medical Diagnosis and Management*, second edition. Philadelphia, PA: Lippincott, Williams & Wilkins; 2001: 47–80.

37. Jenny C, Hymel KP, Ritzen A, Reinert SE, Hay TC. Analysis of missed cases of abusive head trauma. *JAMA*. 1999; 281: 621–6.

38. Keenan HT, Runyan DK, Marshall SW, Nocera MA, Merten DF, Sinal SH. A population-based study of inflicted traumatic brain injury in young children. *JAMA*. 2003; 290: 621–6.

39. Reijneveld S, van der Wal M, Brugman E, Hira Sing R, Verloove-Vanhorick S. Infant crying and abuse. *Lancet*. 2004; 364(9442): 1340–2.

40. Caffey J. On the theory and practice of shaking infants. Its potential residual effects of permanent brain damage and mental retardation. *Am J Dis Child*. 1972; 124: 161–9.

41. Guthkelch AN. Infantile subdural haematoma and its relationship to whiplash injury. *Br Med J*. 1971; 2: 430–1.

42. U.S. Advisory Board on Child Abuse and Neglect. *A Nation's Shame: Fatal Child Abuse and Neglect in the United States*. Washington, DC: U.S. Department of Health and Human Services; 1995. Report No. 5.

43. Alexander R, Smith W, eds. *Abusive Head Trauma: Proceedings of a Consensus Conference*. Funded by Brain Trauma Foundation. Iowa City, IA: University of Iowa; 1991.

44. Ludwig S, Warman M. Shaken baby syndrome: a review of 20 cases. *Ann Emerg Med*. 1984; 13: 104–7.

45. Bruce DA, Zimmerman RA. Shaken impact syndrome. *Pediatr Ann*. 1989; 18: 482–94.

46. Alexander R, Sato Y, Smith W, Bennett T. Incidence of trauma with cranial injuries ascribed to shaking. *Am J Dis Child*. 1990; 144: 724–6 [Abstract].

47. Gilliland MG, Folberg R. Shaken babies – some have no impact injuries. *J Forens Sci*. 1996; 41: 114–16.

48. Duhaime AC, Gennerelli TA, Thibault LE, Bruce DA, Margulies SS, Wiser R. The shaken baby syndrome. A clinical, pathological, and biomechanical study. *J Neurosurg*. 1987; 66: 409–15.

49. Alexander R, Crabbe L, Sato Y, Smith W, Bennett T. Serial abuse in children who are shaken. *Am J Dis Child*. 1990; 144: 58–60.

50. Ewings-Cobb L, Kramer L, Prasad M. Neuroimaging, physical, and developmental findings after inflicted and non-inflicted traumatic brain injury in young children. *Pediatrics*. 1998; 102: 300–7.

51. Starling SP, Holden JR, Jenny C. Abusive head trauma: the relationship of perpetrators to their victims. *Pediatrics*. 1995; 95: 259–62.

52. Levin AV. Ocular manifestations of child abuse. *Ophthalmol Clin North Am*. 1990; 3: 249–64.

53. Sato Y, Yuh WT, Smith WL, Alexander RC, Kao SC, Ellerbroek CJ. Head injury in child abuse: evaluation with MR imaging. *Radiology*. 1989; 173: 653–7.

54. American Academy of Pediatrics, Section on Radiology. Diagnostic imaging of child abuse. *Pediatrics*. 2000; 105: 1345–8.

55. Meservy CJ, Towbin R, McLaurin RL, Myers PA, Ball W. Radiographic characteristics of skull fractures resulting from child abuse. *AJR Am J Roentgenol*. 1987; 149: 173–5.

56. Coant PN, Komberg AE, Brody AS, Edwards-Holmes K. Markers for occult liver injury in cases of physical abuse in children. *Pediatrics*. 1992; 89: 274–8.

57. Suson EM, Klotz D Jr, Kottmeier PK. Liver trauma in children. *J Pediatr Surg*. 1975; 10(3): 411–17.

58. Ledbetter DJ, Hatch EI Jr, Feldman KW, Fligner CL, Tapper D. Diagnostic and surgical implications of child abuse. *Arch Surg*. 1988; 123(9): 1101–5.

59. Price E, Rush L, Perper J, Bell M. Cardiopulmonary resuscitation-related injuries and homicidal blunt abdominal trauma in children. *Am J Forensic Med Pathol*. 2000; 21: 307–10.

60. American Academy of Pediatrics, Section on Radiology: Diagnostic imaging of child abuse. *Pediatrics*. 1991; 87: 262–4.

61. Belfer RA, Klein BL, Orr L. Use of the skeletal survey in the evaluation of child maltreatment. *Am J Emerg Med*. 2001; 19: 122–4.

62. Barsness KA, Cha ES, Bensard DD, et al. The positive predictive value of rib fractures as an indicator of non-accidental trauma in children. *J Trauma-Injury Infect Crit Care*. 2003; 54: 1107–10.

63. Kemp AM, Butler A, Morris S, Mann M, Kemp KW. Which radiological investigations should be performed to identify fractures in suspected child abuse? *Clin. Radio*. 2006; 61: 723–36.

64. Kleinman PK, Nimkin K, Spevak MR, et al. Follow-up skeletal surveys in suspected child abuse. *AJR Am J Roentgenol*. 1996; 167: 893–6.

65. Ellerstein NS, Norris KJ. Value of radiologic skeletal survey in assessment of abused children. *Pediatrics*. 1984; 74: 1075–8.

66. Jaudes PK. Comparison of radiography and radionuclide bone scanning in the detection of child abuse. *Pediatrics*. 1984; 73: 166–8.

67. Zimmerman S, Makoroff K, Care M, et al. Utility of follow-up skeletal surveys in suspected child physical abuse evaluations. *Child Abuse Negl*. 2005; 29: 1075–83.

68. Helfer RE, Slovis TL, Black M. Injuries resulting when small children fall out of bed. *Pediatrics*. 1977; 60(4): 533–5.

69. Nimityongskul P, Anderson L. The likelihood of injuries when children fall out of bed. *J Pediatr Orthop*. 1987; 7: 184–6.

70. Barlow B. Accidents in childhood. *Nurs Mirror Midwives J*. 1977; 144(8): 39–40.

71. Williams RA. Injuries in infants and small children resulting from witnessed and corroborated free falls. *J Trauma*. 1991; 31(10): 1350–2.

72. Musemeche CA, Barthel M, Cosentino C, Reynolds M. Pediatric falls from heights. *J Trauma*. 1991; 31(10): 1347–9.

73. Smith MD, Burrington JD, Woolf AD. Injuries in children sustained in free falls: an analysis of 66 cases. *J Trauma*. 1975; 15(11): 987–91.

74. Chadwick DL, Chin S, Salerno C, Landsverk J, Kitchen L. Deaths from falls in children: how far is fatal? *J Trauma*. 1991; 31(10): 1353–5.

75. Selbst SM, Baker MD, Shames M. Bunk bed injuries. *Am J Dis Child*. 1990; 144(6): 721–3.

76. Mayr JM, Seebacher U, Lawrenz K, Pesendorfer P, Berghold A, Baradaran S. Bunk beds – a still underestimated risk for accidents in childhood? *Eur J Pediatr*. 2000; 159: 440–3.

77. Joffe M, Ludwig S. Stairway injuries in children. *Pediatrics*. 1988; 82(3 Pt 2): 457–61.

78. Mayr JM, Seebacher U, Shimpl G, Fiala F. High chair accidents. *Acta Pediatr*. 1999; 88: 319–22.

79. Waltzman ML, Shannon M, Bowen AP, Bailey MC. Monkeybar injuries: complications of play. *Pediatrics*. 1999; 103: e58.

80. Dowd MD, Fitzmaurice L, Knapp J, Mooney D. The interpretation of urogenital findings in children with straddle injuries. *J Pediatr Surg*. 1994; 29: 7–10.

81. U.S. Consumer Product Safety Commission Baby Walkers. Advance notice of proposed rulemaking. *Fed. Reg*. 1994; 59: 39306–11.

82. Drago DA, Winston FK, Baker SP. Clothing drawstring entrapment in playground slides and school buses. *Arch Pediatr Adolesc Med*. 1997; 151: 72–7.

83. Drago DA, Dannenberg AL. Infant mechanical suffocation deaths in the United States, 1980–1997. *Pediatrics*. 1999; 103: e59.

84. Bernard PA, Johnston C, Curtis SE, King WD. Toppled television sets cause significant pediatric morbidity and mortality. *Pediatrics*. 1998; 102(3): E32.

85. DiScala C, Bartel M, Sege R. Outcomes from television sets toppling onto toddlers. *Arch Pediatr Adolesc Med*. 2001; 155: 145–8.

86. Kemp A, Mott AM, Sibert JR. Accidents and child abuse in bathtub submersions. *Arch Dis Child*. 1994; 70: 435–8.

87. Lavelle JM, Shaw KN, Seidl T, Ludwig S. Ten-year review of pediatric bathtub near-drownings: evaluation for child abuse and neglect. *Ann Emerg Med*. 1995; 25(3): 344–8.

88. Byard RW, Lipsett J. Drowning deaths in toddlers and preambulatory children in South Australia. *Am J Forensic Med Pathol*. 1999; 20(4): 328–32.

89. DiScala C, Barthel M, Sege R. Outcomes from television sets toppling onto toddlers. *Arch Pediatr Adolesc Med*. 2001; 155(2): 145–8.

90. Bernard PA, Johnston C, Curtis SE, King WD. Toppled television sets cause significant pediatric morbidity and mortality. *Pediatrics*. 1998; 102(3): E32.

91. Makoroff KL, Brauley JL, Brander AM, Myers PA, Shapiro RA. Genital examinations for alleged sexual abuse of prepubertal girls: findings by pediatric emergency medicine physicians compared to child abuse trained physicians. *Child Abuse Neglect*. 2002; 26: 1235–42.

92. Adams H. Approach to the interpretation of medical and laboratory findings in suspected child sexual abuse: a 2005 revision. *The APSAC Advisor*. 2005; pp. 7–13.

93. Astrid Heger A, Lynne T, Velasquez O, Bernier R. Children referred for possible sexual abuse: medical findings in 2384 children. *Child Abuse Neglect*. 2002; 26: 645–59.

94. Finkel MA. Anogenital trauma in sexually abused children. *Pediatrics*. 1989; 84: 317–22.

95. McCann J, Voris J, Simon M. Genital injuries resulting from sexual abuse: a longitudinal study. *Pediatrics*. 1992; 89: 307–17.

96. Faller KC. *Interviewing Children about Sexual Abuse: Controversies and Best Practice*. Oxford University Press, USA: 2007.

97. Sorensen T, Snow B. How children tell: the process of disclosure in child sexual abuse. *Child Welfare*. 1990; 70(1): 3–15.

98. Christian CW, Lavelle JM, De Jong AR, et al. Forensic evidence findings in prepubertal victims of sexual assault. *Pediatrics*. 2000; 106(1 Pt 1): 100–4.

99. McCann J, Miyamoto S, Boyle C, Rogers K. Healing of hymenal injuries in prepubertal and adolescent girls: a descriptive study. *Pediatrics*. 2007; 119: e1094–e1106; originally published online Apr 9, 2007.

100. Friedrich WN, Fisher J, Broughton D, et al. Normative sexual behavior in children: a contemporary sample. *Pediatrics*. 1998; 101(4): E9.

101. American Professional Society on the Abuse of Children (1995a), Guidelines for psychosocial evaluation of suspected sexual abuse in young children. (Available from APSAC, 407 South Dearborn Avenue, Suite 1300, Chicago IL 60605).

102. Berenson AB. A longitudinal study of hymenal morphology in the first three years of life. *Pediatrics*. 1995; 95: 490–6.

103. Bays J, Chadwick D. The medical diagnosis of the sexually abused child. *Child Abuse Neglect*. 1993; 17: 91–110.

104. Sinclair KA, Woods CR, Kirse DJ, Sinal SH. Anogenital and respiratory tract human papillomavirus infections among children; age, gender and potential transmission through sexual abuse. *Pediatrics*. 2005; 116: 815–25.

105. Brilliant LC. Perianal Streptococcal dermatitis. *Ame. Fam. Physician*. January; 61(2): 391–3.

106. Siegel RM, Schubert CJ, Myers PA, Shapiro RA. The prevalence of sexually transmitted diseases in children and adolescents evaluated for sexual abuse in Cincinnati: rationale for limited STD testing in prepubertal girls. *Pediatrics*. 1995; 96: 1090–4.

107. Shapiro RA, Makaroff KL. Sexually transmitted diseases in sexually abused girls and adolescents. *Curr. Opin. Obstet. Gyneco*. 2006; 18(5): 492–7.

108. Ingram DM, Miller WC, Schoenbach VJ, Everett VD, Ingram DL. Risk assessment for Gonococcal and Chlamydial infections in young children undergoing evaluation for sexual abuse. *Pediatrics*. 2001; 107(5): E73.

109. Centers for Disease Control and Prevention. Sexually transmitted diseases treatment guidelines 2006. *MMWR Recomm Rep*. 2006; 55(RR11); 1–94.

110. Sullivan PM, Knutson JF. Maltreatment and disabilities: a population-based epidemiological study. *Child Abuse Neglect*. 2000; 24: 1257–74.

111. Bennett S, Baladerian NJ. The International Society for Prevention of Child Abuse and Neglect. Children with disabilities and child maltreatment. The Link: The Official Newsletter of the International Society for Prevention of Child Abuse and Neglect. 2005; 14(2).

112. McMillan JA, Feigin RD, DeAngelis C, Jones MD Jr. (eds.). *Oski's Pediatrics*, Fourth Edition. Philadelphia, PA: Lippincott, Williams & Wilkins 2006.

Quick Reference Pages

Child abuse

Questions to ask in the history of a potentially abused child:

1. Who are you and what is your relationship to the child/adolescent?
2. What is your reason for concern regarding abuse?
   - Is this a referral from a child abuse investigative agency?
   - Have you witnessed the abuse?
   - Did the child/adolescent disclose abuse? If so, to whom was the disclosure made? What are the exact words the child/adolescent used?
3. Who is the suspected perpetrator and what is that person's relationship to the child/adolescent?
4. Does the child/adolescent live with the suspected abuser or have regular contact with that person? Is the child/adolescent safe from the suspected perpetrator now?
5. Are you safe? Do you think your present situation is dangerous?
6. Is there a medical concern such as pain, bruising, bleeding, alteration in mental status or acute change in behavior, or possible pregnancy?
7. When was the last time that the child/adolescent had contact with the suspected perpetrator?

Treatment for sexual assault: For HIV

Recommendations for PEP Assessment of Adolescent Survivors within 72 Hours of Sexual Assault

- Assess risk for HIV infection in the assailant
- Evaluate characteristics of the assault event that might increase the risk of transmission
- Consult with specialist in HIV treatment if PEP is being considered
- If the survivor appears to be at risk for HIV transmission from the assault, discuss antiretroviral prophylaxis including toxicity and lack of proven benefit
- If the survivor chooses to start antiretroviral PEP, provide enough medication to last until the next return visit; re-evaluate the survivor in three to seven days after the initial assessment and assess tolerance of medication
- If PEP is started, perform baseline CBC and serum chemistries; initiation of medication should not be delayed pending results
- Perform HIV antibody test at original assessment; repeat at six weeks, three months, and six months

Treatment for sexual transmitted infections

The decision to provide prophylactic treatment for sexually transmitted infections must be made on a case-by-case basis. Many providers feel more inclined to treat adolescents who present for medical care after an acute sexual assault. The greater concern in adolescents is predicated on many factors including the following:

1. Follow-up may be more difficult in this age group
2. The prevalence of some sexually transmitted infections is high in sexually active women and the visit for medical care after a sexual assault may represent an opportunity that should not be "missed"
3. There is a risk of complications from untreated ascending infections from Chlamydia and Gonorrhea

As a general concept, prophylactic treatment is not generally indicated in pre-pubertal children who have been sexually abused. Treatment, in these instances will be guided by the results of the microbiologic testing.

Consult the Centers for Disease Control website for the most up-to-date recommendations regarding STD prophylaxis. At the time of this publication:

Prophylaxis	Order
Gonorrhea Children less than 45 kg:	☐ **Ceftriaxone** 125 mg intramuscularly in a single dose. ☐ **Spectinomycin** [40 mg/kg (max. 2 gm)]_____mg IM in a single dose. (not recommended for treatment of gonococcal pharyngitis).
Children greater than or equal to 45 kg:	☐ **Cefixime (Suprax®)** 400 mg by mouth in a single dose. (Suspension of 200-mg/5-mL formulation of cefixime oral suspension) ☐ **Ceftriaxone (Rocephin®)** 125 to 250 mg intramuscularly in a single dose. ☐ **Ciprofloxacin (Cipro®)** 500 mg by mouth in a single dose. ☐ **Levofloxacin (Levaquin®)** 250 mg by mouth in a single dose.

Chlamydia
Children less than or equal to 45 kg:
 	
Children greater than or equal to 45 kg and less than 8 years old:
	☐ **Erythromycin base or ethylsuccinate** 50 mg/kg/day by mouth divided into four doses daily for 14 days.
	  Erythromycin _____ _____mg four times daily for 14 days.
	    (Specify base or ethylsuccinate) (Dose)
	☐ **Azithromycin (Zithromax®)** (20 mg/kg) _____mg by mouth in a single dose.

Children greater than or equal to 8 years old:	☐ **Azithromycin (Zithromax®)** 1 gm by mouth in a single dose.
	☐ **Azithromycin (Zithromax®)** 1 gm by mouth in a single dose.
	☐ **Doxycycline (Vibramycin®)** 100 mg twice daily for 7 days.

Bacterial Vaginosis & **Trichomoniasis**	☐ **Metronidazole** 2 gm by mouth in a single dose
Hepatitis B	☐ **Hepatitis B virus vaccine** 1 mL intramuscularly (deltoid) at 0, 1, and 6 months. **and/or** ☐ **Hepatitis B immune globulin** 0.06 mL/kg intramuscularly in a single dose; within 14 days of exposure.
Human Immunodeficiency Virus **Zidovudine (Retrovir®) + Lamivudine (Epivir®) + / – Lopinavir/ritonavir (Kaletra®) for 4 weeks.**	**Zidovudine** ☐ 12 years of age: 160 mg/m^2/dose, 3 times a day, by mouth or 180–240 mg /m^2/dose, by mouth twice daily (max. 200 mg/dose three daily or 300 mg /dose, twice daily. Zidovudine _____mg by mouth _____times daily for 4 weeks. ☐ Greater than or equal to 13 years: 200 mg/dose by mouth 3 times daily, or 300 mg /dose by mouth twice daily. Zidovudine _____mg by mouth _____times daily for 4 weeks. **Lamivudine** ☐ Less than one month of age: 2 mg/kg/dose by mouth twice daily. Lamivudine _____mg by mouth twice daily for 4 weeks. ☐ Less than 37.5 kg in body weight: 4 mg/kg/dose by mouth twice daily. Lamivudine _____mg by mouth twice daily for 4 weeks. ☐ Greater than or equal to 37.5 kg in body weight: 150 mg/dose by mouth twice daily. Lamivudine _____mg by mouth twice daily for 4 weeks. **Lopinavir/ritonavir (Kaletra®)** available as 400mg/100mg/5 mL solution ☐ Children 7 kg to 14 kg and 6 month to 12 years: Kaletra® (12 mg/3 mg per kg per dose) _____mg by mouth twice daily for 4 weeks. ☐ Children 15 kg to 40 kg and 6 month to 12 years: Kaletra® (10 mg/2.5 mg per kg per dose) _____mg by mouth twice daily for 4 weeks. ☐ Children over 40 kg:
Alternative for children 13 years and older and 40 kg or more.	Kaletra® (400 mg/100 mg per dose) _____mg by mouth twice daily for 4 weeks.
	☐ **Lamivudine/Zidovudine (Combivir®)** 1 tablet by mouth twice daily and Tenofovir (**Viread®**) 300 mg by mouth daily.
Emergency Contraception	☐ **Levonorgestrel (Plan B®)** 2 tablets of 0.75 mg. One tablet (0.75 mg) should be taken by mouth within 72 hours after unprotected intercourse. The second tablet (0.75 mg) should be taken 12 hours after the first dose.

Intimate partner violence

Peggy E. Goodman, M.D., M.S., F.A.C.E.P.

Goals and objectives

1. To understand the dynamics of intimate partner violence (IPV) and its effects on patients
2. To recognize the spectrum of clinical (non-traumatic & traumatic) presentations of intimate partner violence
3. To learn appropriate screening, treatment, documentation, and referral of victims of intimate partner violence

Intimate partner violence as a health issue

Intimate partner violence is a significant patient health issue. While IPV was previously treated by law enforcement as a couple's "private matter," it is now clearly recognized that IPV has significant medical ramifications that can extend to other family members, friends, and co-workers, and can affect the health and safety of the general public. In many cases the emergency department (ED) or emergency medical services (EMS) provide these patients' first-line medical assessment.

Epidemiology

The previously used term, "wife-beating," made the assumptions that physical abuse by a male was perpetrated upon a female with whom he cohabited in a current marital relationship. It is now recognized that a much broader definition is necessary to include physical, emotional, sexual, or financial control by one person over another, who are or have previously been in an intimate relationship, regardless of gender, marital, or habitation status.

While data sharing and reporting is often hampered by safety and confidentiality concerns, in the United States, approximately 5.3 million incidents occur annually, affecting approximately 1.8 million individuals, with an annual prevalence of 3 percent, and a lifetime prevalence of 29 percent for women and 22 percent for men.[1,2] This accounts for 47 IPV assaults per 1,000 women and 32 IPV assaults per 1,000 men, with more than 1 million women and 371,000 men stalked by intimate partners each year.[3]

Almost two-thirds of intimate incidents (60% of IPV, 63% of sexual assaults) occurred between 6:00 PM and 6:00 AM, when resources other than the emergency department are not readily available.[4] In 2002, 76 percent of IPV homicide victims were female and 24 percent were male.[5] Two-thirds (67%) of these homicides were committed with firearms, 13 percent with knives, 5 percent with blunt objects, and 16 percent by other means (strangulation, burns, motor vehicle crashes, and other miscellaneous mechanisms).[6] Of the women physically assaulted, 30.2 percent said they received medical treatment; 61.4 percent were treated in an emergency department, 22.3 percent received other outpatient services; and 15.1 percent were admitted to the hospital. More than half (52.8%) also received treatment from a physician outside of a hospital setting, while 17.5 percent received care by EMS personnel. Similarly, 37.1 percent of the men injured received medical care; 85.7 percent went to a hospital for treatment; and two-thirds of these (66.7%) were treated in an emergency department. These health care interventions cost over 4.1 billion dollars; even when a patient had personal health insurance, it might not have been declared if the policy was in the name of the abuser.[2,3,7]

Dynamics of intimate partner violence

One of the great frustrations and areas of misunderstanding is lack of insight into why these situations and relationships continue. "Why don't they just leave?" is a frequent question thought to address the issue of IPV. This is a complex problem, with financial, cultural, social, religious, and safety aspects that require consideration. Asking this question reflects to the patient that you are unfamiliar with the complexity of abuse, and decreases the likelihood that they will trust you enough to disclose further issues.

It is important to recognize that the abuser is a person they now or previously loved, and with whom they entered into a commitment. Abusers use a number of mechanisms to maintain their control over a victim. In most cases, psychological methods are sufficient to maintain control over their victim. These have been described in the Duluth Domestic Abuse Intervention Project (DAIP) "Power and Control Wheel" (Figure 2.1).[8]

- Intimidation occurs, in both obvious and subtle ways. Behaviors such as display of weapons, destruction of personal property, and abuse of pets relay the message, "I can hurt you or things you treasure."

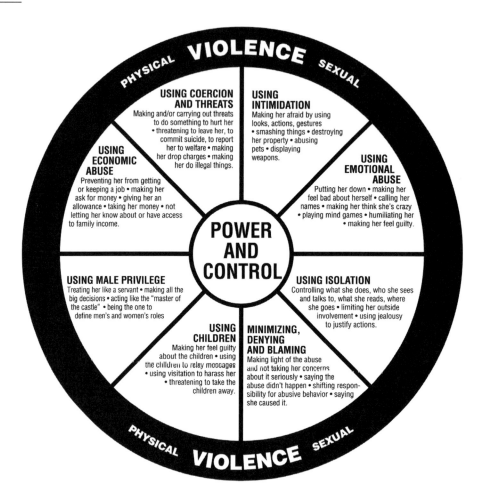

Figure 2.1   Duluth Power and Control Wheel

- Emotional abuse, such as name-calling, destroys self-esteem and leads the victim to believe they caused and deserve the abuse.
- Isolation is a challenging component of abuse because it prevents the victim from accessing resources, and keeps them from sources of support. In many cases, the abuse is long-standing and intergenerational, so that it is their familial norm with no external indications that this is a dysfunctional relationship. Family, cultural, and religious beliefs within the community may exert subtle or overt pressure to

remain in the relationship "for the sake of the kids" or "until death do you part," with sanctions against divorce or otherwise ending the relationship.[7]

- Minimizing, denying, and blaming is an attempt to normalize the abusive behavior, (e.g., "all couples fight") or again, leading the victim to believe they are responsible for the abuse they suffer.

- Using children is often a complex form of manipulation. Even when the children are not physically abused, they are often forced to choose between two people they love; often perceived as a "strong" perpetrator and a "weak" victim; they may aspire or identify with either trait, leading to bullying, victimization, or hopefully, empathy. The children may be told that one parent is "bad" and the other "good," and may be caught in the middle of custody issues.

- Economic abuse is a challenging situation that often prevents leaving an abusive situation. Financial control by the dominant partner may leave the victim with no knowledge of the couple's finances, no bank account, no personal property, no transportation, no personal funds, no insurance, no credit history, and great difficulty obtaining these in a time of crisis.

- Male privilege is a very subjective standard; some cultures are patriarchal, with more traditional gender roles, but even these advocate behaviors of protection and providing a "good living," rather than of abuse and servitude.[9,10]

- Coercion and threats tie in with other aspects of intimidation and blaming. Threatening homicide and/or suicide, threatening harm to children, pets, friends, or relatives if the victim doesn't comply with the abuser's wishes can be very persuasive tools to keep a victim in line. Threats of "outing" homosexual victims, reports to immigration or law enforcement of minorities, or public disclosures about "prominent" members of society (e.g., teachers, religious leaders, public officials) also maintains silence by victims.[7,11,12]

A "Cycle of Violence" has been described, with three phases to the interpersonal relationship:

- The tension-building phase, during which the abuse occurs;
- The explosion phase, when a specific argument or assault occurs;
- The honeymoon phase, when the abuser convinces the victim that the incident was an exception rather than the rule, and displays behavior to enhance and continue the relationship.

Unfortunately, these cycles are of unpredictable duration, and the degree and severity of escalation are likewise unpredictable.[13] The combination of control factors often makes it difficult to leave, and once a victim leaves, he or she may return numerous times. Often, a specific event, particularly affecting children, pets, or family, rather than the victim, are the event that will result in a decision to leave.

Leaving an abusive relationship is the most dangerous time for the victim.[14] Loss of control of the victim by the abuser may lead to the sentiments of "nothing left to lose" or "if I can't have her/him, no one else will," increasing the incidence of extreme behavior, such as harassment, stalking, and murder or murder/suicide.

Failure to understand the dilemmas faced by victims often results in frustration for well-meaning providers. They may then label the victims as "non-compliant" or "weak" for not leaving, and become less likely to help current or future victims, perceiving it as a "waste of time."[15]

Clinical presentations of intimate partner violence

"Battering" or physical injury is the stereotypic presentation of IPV, however, physical injuries are the presenting complaint in only approximately 20 percent of victims. The majority of IPV victims are likely to present with emotional or medically related symptoms that are less obviously abuse-related.[16–20] Survivors of intimate partner violence suffer greater long-term morbidity and mortality than women who were not abused.[1,21]

These presentations cover the spectrum of medical illness, and include:

- Psychiatric illnesses, such as depression, anxiety, somatization disorder, post-traumatic stress disorder, and eating and sleeping disorders.[22–26] Suicidal or homicidal behaviors may occur if the victim sees them as the "only way to stop the abuse;"
- Abuse of mood-altering or pain-relieving substances including alcohol, tobacco, caffeine, cocaine, opiates, benzodiazepines, and antidepressants;[27,28]
- Chronic pain syndromes, such as headaches, abdominal pain, and pelvic pain;
- Neurologic symptoms such as headaches, fatigue, weakness, dizziness, and malaise;
- Respiratory complaints, such as hyperventilation syndromes, and exacerbation of pre-existing asthma, congestive heart failure (CHF), or chronic obstructive pulmonary disease (COPD);[29]
- Cardiac complaints such as palpitations and chest pain, thought to be related to excessive catecholamine release;
- Functional gastrointestinal disorders, such as chronic nausea, irritable bowel syndrome, chronic abdominal pain, and esophageal reflux;[30,31]
- Infectious disorders, particularly HIV, herpes, and other sexually transmitted diseases from non-consensual or coerced intercourse;[32,33]
- Gynecologic disorders including chronic pelvic pain and dyspareunia.[34]

- Pregnancy complications, such as failure to thrive, premature rupture of membranes, and pre-term labor may be due to a combination of factors including poor prenatal care, poorly controlled chronic disease, and substance abuse;[35–37]
- Medication "non-compliance" or the "difficult patient," who misses appointments, does not take medications, and does not follow a care plan as previously prescribed. The abuser may be withholding needed medications causing the patient to become more ill, may cancel appointments and refuse to let them seek follow-up medical care.[38] Often, the patient is blamed for "their" failure to follow through, when they may be embarrassed or afraid to disclose the true reason for their inability to comply.

Some patients present with vague medical complaints, such as malaise or general "ill-being," which are not clearly related to abuse. In some cases, this is deliberate because the patient needed a reason to seek medical attention without raising suspicion by the partner, and in other cases, they themselves may not recognize that their symptoms are manifestations of stress-related syndromes.

Injuries can be inflicted on any part of the body, although some are more characteristic than others. The head and neck are most commonly injured, followed by areas that are concealed by hair or clothing.

- The mandible, zygoma, nasal, and other facial fractures are the most common injuries, with injury to the temporomandibular joint (TMJ), dental loss, tympanic membrane perforation, and lens dislocations as other notable injuries.[39–43]
- Non-lethal strangulation (manual asphyxiation) is a deceptively benign injury, with 20 percent reporting only pain, 42 percent with no visible injury, and the remaining 38 percent with generally "minor-appearing" contusions, abrasions, ligature marks, or finger impressions. Initially, venous blood flow from the brain is occluded, leading to increased intracranial pressure, followed by occlusion of arterial flow to the brain, which can cause ischemic, or "stroke-like" symptoms. Airway occlusion, mistakenly referred to as "choking," rarely occurs, due to the excessive force needed to compress the tracheal cartilages that maintain airway patency. The symptoms are often subtle, such as hoarseness, difficulty swallowing, dizziness, and syncope, which may be incorrectly attributed to anxiety or "hysteria," rather than the development of traumatic laryngeal edema or neurologic sequelae from transient anoxia or traumatic brain injury.[44–46]
- Central injuries, particularly of the breasts, abdomen, and genitals, are strongly suggestive of intentional injury, since they are covered by clothing, and are usually shielded by the extremities when unintentional injuries (e.g., falls) occur.
- Patterned injuries, such as cigarette burns, immersion burns, ligature marks, and belt or whip marks, are easily differentiated from random "accidental" injuries.

Defensive wounds, such as forearm injuries from blocking an attack ("nightstick fracture") also indicate the intentional nature of the injury.

- Approximately 16 percent of pregnant women report abuse during their current or a prior pregnancy, and it is second only to motor vehicle crashes as a leading cause of miscarriage and maternal death. The approximate IPV prevalence in pregnancy is 3.9 to 8.3 percent.[47] This makes it more common than gestational diabetes (1.4–6.1%) and as common as pre-eclampsia (2–7%).[48,49] Placental abruption, feto-maternal hemorrhage, amniotic fluid embolism, disseminated intravascular coagulation, and uterine rupture are all consequences of blunt uterine trauma. Penetrating abdominal trauma in the second and third trimesters is more likely to injure the uterus and fetus, relatively sparing the mother's abdomen.[36,40,51]

- Musculoskeletal injuries, such as sprains and contusions of the extremities are common injuries. When recurrent injuries occur, and are attributed to "clumsiness," or the injury is not consistent with the reported mechanism, abuse should be suspected.

- When evaluating patients injured in motor vehicle crashes, one should consider whether the patient was a driver attempting to flee from abuse, attempting to commit suicide or homicide, or was pushed or thrown from the vehicle by another occupant.

Evaluation and management of victims of intimate partner violence

Because abuse is rarely obvious, all patients should be evaluated for illness or injury related to IPV. The main components of evaluation are screening, examination, treatment, documentation, and referral. Depending on the clinical setting and the severity and acuity of abuse, different components may be more pressing and detailed during a particular health care encounter.

Screening

Screening for abuse is recommended by most professional medical societies, including the American Medical Association (AMA), American College of Emergency Physicians (ACEP), American Academy of Pediatrics (AAP), American College of Obstetricians and Gynecologists (ACOG), American Academy of Family Practitioners (AAFP), and the American College of Physicians (ACP).

The US Preventive Services Task Force (USPTF) reported that they had insufficient evidence to recommend for or against screening for child, partner, or elder abuse and neglect. This conclusion was based on the lack of good studies to determine the accuracy of screening tools; lack of data-sharing among law enforcement, health care, and social services; "invisibility" of many victims due to isolation

---

"RADAR"

Remember to ask about abuse.

Ask direct questions ("Have you been hit, pushed, or threatened by someone with whom you've been in a relationship?").

Document the interview objectively.

Assess patient safety before they leave the clinical setting.

Refer the patient to any appropriate resources necessary (in many cases, referral to the local intimate partner violence program will act as a gateway to additional social and legal services).

Figure 2.2   "RADAR" Mnemonic Alpert E J. *Annals of Internal Medicine*. 1995; 123: 774–81.

by their abuser; and difficulty obtaining good follow-up of these victims. However, screening does appear to be justifiable based on a high prevalence of undetected abuse, risk of long-term consequences, and low cost and low risk from screening.[52–54]

Since there is no typical victim, many recommend "universal," rather than "targeted," screening of patients. This is also safer for the abuse victim, since they will not be lead to believe that their behavior "gave away" the secret of their abuse. While some physicians argue that screening is time consuming, there are a number of brief screening methods that add minimal length to a patient interview. Three of the most-commonly used are: "RADAR" (Figure 2.2),[55] "HITS" Scale (Figure 2.3),[56] and the Partner Violence Screen (Figure 2.4).[57]

Screening for abuse is recommended for any new patient visit, during annual exams in primary care clinics, during prenatal visits, at least once per trimester during pregnancy, and at least once post-partum.[58] Additional screening should occur if there are signs or other suspicions of abuse. Caregivers of children should be screened for partner violence when children are medically evaluated, and adolescents should be interviewed without a parent, other caregiver, or significant other present.

"HITS"

How often does your partner:

Hit

Insult

Threaten or

Scream at you?

Figure 2.3   "HITS" Scale Sherin KM, Sinacore JM, Li XQ, Zitter RE, Shakil A. HITS: a short domestic violence screening tool for use in a family practice setting. *Family Medicine. 1998*; 30(7): 508–12.

Partner Violence Screen

Have you been hit, kicked, punched, or otherwise hurt by someone within the past
    year? If so, by whom?

Do you feel safe in your current relationship?

Is there a partner from a previous relationship who is making you feel unsafe now?

Figure 2.4   Partner Violence Screen Feldhaus KM, Koziol-McLain J, Amsbury HL, Norton IM,
Lowenstein SR, Abbott JT. Accuracy of 3 brief screening questions for detecting partner
violence in the emergency department. *Journal of the American Medical Association*.
1997; 277(17): 1357–61.

All patients should be screened privately, away from their significant other. Some
partners wish to stay with the patient to provide emotional support, but partners
who adamantly refuse to leave, are openly disparaging toward the patient, or answer
questions on the patient's behalf may be showing signs of excessive control. Some
victims may insist that their partners stay in order to allow the abuser to witness the
interaction, so that they cannot be accused later of disclosing anything "improper"
to the health care provider. Additional requests can be made "to respect the privacy
of the patient," and attempts can be made to interview the patient in private in
another part of the facility, such as the Radiology Department, or to send the
partner to address a registration or billing issue, but care must be taken not to
jeopardize the patient's safety.

Certain groups at higher risk of abuse, such as disabled or dependent adults,
are more challenging to screen, because their baseline level of mental or physical
function may be known only to their caregiver, who may also be their abuser. If the
patient is unable to provide necessary information, and the caregiver's report of
events is suspicious, obtaining additional information from another source, such
as a nursing home attendant or other family member may be helpful to determine
if abuse or neglect are occurring. Some elder abuse is in fact "chronic intimate
partner violence" that was better hidden when the patient was younger or healthier,
and is now only evident as the patient becomes more frail and unable to care for
themselves.

If the patient is non-English speaking, a neutral third-party interpreter should
be used instead of a family member or friend. In smaller community settings it is
important to recognize that the abuse victim or perpetrator may be well-known in
the community and even their presence in an office or ED waiting room might be
a significant deterrent to disclosure.

Abuse awareness does not necessarily need to be limited to medical staff; abusive
behavior may occur in front of office or housekeeping staff while being hidden

from the medical staff. Staff members witnessing or overhearing abusive behavior should be encouraged to report it to the medical staff for further evaluation.

Screening questions should be kept gender-neutral, to encourage disclosure of abuse in same-sex relationships. The victim should be assured that they do not deserve to be abused, and that abuse is wrong. When discussing abuse and the patient's response to it, avoid characterizing it as "abnormal" behavior, since the behavior is very likely to be a modeled response from familial or cultural influences. Suggesting there are safer, less violent alternatives is less likely to cause them to become defensive and inhibit disclosure. Letting the patient know that you have concerns about their well-being and safety, and that you are available if they choose to discuss the issue in the future, increases the possibility of discussion when they need assistance.[59,60]

Examination

When obtaining a medical history, determining the timing of symptoms related to stressors may be helpful in identifying abuse as the underlying etiology, such as pelvic pain that only occurs on weekends, and resolves when the partner is too busy with work during the week. Delays in seeking medical attention may occur if the victim is unable to escape until the abuser goes to work, which might take several hours to days if the incident occurred at night or on a weekend. A history of stress-related illness, such as panic attacks, palpitations, eating or sleeping disorders, and the degree of control of chronic disease, may also provide clues to underlying abuse, even if the patient does not make this connection.

The physical examination should be detailed, particularly when examining areas that can conceal injuries, such as the scalp, the external auditory canal, retroauricular area, the mouth, the perineum, and areas normally covered by undergarments or clothing. If the evaluation occurs soon after an abuse incident, there may be few indications of physical trauma, since erythema, edema, and ecchymoses develop over time. Injuries that do not correspond to the reported mechanism, injuries in multiple stages of healing, recurrent injuries, and patterned injuries should be followed up with questions acknowledging that you recognize these as potential signs of abuse. This gives the patient another opportunity to disclose the abuse, and demonstrates to them that this is an area with which you are familiar.

Treatment

Treatment of IPV-related illness often hinges on the recognition of abuse as the etiology of the symptoms. Many patients have had extensive neurologic, cardiac, and gastrointestinal work-ups, only to be told that they have "nothing" wrong with them. Addressing underlying depression, anxiety, reproductive concerns, and substance abuse may decrease symptomatology and result in an improved sense of well-being.

When medications are necessary, particularly for chronic illness and infections, maximizing treatment in the clinical setting is preferred. This decreases the risk of problems in obtaining and accessing these medications, or other interference in treatment by the abuser.

Injuries resulting from IPV should be addressed according to established trauma standards of care. Documentation on body diagrams or with photographs should be as detailed as possible and included as part of the medical record if possible, according to institutional regulations.

Whenever possible, care should be taken to preserve and secure evidence. Tears, holes, or stains on clothing may all be evidence of the assault and tied to a weapon or specific injury, and should not be cut through or otherwise compromised. Pulled hair, torn, bloody, or dirty clothes, and belts or other items used as ligatures might all be forms of evidence, and should be turned over to law enforcement as soon as possible in accordance with local requirements.

Complaints suggesting specific injuries, such as injury to the gravid abdomen or strangulation, should be evaluated thoroughly even in the absence of obvious clinical findings, because of the delay in development of findings, and potentially high morbidity from complications such as laryngeal edema or placental abruption.

Documentation

Proper documentation of abuse can help both the victim and the person trying to help the victim. The most useful chart, whether documenting continuing medical care or being referred to in a courtroom, is one that is clearly written, detailed, stated in objective language, uses direct quotes from the patient, and has visual documentation whenever possible. Even if the patient decides not to prosecute an assault, a chart documenting "my boyfriend Bob Smith pushed me down the stairs on January 5" can validate the episode more effectively than "I got pushed by my boyfriend one night." Additional information such as photographs, police reports, or witness accounts can help substantiate the victim's report even when they are unable or unwilling to do so.

A body injury map (Figure 2.5), sketches, diagrams, or photographs can be used to document injuries, even though some may not be initially evident. Many law enforcement jurisdictions have mechanisms for taking repeat photographs several days after an incident that demonstrate more obvious injuries.

Before the patient leaves the health care setting, a safety assessment should be performed and a safety plan (Figure 2.6) filled out or given to the patient to fill out.

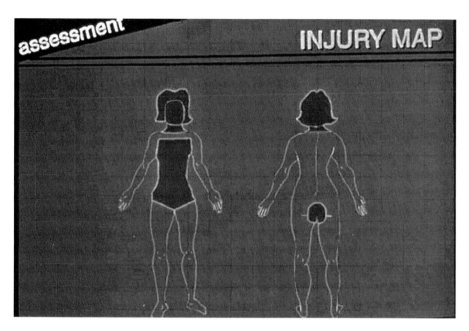

Figure 2.5   Sample body injury map (red areas are those more frequently injured)

Safety Plan

1. Move to a room with more than one exit, avoiding rooms with potential weapons (e.g., kitchen knives).
2. Know the quickest route out of your home.
3. Know the quickest route out of your workplace. Find out what resources they have to protect employees.
4. Pack a bag with essential clothes, valuables, and documents for you and each of your children. Keep it hidden but make it easy to grab quickly.
5. Tell your neighbors about your abuse and ask them to call the police when they hear a disturbance.
6. Have a code word to use with your kids, family, and friends when you need help.
7. Have a safe place selected in case you ever have to leave.
8. Use your instincts.
9. You have the right to protect yourself and your kids.

Figure 2.6   IPV Safety Plan

Many victims of IPV homicide, or "femicide," have had interactions with health care providers in the 12 months prior to their death, without assessment of their safety or development of a safety plan. Appropriate questions include, "Do you feel safe leaving here?" "Do you have a safe place to go?" "Do you have someone you can stay with or who can stay with you?" "Does the abuser have access to your residence?" and "Have you changed the locks on your home?" These allow the patient to focus on specific steps that they may need to take to decrease risk of further abuse or injury. Even if law enforcement has taken the abuser into custody, preliminary hearings often result in release in less than 72 hours, with return of the abuser to the community or home.

Overall, intimate partner homicide accounts for approximately 40 to 50 percent of US femicides, but only 6 percent of male homicides. Sixty-seven to 80 percent of intimate partner homicides involved physical abuse of the female by the male before the murder. Separating from an abusive partner after living together was associated with a higher risk of femicide, as was ever leaving or asking the partner to leave.[14] Therefore, it is essential to identify women at risk. A danger assessment (Figure 2.7) should be included, to determine if the patient is at high risk of lethal IPV based on certain characteristics of the abuser, particularly if there is escalating abuse, substance abuse, access to firearms, or prior threats, assaults, or stalking.[61]

DANGER ASSESSMENT

Several risk factors have been associated with increased risk of homicides (murders) of women and men in violent relationships. We cannot predict what will happen in your case, but we would like you to be aware of the danger of homicide in situations of abuse and for you to see how many of the risk factors apply to your situation.

Using the calendar, please mark the approximate dates during the past year when you were abused by your partner or ex-partner. Write on that date how bad the incident was according to the following scale:

1. Slapping, pushing; no injuries and/or lasting pain
2. Punching, kicking; bruises, cuts, and/or continuing pain
3. "Beating up"; severe contusions, burns, broken bones
4. Threat to use weapon; head injury, internal injury, permanent injury
5. Use of weapon; wounds from weapon

(If **any** of the descriptions for the higher number apply, use the higher number.)

Mark "Yes" or "No" for each of the following. ("He" refers to your husband, partner, ex-husband, ex-partner, or whoever is currently physically hurting you.)

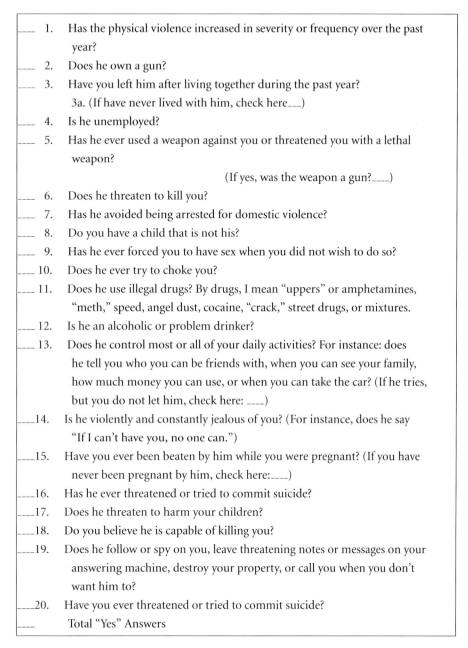

1. Has the physical violence increased in severity or frequency over the past year?
2. Does he own a gun?
3. Have you left him after living together during the past year?
    3a. (If have never lived with him, check here____)
4. Is he unemployed?
5. Has he ever used a weapon against you or threatened you with a lethal weapon?
    (If yes, was the weapon a gun?____)
6. Does he threaten to kill you?
7. Has he avoided being arrested for domestic violence?
8. Do you have a child that is not his?
9. Has he ever forced you to have sex when you did not wish to do so?
10. Does he ever try to choke you?
11. Does he use illegal drugs? By drugs, I mean "uppers" or amphetamines, "meth," speed, angel dust, cocaine, "crack," street drugs, or mixtures.
12. Is he an alcoholic or problem drinker?
13. Does he control most or all of your daily activities? For instance: does he tell you who you can be friends with, when you can see your family, how much money you can use, or when you can take the car? (If he tries, but you do not let him, check here: ____)
14. Is he violently and constantly jealous of you? (For instance, does he say "If I can't have you, no one can.")
15. Have you ever been beaten by him while you were pregnant? (If you have never been pregnant by him, check here:____)
16. Has he ever threatened or tried to commit suicide?
17. Does he threaten to harm your children?
18. Do you believe he is capable of killing you?
19. Does he follow or spy on you, leave threatening notes or messages on your answering machine, destroy your property, or call you when you don't want him to?
20. Have you ever threatened or tried to commit suicide?
____ Total "Yes" Answers

Thank you. Please talk to your nurse, advocate, or counselor about what the Danger Assessment means in terms of your situation.

Figure 2.7 IPV Danger Assessment Campbell JC. Danger Assessment. 2003 http://dangerassessment.com.

Referral

Due to the multidisciplinary nature of intimate partner violence, there are many potential referrals that can be made to help the patient find options that are safer and healthier than their current situation. Many health care providers avoid screening for abuse because they are: concerned about the amount of time necessary to make referrals, unsure of their legal obligations, unfamiliar with their local resources, or frustrated by the high percentage of patients who are either lost to follow-up or return repeatedly with similar abuse-related issues.[15] Even providers aware of the possibility of abuse do not want to make the time investment that may interfere with the efficient running of their practice, or expose themselves to increased involvement with the legal system.

In many areas, becoming acquainted with the services offered by the local family violence program will address these concerns. Although physicians want to "cure the patient," and believe they should be able to take care of the problem themselves, this can be a chronic process requiring expertise from multiple areas. While physicians think nothing of referring a patient with heart disease to a cardiologist or with appendicitis to a surgeon, they do not feel as comfortable referring victims of intimate partner violence to advocates who routinely work in this field.

Many family violence programs provide more than "shelter." Services may include, but are not limited to:

- Legal counseling, including information on obtaining protective orders
- Peer group counseling
- Job training or emergency financial assistance
- Displaced homemaker programs and other social services
- Transportation to court, work, or medical appointments
- Referrals to substance abuse programs
- Crisis intervention for sexual assault
- Programs specific to gay, lesbian, bi-gender, and transsexual clients
- Programs for non-English speaking or immigrant clients
- Emergency shelter or relocation assistance
- Advocates who accompany the client to court for emotional support
- Special programs for elder clients, disabled clients, and children
- Abuser treatment programs
- Personal safety classes

Once familiar with the services provided by the local program, referring the patient there, or calling directly from the health care facility (with the patient's permission), can direct the patient to the appropriate social and legal resources, often with little additional time or effort required by the physician. If there is no easily identifiable local family violence program, the physician or patient can call the National Domestic Violence Hotline, 1-800-799 SAFE (7233) for information.

When medical consults are necessary, obtaining them before the patient leaves the health care facility is helpful, due to difficulties the patient might have calling for an appointment, obtaining transportation, obtaining prescriptions, and avoiding interference or monitoring by the abuser. This allows you to inform the consultant of the history of abuse and any other concerns you have regarding the patient's ability to comply with the treatment plan.

If arranging counseling for the patient, current recommendations suggest that each partner attend peer group counseling related to their perspective, so that abusers are in counseling with other abusers and victims are with other victims of abuse. While wide variations in composition of group, group leadership, and length of counseling varies, these seem to provide better opportunities for the couple to be with others in similar situations undergoing the process from abuse to safety. Couples counseling is not recommended in cases of intimate partner violence. Due to the power inequity within the relationship, the abuser will likely resent interference in the relationship, deny the abuse, refuse to attend the sessions, and be angered with the victim for the disclosure leading to the counseling, resulting in increased abuse and intimidation.

Mandatory reporting of intimate partner violence is a controversial issue that varies widely from state to state. It is critical to understand the requirements for your jurisdiction in order to comply with state laws while advocating for your patient. Most states require reporting of injuries caused by firearms or knives, however, laws are not always clear on what other injuries must be reported, or to whom. Some states require reporting of "illness or injury resulting from a criminal act," although medical personnel rarely have the training to determine this, particularly if the patient denies abuse. Some states require reporting of only physical injuries, not emotional abuse. Some states require reporting to law enforcement, although others require reporting only to social service agencies, and one state requires referral to social services, but not reporting.

The current studies of mandatory reporting show both positive and negative outcomes, without overwhelming evidence to support either extreme.[62,63] Positive results of mandatory reporting include: documentation of abuse, data to improve funding and resource allocation, and improvement of social services to include services for children who are abused or witness IPV. Consequences of mandatory reporting include compromise of patient autonomy and confidentiality, and possible escalation of violence by abusers who have been reported. As a result of these contradictions, and the possible, although inconclusive concerns about patient safety, mandatory reporting of intimate partner violence is not currently recommended by the major medical organizations such as the AMA, ACEP, ACOG, or AAFP.

References

1. Coker AL, Davis KE, Arias I, Desai S, Sanderson M, Brandt HM, et al. Physical and mental health effects of intimate partner violence for men and women. *American Journal of Preventive Medicine*. 2002; 23(4): 260–8.

2. NCIPC 2003. *Costs of Intimate Partner Violence Against Women in the United States*. http://www.cdc.gov/ncipc/pub-res/ipv_cost/ipv.htm.

3. Tjaden P, Thoennes N. *Extent, Nature, and Consequences of Intimate Partner Violence: Findings from the National Violence Against Women Survey*. Washington (DC): Department of Justice (US); 2000. Publication No. NCJ 181867. http://www.ojp.usdoj.gov/nij/pubs-sum/181867.htm.

4. Birnbaum A, Calderon Y, Gennis P, Rao R, Gallagher EJ. Intimate partner violence: diurnal mismatch between need and availability of services. *Academic Emergency Medicine*. 1996; 3(3): 246–51.

5. Fox JA, Zawitz MW. *Homicide Trends in the United States*. Washington (DC): Department of Justice (US); 2004. http://www.ojp.usdoj.gov/bjs/homicide/homtrnd.htm.

6. Rennison C. *Intimate Partner Violence, 1993–2001*. Washington (DC): Bureau of Justice Statistics, US Department of Justice; 2003. Publication No. NCJ 197838.

7. Lipsky S, Caetano R, Field CA, Larkin GL. The role of intimate partner violence, race, and ethnicity in help-seeking behaviors. *Ethnicity & Health*. 2006; 11(1): 81–100.

8. Domestic Abuse Intervention Project, http://www.duluth-model.org.

9. Edelson MG, Hokoda A, Ramos-Lira L. Differences in Effects of Domestic Violence Between Latina and Non-Latina Women. *Journal of Family Violence*. 2007; 22: 1–10.

10. Valente SM. Evaluating Intimate Partner Violence. *Journal of the American Academy of Nurse Practitioners*. 2002; 14(11): 505–13.

11. Barnes PG. It's Just a Quarrel. *American Bar Association Journal*. 1998 (Feb); 24–5.

12. Halpern CT, Young ML, Waller MW, Martin SL, Kupper LL. Prevalence of partner violence in same-sex romantic and sexual relationships in a national sample of adolescents. *Journal of Adolescent Health*. 2004; 35(2): 124–31.

13. Walker LE. *The Battered Woman*. New York: Harper & Row, 1979.

14. Campbell JC, Webster D, Koziol-McLain J, Block C, Campbell D, Curry MA, et al. Risk factors for femicide in abusive relationships: results from a multisite case control study. *American Journal of Public Health*. 2003; 93(7):1089–97.

15. Taft A, Broom DH, Legge D. General practitioner management of intimate partner abuse and the whole family: qualitative study. *British Medical Journal*. 2004; 328(7440): 618.

16. Abbott J. Injuries and illnesses of intimate partner violence. *Annals of Emergency Medicine*, 1997; 29(6): 781–5.

17. Campbell JC. Health consequences of intimate partner violence. *Lancet*. 2002; 359(9314): 1331–6.

18. Fisher JW, Shelton AJ. Survivors of domestic violence: demographics and disparities in visitors to an interdisciplinary specialty clinic. *Family & Community Health*. 2006; 29(2): 118–30.

19. Goodman PE, Capps J. Not in my practice. A look at the pervasive consequences of domestic violence. *North Carolina Medical Journal.* 1997; 58(5): 310–4.

20. Muelleman RL, Lenaghan PA, Pakieser RA. Nonbattering presentations to the ED of women in physically abusive relationships. *American Journal of Emergency Medicine.* 1998; 16(2): 128–31.

21. Nicolaidis C, Curry M, McFarland B, Gerrity M. Violence, mental health, and physical symptoms in an academic internal medicine practice. *Journal of General Internal Medicine.* 2004; 19(8): 819–27.

22. Budd G. Disordered eating: young women's search for control and connection. *Journal of Child & Adolescent Psychiatric Nursing.* 2007; 20(2): 96–106.

23. Csoboth CT, Birkas E, Purebl G. Living in fear of experiencing physical and sexual abuse is associated with severe depressive symptomatology among young women. *Journal of Women's Health.* 2005; 14(5): 441–8.

24. Forte T, Cohen MM, Du Mont J, Hyman I, Romans S. Psychological and physical sequelae of intimate partner violence among women with limitations in their activities of daily living. *Archives of Women's Mental Health.* 2005; 8(4): 248–56.

25. Mezey G, Bacchus L, Bewley S, White S. Domestic violence, lifetime trauma and psychological health of childbearing women. *BJOG: An International Journal of Obstetrics & Gynaecology.* 2005; 112(2): 197–204.

26. Pico-Alfonso MA, Garcia-Linares MI, Celda-Navarro N, Blasco-Ros C, Echeburua E, Martinez M. The impact of physical, psychological, and sexual intimate male partner violence on women's mental health: depressive symptoms, posttraumatic stress disorder, state anxiety, and suicide. *Journal of Women's Health.* 2006; 15(5): 599–611.

27. Greenfield SF, Manwani SG, Nargiso JE. Epidemiology of substance use disorders in women. *Obstetrics & Gynecology Clinics of North America.* 2003; 30(3): 413–46.

28. Weinsheimer RL, Schermer CR, Malcoe LH, Balduf LM, Bloomfield LA. Severe intimate partner violence and alcohol use among female trauma patients. *Journal of Trauma-Injury Infection & Critical Care.* 2005; 58(1): 22–9.

29. Wright RJ. Health Effects of Socially Toxic Neighborhoods: The Violence and Urban Asthma Paradigm. *Clinics in Chest Medicine.* 2006; 27(3): 413–21.

30. Bhatia V, Tandon RK. Stress and the gastrointestinal tract. *Journal of Gastroenterology & Hepatology.* 2005; 20(3): 332–9.

31. Drossman DA, Talley NJ, Leserman J, et al. Sexual and physical abuse and gastrointestinal illness: Review and recommendations. *Annals of Internal Medicine.* 1995; 123: 782–94.

32. Galvan FH, Collins R, Kanouse DE, Burnam MA, Paddock SM, Beckman R, Mitchell SR. Abuse in the close relationships of people with HIV. *AIDS & Behavior.* 2004; 8(4): 441–51.

33. Garcia-Linares MI, Sanchez-Lorente S, Coe CL, Martinez M. Intimate male partner violence impairs immune control over herpes simplex virus type 1 in physically and psychologically abused women. *Psychosomatic Medicine.* 2004; 66(6): 965–72.

34. John R, Johnson JK, Kukreja S, Found M, Lindow SW. Domestic violence: prevalence and association with gynaecological symptoms. *BJOG: An International Journal of Obstetrics & Gynaecology.* 2004; 111(10): 1128–32.

35. Coker AL, Sanderson M, Dong B. Partner violence during pregnancy and risk of adverse pregnancy outcomes. *Paediatric and Perinatal Epidemiology*. 2004; 18(4): 260–9.

36. El-Kady D, Gilbert WM, Anderson J, Danielsen B, Towner D, Smith LH. Trauma during pregnancy: an analysis of maternal and fetal outcomes in a large population. *American Journal of Obstetrics & Gynecology*. 2004; 190(6): 1661–8.

37. Jasinski JL. Pregnancy and intimate partner violence: a review of the literature. *Trauma Violence & Abuse*. 2004; 5(1): 47–64.

38. McCloskey LA, Williams CM, Lichter E, Gerber M, Ganz ML, Sege R. Abused women disclose partner interference with health care: an unrecognized form of battering. *Journal of General Internal Medicine*. 2007; 22(8): 1067–72.

39. Bhandari M, Dosanjh S, Tornetta P 3rd, Matthews D. Violence Against Women Health Research Collaborative. Musculoskeletal manifestations of physical abuse after intimate partner violence. *Journal of Trauma-Injury Infection & Critical Care*. 2006; 61(6): 1473–9.

40. Halpern LR, Dodson TB. A predictive model to identify women with injuries related to intimate partner violence. *Journal of the American Dental Association*. 2006; 137(5): 604–9.

41. Le BT, Dierks EJ, Ueeck BA, Homer LD, Potter BF. Maxillofacial injuries associated with domestic violence. *Journal of Oral & Maxillofacial Surgery*. 2001; 59(11): 1277–83; discussion 1283–4.

42. Gwinn C, McClane GE, Shanel-Hogan KA, Strack GB. Domestic violence: no place for a smile. *Journal of the California Dental Association*. 2004; 32(5): 399–409.

43. Huang V, Moore C, Bohrer P, Thaller SR. Maxillofacial injuries in women. *Annals of Plastic Surgery*. 1998; 41(5): 482–4.

44. Hawley DA, McClane GE, Strack GB. A review of 300 attempted strangulation cases Part III: injuries in fatal cases. *Journal of Emergency Medicine*. 2001; 21(3): 317–22.

45. McClane GE, Strack GB, Hawley D. A review of 300 attempted strangulation cases Part III: clinical evaluation of the surviving victim. *Journal of Emergency Medicine*. 2001; 21(3): 311–5.

46. Strack GB, McClane GE, Hawley D. A review of 300 attempted strangulation cases. Part I: criminal legal issues. *Journal of Emergency Medicine*. 2001; 21(3): 303–9.

47. Gazmararian JA, Lazorick S, Spitz AM, Ballard TJ, Saltzman LE, Marks JS. Prevalence of violence against pregnant women: a review of the literature. *Journal of the American Medical Association*. 1996; 275(24): 1915–20.

48. Jovanovic L, Pettitt DJ. Gestational diabetes mellitus. *Journal of the American Medical Association*. 2001; 286(20): 2516–18.

49. Sibai B, Dekker G, Kupferminc M. Pre-eclampsia. *Lancet*. 2005; 365(9461): 785–99.

50. Grossman NB. Blunt trauma in pregnancy. *American Family Physician*. 2004; 70(7): 1303–10.

51. Shah AJ, Kilcline BA. Trauma in pregnancy. *Emergency Medicine Clinics of North America*. 2003; 21(3): 615–29.

52. Anglin D, Sachs C. Preventive care in the emergency department: screening for domestic violence in the emergency department. *Academic Emergency Medicine*. 2003; 10(10): 1118–27.

53. Nelson HD, Nygren P, McInerney Y, Klein J. Screening Women and Elderly Adults for Family and Intimate Partner Violence: A Review of the Evidence for the U.S. Preventive Services Task Force. *Annals of Internal Medicine*. 2004; 140(5): 387–96.

54. Punukollu M. Domestic violence: screening made practical. *Journal of Family Practice*. 2003; 52(7): 537–43.

55. Alpert EJ. *Annals of Internal Medicine*. 1995; 123: 774–81.

56. Sherin KM, Sinacore JM, Li XQ, Zitter RE, Shakil A. HITS: a short domestic violence screening tool for use in a family practice setting. *Family Medicine*. *1998*; 30(7): 508–12.

57. Feldhaus KM, Koziol-McLain J, Amsbury HL, Norton IM, Lowenstein SR, Abbott JT. Accuracy of 3 brief screening questions for detecting partner violence in the emergency department. *Journal of the American Medical Association*. 1997; 277(17): 1357–61.

58. Shadigian EM, Bauer ST. Screening for partner violence during pregnancy. *International Journal of Gynaecology & Obstetrics*. 2004; 84(3): 273–80.

59. Battaglia TA, Finley E, Liebschutz JM. Survivors of intimate partner violence speak out: trust in the patient–provider relationship. *Journal of General Internal Medicine*. 2003; 18(8): 617–23.

60. McCauley J, Yurk RA, Jenckes MW, Ford DE. Inside "Pandora's box": abused women's experiences with clinicians and health services. *Journal of General Internal Medicine*. 1998; 13(8): 549–55.

61. Campbell JC. Danger Assessment. 2003; http://dangerassessment.com.

62. Chang JC, Cluss PA, Ranieri L, Hawker L, Buranosky R, Dado D, McNeil M, Scholle SH. Health care interventions for intimate partner violence: what women want. *Womens Health Issues*. 2005; 15(1): 21–30.

63. Gupta M. Mandatory reporting laws and the emergency physician. *Annals of Emergency Medicine*. 2007; 49(3): 369–76.

64. Warshaw C, Ganley AL. *Improving the Health Care System's Response to Domestic Violence: a Resource Manual for Health Care Providers*. San Francisco: Family Violence Prevention Fund, 1998.

65. Bacchus L, Mezey G, Bewley S. Experiences of seeking help from health professionals in a sample of women who experienced intimate partner violence. *Health & Social Care in the Community*. 2003; 11(1): 10–18.

66. Centers for Disease Control and Prevention; National Center for Injury Prevention and Control. Costs of Intimate Partner Violence Against Women in the United States. Atlanta GA: March 2003. http://www.cdc.gov/ncipc/pub-res/ipv_cost/ipv.htm.

67. Centers for Disease Control and Prevention; National Center for Injury Prevention and Control. *Costs of Intimate Partner Violence Against Women in the United States*. Atlanta GA. Measuring Intimate Partner Violence Victimization and Perpetration: A Compendium of Assessment Tools. October 2006. http://www.cdc.gov/ncipc/IPVp/Compendium/Measuring_IPV_Victimization_and_Perpetration.htm.

68. Sharps PW, Koziol-McLain J, Campbell J, McFarlane J, Sachs C, Xu X. Health care providers' missed opportunities for preventing femicide. *Preventive Medicine*. 2001; 33(5): 373–80.

69. Sutherland C, Bybee D, Sullivan C. The long-term effects of battering on women's health. *Womens Health*. 1998; 4(1): 41–70.

70. Wadman MC, Muelleman RL. Intimate partner violence homicides: ED use before victimization. *American Journal of Emergency Medicine*. 1999; 17(7): 689–91.

Quick Reference Pages

Domestic violence acute care checklist

Following these steps will ensure the expedient and comprehensive care of patients reporting domestic violence. Some patients may not require all of these interventions, and other patients may require interventions not listed. Examiners must use their clinical judgment in following this outline, including the time line. Any questions, contact _____ at: _____.

		Y	N
1	Patient identified at triage and brought into private room		
2	Contact Social Worker or advocate		
3	Consent patient for care and treatment, including possible photographs		
4	Emergent medical care as required (implied consent if victim unable to give verbal/written consent secondary to trauma)		
5	Determine if sexual assault has also occurred within 96 hours. See sexual assault checklist as appropriate		
6	**Treat Pain**		
7	Ask patient: Patient threatened with homicide?		
	Weapon involved?		
	Escalation of violence?		
	ETOH or drug use by abuser?		
	Abuser in patient's home?		
	Have children witnessed the abuse or been abused?		
	Are police involved; if not, does victim want to contact the police now?		
8	Obtain history both medical and of assault. Note from history places to be examined for injury		
9	Physical exam including head-to-toe survey		
10	Write history/findings: give history of abuse in patient's words, and detailed descriptions of injuries including #, type, size, location, color, and likely causes (i.e., handprint)		
11	Draw pictures on traumagrams		
12	Photographs		
13	X-rays, *if required medically*		
14	**Wound care and any other required treatment**		
15	Determine if patient has SAFE PLACE TO GO. DO NOT DISCHARGE PATIENT TO UNSAFE ENVIRONMENT UNLESS THAT IS HIS/HER CHOICE. Admit patient for safety if no other option can be found		
16	Social Work referral order if patient consents and no social worker saw the patient in the ED		

17 SAFE, REACHABLE PHONE NUMBER ON REFERRAL IS OF
   PARAMOUNT IMPORTANCE

18 If patient is discharged, and it is safe to do so, give Discharge Instructions
   including WOUND CARE

19   Victim's Rights Sheet (required by law–*if safe for patient*)

20   Domestic Violence Hotline #

21   Follow-up care referrals

MD_____   RN_____

Discharge review

Have the following been provided?

1. Screening for possible abuse (see Figures 2.2–2.4)
2. Treatment for acute medical problems
3. Assessment and addressing of acute psychiatric risk, and evaluation and referral for mental health needs
4. Assessment of pattern and impact of abuse
5. Appropriate documentation and evidence collection
6. Validating
7. Safety assessment and plan (see Figure 2.6)
8. Information about domestic violence in verbal and written form
9. Options for shelter, legal assistance, and counseling
10. Appropriate follow-up care (or referral) for medical, psychological, and advocacy needs
11. Assurance of confidentiality

Figure 2.8   Discharge Review (Adapted from Warshaw C, Ganley AL. *Improving the Health Care System's Response to Domestic Violence: a Resource Manual for Health Care Providers.* San Francisco: Family Violence Prevention Fund, 1998.)

Intimate Partner Violence Guide

Intimate partner violence – deliberate use of physical, sexual, or psychological abuse or intimidation to control another person in a family, dating, or household relationship.

SCREEN (all patients, in private; suggested questions):
   1)   Do you feel safe in your current relationship?
   2)   Did someone cause your injuries or trigger your illness?

HISTORY (clues):

   1)   Reluctance to speak in front of partner, evasiveness

2)   History inconsistent with injury/illness

3)   Multiple episodes of "clumsiness," miscarriages

4)   Stress-related symptoms, vague complaints

5)   History of suicide attempts, substance abuse

6)   Delay in seeking medical attention, non-compliance

PHYSICAL (clues):

1)   Excess clothing/accessories/makeup covering injuries

2)   Injuries in patterns/multiple stages of healing

3)   Injuries during pregnancy

4)   Injuries in central areas (face, neck, abdomen, genitals)

5)   Injuries in protected areas (behind ears, under breasts)

6)   Defensive injuries

TREAT

1)   Expose patient to check for occult injuries

2)   Maximize current treatment, minimize prescriptions, MD referrals

3)   Relay concerns to consultants

4)   Recognize personal/professional biases/limitations

5)   Provide message that abuse is not deserved or acceptable

6)   Assess safety, provide information to develop safety plan

DOCUMENT

1)   Use patient's exact words when possible

2)   Detailed descriptions of injuries, with body map or photos

3)   Document treatment, consults, referrals, prescriptions, follow-up

REFERRALS

1)   If partner cancels appointments, consider it a "red flag"

2)   Hospital, City, County Dept. of Social Service

3)   Child Protective Services, if applicable

4)   Local family violence program/"shelter"

5)   Legal Aid Society, Bar Association

6)   Law enforcement (police dept., sheriff's dept.)

7)   The National Domestic Violence Hotline, 1-800-799 SAFE (7233)

Figure 2.9   IPV Guide

Permission to use danger assessment

Thank you for your interest in the Danger Assessment instrument. The challenge for those who encounter abused women is to identify those with the highest level of danger. The "Danger Assessment" instrument has been used by law enforcement, health care professionals, domestic violence advocates, and researchers for 25 years.

To use the Danger Assessment to its fullest extent, a scoring system, which has been updated and validated, is available to interpret the Danger Assessment results. The Danger Assessment is best used by a person certified to administer the assessment and interpret the scoring system. Certification programs in various formats can be found at www.dangerassessment.com.

There is no charge and no further permission needed for the use of this instrument as long as the reference is properly cited (see below). However, it has a copyright to indicate that it may *not* be *changed* in any way without specific permission from me.

There is a charge to become certified to use the scoring system; see the rest of the website for details.

The Danger Assessment is a project in process. It is continually being checked for accuracy and usefulness. In light of that, we ask that you share the results of any research (raw or coded data) which is conducted using the instrument. The following information would be extremely valuable:

• an approximate number of women with whom the instrument was used,
• a description of their demographics,
• their mean score, and
• the setting in which the data was collected.

Comments (positive and negative) and suggestions for improvement from battered women themselves, advocates, and professionals who are involved in its use are also being collected. Please send this information to the address below.

I look forward to your feedback regarding the Danger Assessment.

Sincerely,
Jacquelyn C. Campbell, PhD, RN, FAAN
Anna D. Wolf Chair
Associate Dean for Faculty Affairs
525 N. Wolfe Street
Baltimore, MD21205
www.dangerassessment.com
jcampbell@dangerassessment.com

Danger assessment reference list

Block CR., Engel B, Naureckas SM, RiordanKA. The Chicago women's health risk study: Lessons in collaboration. *Violence Against Women.* 1999; 5: 1158–77.

Browne A. (1987). *Battered Women Who Kill.* New York: Free Press.

Browne A, Williams K, Dutton D. (1998). Homicide between intimate partners. In: *Homicide: A Sourcebook of Social Research*, edited by M. D. Smith and M. Zahn, Thousand Oaks, CA: Sage, p. 149–64.

Campbell JC. (1995). *Assessing Dangerousness.* Newbury Park: Sage.

Campbell JC. (1992). "If I can't have you, no one can": Power and control in homicide of female partners. In: *Femicide: The Politics of Woman Killing*, edited by J. Radford and D. E. H. Russell, New York: Twayne, p. 99–113.

Campbell JC. Misogyny and homicide of women. *Advances in Nursing Science.* 1981; 3: 67–85.

Campbell JC. Nursing assessment for risk of homicide with battered women. *Advances in Nursing Science.* 1986; 8: 36–51.

Campbell DW, Campbell JC, King C, Parker B, Ryan J. The reliability and factor structure of the index of spouse abuse with African-American battered women. *Violence and Victims.* 1994; 9: 259–74.

Campbell JC, Sharps P, Glass N. (2000). Risk Assessment for Partner Homicide. In: *Clinical Assessment of Dangerousness: Empirical Contributions*, edited by G. F. Pinard and L. Pagani, New York: Cambridge University Press.

Campbell JC, Soeken K, McFarlane J, Parker B. (1998). Risk factors for femicide among pregnant and nonpregnant battered women. In: J. C. Campbell (Ed.), *Empowering Survivors of Abuse: Health Care for Battered Women and Their Children* (pp. 90–7). Thousand Oaks, CA: Sage.

Campbell JC, Webster D. (submitted). The Danger Assessment: Psychometric support from a case control study of intimate partner homicide.

Campbell JC, Webster D, Koziol-McLain J, et al. (2003). Assessing risk factors for intimate partner homicide. *National Institute of Justice Journal.* (250): 14–19. (Full Text: http://ncirs.org/pdffiles1/irOOQ250e.pdf)

Campbell JC, Webster D, Koziol-McLain J, et al. Risk Factors for Femicide in Abusive Relationships: Results from a Multi-Site Case Control Study. *American Journal of Public Health.* 2003; 93(7): 1089–97.

Diaz-Olavarrieta C, Campbell JC, Garcia de la Cadena Campbell JC, Webster D. (submitted). The Danger Assessment: Psychometric support from a case control study of intimate partner homicide.

C, Paz F, Villa A. Domestic violence against patients with chronic neurologic disorders. *Archives of Neurology.* 1999; 56: 681–85.

Fagan J A, Stewart DE, Hansen K. (1983). Violent men or violent husbands? Background factors and situational correlates. In: R. J. Gelles, G. Hotaling, M. A. Straus, & D. Finkelhor (Eds.), *The Dark Side of Families* (pp. 49–68). Beverly Hills: Sage.

Ferraro KJ, Johnson JM. How women experience battering: The process of victimization. *Social Problems.* 1983; 30: 325–39.

Goodman L, Dutton M, Bennett M. Predicting repeat abuse among arrested batterers: use of the danger assessment scale in the criminal justice system. *J. Interpers. Violence*. 1999; 15: 63–74.

Heckert DA, Gondolf EW. Battered women's perceptions of risk versus risk factors and instruments in predicting repeat reassault. *J. Interpers. Violence*. 2004; 19(7): 778–800.

Heckert DA, Gondolf EW. (2001). Predicting levels of abuse and reassault among batterer program participants. Paper presented at the American Society of Criminology, Atlanta, GA.

McFarlane J, Campbell JC, Sharps P, Watson K. Abuse during pregnancy and femicide: urgent implications for women's health. *Obstet. Gynecol*. 2002; 100: 27–36.

McFarlane J, Campbell JC, Watson K. Intimate Partner Stalking and Femicide: urgent implications for women's safety. *Behavioral Sciences and the Law*. 2002; 20: 51–68.

McFarlane J, Campbell JC, Wilt S, et al. Stalking and intimate partner femicide. *Homicide Studies*. 1999; 3(4): 300–16.

McFarlane J, Parker B, Soeken K, Bullock L. Assessing for abuse during pregnancy: Severity severity and frequency of injuries and associated entry into prenatal care. *JAMA*. 1992; 267: 3176–8.

McFarlane J, Parker B, Soeken K. Abuse during pregnancy: associations with maternal health and infant birth weight. *Nursing Research*. 1996; 45: 37–42.

McFarlane J, Soeken K, Campbell JC, Parker B, Reel S, Silva C. Severity of abuse to pregnant women and associated gun access of the perpetrator. *Public Health Nurs*. 1998; 15(3): 201–6.

McFarlane J, Soeken K, Reel S, Parker B, Silva C. Resource use by abused women following an intervention program: Associated severity of abuse and reports of abuse ending. *Public Health Nursing*. 1997; 14: 244–50.

Parker B, McFarlane J, Soeken K. Abuse during pregnancy: Effects on maternal complications and birth weight in adult and teenage women. *Obstetrics & Gynecology*. 1994; 84: 323–8.

Roehl J. Guertin K. (1998) Current use of dangerousness assessments in sentencing domestic violence offenders, Pacific Grove, CA: State Justice Institute.

Sharps PW, Koziol-McLain J, Campbell JC, et al. Health Care Providers' Missed Opportunities for Preventing Femicide. *Prev.Med*. 2001; 33: 373–80.

Silva C, McFarlane J, Soeken K, et al. Symptoms of post-traumatic stress disorder in abused women in a primary care setting. *Journal of Women's Health*. 1997; 6: 543–52.

Stuart EP, Campbell JC. Assessment of patterns of dangerousness with battered women. *Issues Mental Health Nursing*. 1989; 10: 245–60.

Weisz A, Tolman R, Saunders DG. Assessing the risk of severe domestic violence: The importance of survivor's predictions. *Journal of Interpersonal Violence*. 2000; 15: 75–90.

Williams K, Conniff E. (2001). Legal Sanctions and the Violent Victimization of Women. Paper presented at the American Society of Criminology, Atlanta, GA.

Sexual assault

Laura Melville, M.D.

Chapter objectives

1. Understand the purpose of a forensic rape exam
2. Be able to perform a forensic rape exam
3. Be able to provide high quality medical care for a victim of sexual assault
4. Provide resources for both immediate referral and continued learning by the health care professional

The sexually assaulted patient

Sadly, it is guaranteed that every physician will work with a patient who has been sexually assaulted. It is commonly estimated that around 20 percent of women and 3 percent of men will be sexually assaulted during their lifetime.[1,2] Sexual assault occurs worldwide, with youth, poverty, and living in a conflict area contributing to the risk of being victimized.[1] Depending on your specialty you may treat victims acutely or in follow-up. Even if you never perform a forensic rape exam immediately following the attack, it will be helpful to know what the exam entails and how it may impact your patient. If you are an emergency physician, ob/gyn, or pediatrician, you may be called upon to collect forensic evidence as part of the acute care of a sexual assault victim. The quality of the care you provide can have far-reaching effects for the patient – physically, legally, and psychologically. There is evidence that the patient's experience of the health care interaction can impact the development of post-traumatic stress disorder (PTSD) in the future.[3]

Reviews of the National Ambulatory Care Database illustrate the need for better training and management in the care of sexually assaulted patients. Analysis of this large database identifies serious deficits in the provision of basic medical care to sexual assault victims, including proper STD prophylaxis, pregnancy testing, emergency contraception, and follow-up for HIV testing. In a review of emergency department (ED) visits in 2003, Straight and Heaton reported that only 6.7 percent of ED visits for sexual assault or molestation included coding for appropriate antibiotics.[4] These numbers may be biased by the fact that coding may not reflect details of the visit (i.e., assault occurred out of the appropriate time frame for antibiotics or the patient refused) but this number is so low it is hard to fathom.

Forensic evidence is ephemeral, and once lost cannot be reacquired. There are several types of mistakes an examiner may make:

1) Not realizing it is necessary or appropriate or wanting to spend the time/effort to collect forensic evidence.
2) Collecting the evidence poorly.
3) Neglecting parts of the exam that are unpleasant but necessary.
4) Not properly securing evidence such that it is admissible in court.

One example of this type of error is if the examining physician decides a rape kit is not necessary because the patient has showered, or she is not reporting to the police. Showering may not destroy all evidence, and it is important to obtain evidence as soon as possible, while allowing the victim to take her time to decide about involving law enforcement. Most hospitals in the United States will hold a rape kit for anywhere from 30 to 90 days.

How you perform this exam is psychologically crucial to the patient. As mentioned, there is literature suggesting that if the exam process is experienced as a re-traumatization, the risk of PTSD or other long-term sequelae is greater.[3] There are several ways to minimize this kind of re-traumatizing:

1) Approach the patient with extra sensitivity, including acknowledging the situation that brings him/her to you.
2) Set aside the amount of time necessary to complete the exam without imparting a sense of being rushed or "under the gun." Your chart rack is your problem, not the patient's.
3) Do not be judgmental. This not only means that you should not treat the sex worker like she cannot be a rape victim, it means that you are not there to *judge* the situation at all. You do not need to determine the "truth." Let this understanding liberate you to provide the best care possible in response to what your patient tells you happened to her.
4) Have at least some idea of how to properly use a rape kit BEFORE you need to collect one for a patient. Many patients report that the worst part of their experience was seeing the doctor open the kit and struggle with the instructions. If you don't regularly treat these patients, try to read through a chapter like this twice a year, or take a SAFE (Sexual Assault Forensic Examiner) class, so that you will already be familiar with the steps. This kind of class can give you a great deal of information and understanding in a very focused and intensive manner. The instructor will also know what your local legal issues and resources are, and can help you plan referrals.

An examination after a sexual assault will never be a pleasant experience, but a non-judgmental, kind, and competent exam can start your patient on the road to taking back control and beginning to heal.

The examiner's role

Understanding your role as the person examining the patient will go a long way toward ensuring that you "do no harm." First, as stated above, you are not there to determine "the truth." That is up to law enforcement and the judicial system. You are there to provide medical care and comfort, collect forensic evidence, and determine if the physical exam findings are *consistent with* the patient's reported history. With this in mind, remember that an atraumatic, or "normal" exam, is the most common finding in patients who are rape survivors, particularly when the patient's evaluation does not include a culposcopic exam. Additionally, there is no "normal" affect for a rape victim. Victims may appear tearful, anxious, detached, or angry. She may make jokes, or be quite hostile with staff. Essentially, almost any finding is "consistent with" the possibility of sexual assault. It is only important to note this affect, not determine what it means. If the patient is hostile, demanding, or otherwise "difficult," try to remember that this may be a defensive reaction to trauma. Be flexible about rules and policies if possible, and try to remain calm and sympathetic even if your patient is reacting negatively to you.

Types of victims

For the purpose of this chapter we will consider post-pubescent adolescents and adults only. The issue of child sexual abuse/assault is addressed in a separate chapter. If at all possible, specially trained examiners should care for a child victim. The majority of adolescent and adult victims will be female, but males are reporting sexual assault more today than in the past. We will often use the pronoun "she," but it is important to be aware of some issues that are specific to the male victim. There is very little research in this area but it is estimated that around 1 to 3 percent of men will experience sexual assault in their lifetime.[5] Male and female children are physically abused and neglected at about the same rate, however, there is still a threefold greater risk for females. Males may be more likely to be victimized as children than as adults, but as there is perhaps more social stigma associated with an adult male reporting sexual assault it becomes very difficult to be confident in numbers based on reporting. Approximately one-third of female victims are believed to report their assault.[1,2,4,6] When men do report sexual assault, males almost exclusively report assault by male assailants. They are more likely to sustain non-genital injuries and anal injuries, and may be somewhat less likely to know their assailants.[5]

Lesbian, gay, and transgender victims are likely to feel the additional burden of worry that their gender status or sexual orientation will become the focus of any health care interactions, rather than the actual assault. They may fear that they will be treated as if they are not really victims, especially if the assault occurred in the context of a date or intimate partner relationship. Transgender individuals in particular often experience cruelty in the hospital setting, as staff struggles (often loudly) with issues such as placing the patient in male or female rooms, and what pronoun to use. Encourage your staff to make extra efforts to be sensitive, and identify the patients with the gender they identify themselves. Whatever the clinicians' opinions or beliefs are in this area, it is pointless and egregious to inflict pain on patients based on their appearance or presentation.

Elderly victims may also have issues complicated by society's stereotypes of the elderly, such as their desexualization. As with their younger counterparts, the elderly can be involved in abusive intimate relationships, be assaulted by a casual acquaintance or a stranger, and like children, a caretaker or someone in a position of trust may sexually abuse them. Physically they are more susceptible to injury; without estrogen, vaginal tissue becomes thin, atrophic, and therefore more likely to tear.[1,7]

Other victims who may require the clinician to be extra thoughtful, or engage additional support services, include sex workers, homeless persons who may also have drug, alcohol, or psychiatric issues, and patients who are developmentally delayed or cognitively impaired. Patients in the last category may require a great deal of help to cope with the process of disclosure and examination.

Initial approach and ABCs

Of course, emergent medical issues, while rare, will take priority in a sexual assault case as with any other. Airway compromise, severe trauma, hemodynamic instability, and altered mental status must be addressed prior to any examination specific to sexual assault. In fact, if there is this severity of injury, it may be that the team has not considered sexual assault. This is very important, especially in the case of altered mental status that appears to be secondary to some form of intoxication, including severe alcohol intoxication. Alcohol is by far the most common drug deliberately used to incapacitate a victim; also, drugs such as benzodiazepines and gamma-hydroxybutyrate (GHB) cause the patient to appear drunk, and are often in combination with alcohol, contributing to this effect.[1,2]

Consent to treat

For the vast majority of cases, consent will be a straightforward issue of asking the patient for her permission so that you may conduct the examination and obtain signatures on the appropriate paperwork. The situation of acute intoxication or other physical inability to give proper consent can be very distressing for clinicians. We use the implied consent doctrine to generally treat people who come to the emergency room (ER) altered or severely injured. This doctrine states that medical treatment is lawful "under the doctrine of implied consent when a medical emergency requires immediate action to preserve the health or life of the patient." (Allore v. Flower Hospital, 121 Ohio App. 3d 229, 236, 699 N.E. 2d 560, 564 (1997)). In the case of a rape kit, clearly, life and limb are not threatened, but the ability to prosecute a case decreases rapidly with time up to the 96-hour limit of DNA detection. This issue is being seriously debated in medical and legal circles; hopefully, a consensus will be forthcoming. In the mean time, it would be advisable to contact your hospital's ethics and legal department in order to help guide you through a difficult case. If another crime is being investigated (i.e., the patient was stabbed or shot) this can affect the decision. Even if a rape kit is not specifically collected, steps can be taken to preserve some of the evidence, such as placing clothes in labeled paper bags, ensuring that undergarments are not lost, and carefully documenting all physical findings that may be relevant.

In the case of cognitive inability to consent that is not related to intoxication, there are a number of agencies that can provide assistance, via phone consultation, or in some cases, a worker will come to the facility where the patient is being evaluated. Often, consent can be obtained using language that is appropriate to the patient's cognitive age level. For example "you came here because you were worried that you might have something wrong down there. We want your permission to check your private parts and the rest of your body to be sure that you were not hurt, to take care of you if you were hurt, and to try to help if you decide to talk with the police about what happened to you."

If the patient is not English speaking, the examiner should be able to speak the patient's native language well. Otherwise, a translator should be assigned who remains with the patient throughout her interaction with medical providers. If this person is also the rape advocate, this is ideal. However, the victim should never be in a position of not being able to communicate her needs.

In the following descriptions of the materials needed and methods used, the New York State Protocol for the Acute Care of Adult Patients Reporting Sexual Assault is used as the main reference. There is some minor variation from state to state, but all kits collect the same types of evidence – they were developed to facilitate the consistent prosecution of sex crimes throughout the country.

Necessary materials

In order to provide acute care for a sexual assault victim you must have certain minimum equipment. If you are office-based and cannot maintain these items, you must refer your patient to another site. Your patient will have come to you because

Table 3.1 Materials necessary for examining a rape victim

Required materials for examining a sexual assault victim	Additional materials to enhance exam quality
1. Private exam room with Gyn capabilities	1. Culposcope
2. Private bathroom	2. Toluidine blue dye
3. Gowns for examination	3. Camera
4. Replacement clothing	4. Dedicated "gyn trauma" room with attached bathroom
5. Approved rape kits	5. Specimen drier
6. Ability to draw and analyze blood and urine	6. On-call advocates
7. Antibiotics to prevent sexually transmitted diseases	7. On-call forensic examiners
8. Antiretroviral drugs to prevent transmission of HIV	8. Internet access
9. Materials to provide care for genital and non-genital injuries	
10. Speculum	
11. Light source	
12. Wood's lamp	
13. Area for specimens to dry	

she trusted you – use this opportunity to reassure her she is making the right choice to be examined, and that you want her to get the best possible exam. You may send her by ambulance to an ER or a site dedicated to providing forensic exams for sexual assault patients. Several states offer site-based care; however, most often, care is provided in an emergency department. In the best case, a trained sexual assault forensic examiner will perform the exam. This can be a nurse, physician's assistant (PA), or doctor who has undergone a standardized training program. In many hospitals, a physician trained in emergency medicine will perform the exam, and in other hospitals, an ob/gyn is called to the ER to perform the exam. If you are aware of the resources around you, it will be possible to send your patient to the best location. If your patient has presented outside the time frame where a forensic exam is indicated (up to 96 hours in most states), a physical exam and treatment to prevent STDs, including HIV and Hepatitis B, is indicated.

The items needed are listed above. In order to adequately examine a patient you must be able to perform both a genital and non-genital exam. A pelvic exam is essential in both acute rape cases and patients with delayed presentations.

In the setting of an emergency department, many states require that minimum standards are met, including private GYN rooms, with access to a bathroom, availability of 24-hour advocates of some type, provision of emergency contraception, and the like. It is prudent to know what your state and local requirements are, as well as what resources are available.

It is extremely helpful to have a clear, written, easily accessible policy in any acute care setting. If trained examiners are not available on call, standardized orders, data sheets, and protocol "checklists" can be very helpful in ensuring the best quality care.

In settings where patients are triaged by acuity, rape victims should be made high-priority patients. They should not have to wait in public waiting areas. Immediately upon identification, the patient should be taken to a private area, preferably the room in which she will be examined. An advocate should be called immediately. Ideally, this person is trained as a rape advocate, and is there specifically to provide support for the patient to whatever degree that patient requires, including staying with the patient throughout the exam. These rape advocates are often non-medical community volunteers, and they receive standardized training as well as ongoing education and supervision. If there is no rape advocate available, staff such as the social worker can serve in this capacity, but they are less likely to be able to stay with the patient throughout her process.

Ideally, exam rooms should be private (doors, not curtained areas) and wheel-chair accessible, with direct access to a bathroom, including a shower. If clothing is to be collected, a change of clothes must be provided. Real clothing, not paper scrubs, is preferred, including brand new (not previously used) underwear and bras. Have a few items appropriate for men.

Patients who present within 96 hours of being assaulted should be encouraged to hold urine until after the forensic exam if they are not too uncomfortable. If need be, the pelvic portion of the exam can be done immediately, and then time given for the patient to urinate before continuing. If drug-facilitated sexual assault (DFSA) is suspected, it is crucial to collect that first urine sample.

The clinician who will be examining the patient should introduce his or herself to the patient as immediately as possible. Let her know who you are, and what the immediate plan is. For example, you might inform her that you will be her doctor, that an advocate is on the way, and that a nurse will be in shortly to draw blood. Ask if she needs anything immediately. Be sure to acknowledge the situation and reinforce her decision to be treated. Say something like "I am very sorry that this happened to you, but I am very glad that you were able to come to the hospital so we can treat you. That takes a lot of courage." If you are not immediately starting the exam, let her know when you expect to begin.

Often we think of the medical exam as history, physical, lab tests, treatment, and discharge or admission. In the case of a rape victim (as with all victims of abuse), it is important to be flexible about the order of things. One example of how this is important is when considering the possibility of oral assault. In a patient who presents within the 96-hour time frame for a forensic exam, ask about oral assault immediately. Routinely collect evidence from the mouth immediately, rather than allow the patient to go through giving the history and other steps until you get to that part of the forensic exam. Imagine how humiliated a patient might feel who is telling you his/her story before having a chance to clean his/her mouth. Open the rape kit, collect oral evidence (usually with swabs), and then offer toothbrush/toothpaste and/or something to drink to the patient. This may be inconvenient, because you must now ensure the chain of evidence remains unbroken for this kit, but it is a huge step in making the victim more comfortable. At this point you may begin to get the history from the patient.

History of events

The history obtained by the examiner should be directed at informing the medical exam. The examiner should note in general terms when and where the attack occurred, the number of assailants involved, if the perpetrator(s) is/are known to the victim, what elements of force or coercion were involved, and ways in which the victim attempted to stop the perpetrator. (See Figure 3.1 for examples.)

The first history gives details of clothing but not information about force and resistance, and is not specific about what the patient means by "rape." The second history gives how the patient was maneuvered into a vulnerable position, the

Inappropriate history	Patient alleges that perp in a green and tan striped cotton polo shirt and jeans grabbed her arm then put his arm around her neck and choked her. She states he then raped her. She states they met at a party and left together.
Appropriate history	Patient reports that person who raped her was someone she met at party earlier. He walked out of the apartment with her and suggested they take the stairs. In the stairway he tried to kiss her and she told him "I don't want to." She said "no" several more times as he grabbed her arm, choked her with a forearm. She states he told her he would kill her if she screamed. He pushed her to the ground. She thinks she hit her head. He then "put it in me" (vaginal penetration). She is not sure if he ejaculated. She reports soreness to the back of her head, her throat, and her vaginal area.

Figure 3.1   Examples of appropriate and inappropriate history documentation.

Table 3.2 Signs of drug-facilitated sexual assault. From the protocol for the acute care of adult patients reporting sexual assault. New York State Department of Health, November 2004.

Signs that your patient may have been drugged

- If the patient remembers taking a drink but cannot remember what happened for a period of time after he/she consumed the drink.
- If the patient feels as though someone had sex wih him/her, but cannot recall any or all of the incident.
- If the patient feels a lot more intoxicated then his/her usual response to the amount of alcohol he/she consumed.
- If the patient woke up feeling very hung over or "fuzzy," experiencing memory lapse, and cannot account for a period of time.
- If the patient wakes up in a strange or different location and does not know how he/she got there.
- If the patient's clothes are absent, inside out, disheveled, or not his/hers.
- If the patient has "snapshots" or "cameo memories."

elements of force used, and the patient's words and medical terms for the assault. Also the areas of pain are reported. This then informs the physical exam – the examiner knows to check the back of her head, and can report bruises or lacerations. If there are no other findings, it can still be noted that this is an area of soreness. Pain and tenderness can be noted again on a body diagram. Also, the patient's own language is used, and then the meaning, as obtained from the patient, is given to clarify.

Lastly, any actions the patient has taken since the assault should be noted in the history, including vomiting, urinating, brushing teeth, changing cloths, showering, and/or douching.

Throughout the history, the clinician should take opportunities to reinforce the survivor that "she did nothing to make this happen, she did not deserve to be assaulted, she made the best choices she could to protect herself," and, by being with the clinician now, "she is again showing great strength and courage in caring for herself."

Drug-facilitated sexual assault (DFSA)

It is important to determine early in the patient's history if there is a possibility of drug-facilitated sexual assault (DFSA). Clues to this possibility include snapshot memories, blackouts, and unexplained circumstances (see Table 3.2).

This information must be obtained early to ensure that the patient's first urine sample is collected. In some states there is a separate DFSA kit, with its own urine and blood containers. If you do not have this kind of kit, the testing requires a urine sample and two grey-topped blood tubes. The majority of hospitals and private labs do not test for all the substances used in DFSA, such as flunitrazepam (rohypnol) and gamma-hydroxybutyrate (GHB), and cannot detect other drugs at the trace levels necessary to confirm drugging. Generally, the analysis will be done by a medical examiner's office at the request of the police or the district attorney's office. Often, this means a patient must make a police report in order to find out if she tests positive. Some victims will be upset by this, wanting to know "if anything actually happened" before pressing charges. It may be helpful for these victims to talk with the Special Victims detectives via phone before making a decision. They can sometimes allay the victim's fears that as soon as they make a report, the person they suspect will be summarily arrested. If Special Victims detectives are notified first, they may respond in person, or contact the officers who will be dispatched. The usual protocol when the situation is unclear is that work is done to try to get more information about what happened, such as staging a recorded phone conversation between the two parties. The possible victim is coached on how to try to get the other person to tell her what happened. In many of these cases it is not necessary to find "date rape drugs" in the victim. A person must be capable of consent for sexual activity to be consensual. If the victim is passed out from too much alcohol, she is not able to consent to sex.

Past medical history

All the usual elements of the past medical history can be included, but it is advisable to leave out details of previous STDs and pregnancies especially in an acute situation. This has no bearing on the current event and, sadly, rape shield laws are not adequate to prevent this type of information from being used to imply that the patient was not raped because she is promiscuous. An exception to this guideline might be if trafficking is suspected or if some other long-term abuse situation is involved. In that case, STDs and pregnancies may be the result of this abuse. This would be particularly true in a child or adolescent, where even "promiscuity" is often a symptom of sexual abuse. It is important to ask about general medical problems, last menstrual period, current medications, and last episode of consensual sex. This last piece of information may seem potentially inflammatory but it is very important because if sperm, semen, or DNA is identified, the consensual partner may need to be tested to rule him out as the source.[2]

Contents of the rape kit

The sexual assault evidence collection kit was developed in the 1970s by a former detective-turned-forensic-scientist Louis R Vitullo. The kits are still occasionally referred to as "Vitullo kits," or more commonly, "rape kits." They vary slightly from state to state, but all have essentially the same materials. This includes:

1. Sealable envelopes.
2. Gloves.
3. Cotton-tipped swabs for taking samples from the mouth, vagina, and anus, as well as for swabbing any bite marks or possible bodily fluids elsewhere on the victim. This is done for the purpose of collecting spermatozoa, semen, or saliva from the assailant.
4. Slides for swabbing the above samples onto, and slide holders to maintain the slides in. Slides are never stained or fixed as they might be for diagnostic exams.
5. Packaging for collection of underwear, and possibility of documenting other clothing collected.
6. Materials for collecting debris from the patient's body during the process of disrobing as well as directly from her body when she is undressed.
7. Items such as wooden sticks to allow the collection of material from under a victim's fingernails.
8. Comb for collection of foreign hairs from the pubic area.
9. Papers for the above materials to be collected into.
10. Instructions for collecting pulled hair standards from the head and pubic area.
11. Buccal swab for collection of DNA standard from the patient's cheek cells.
12. Seals for items that go in the kit, and for the outside of the kit.
13. Paperwork including body diagrams (often called *traumagrams*), consent forms, and documentation of chain of custody.

In some states the paperwork for law enforcement is returned to the kit, while in others, the paperwork stays with the medical chart and goes to law enforcement if requested. It is always necessary to generate many patient labels for the envelopes and some of the materials inside. This material is contained in a box that is sealed, and that must be unsealed, used, and resealed. Some documentation of the chain of command will be on the kit. If a patient is having a kit done but not reporting to the police, the facility is obligated to securely maintain the kit for a minimum of 30 days. Therefore, it would not be advisable for someone with an office-based practice to perform a rape kit unless there are unusual circumstances (i.e., you are the patient's ob/gyn and she states she will only allow *you* to do the exam) and the kit will be immediately given to law enforcement. In a hospital or center for treating sexual assault patients, the kits are maintained in a secure location and refrigerated until they are either turned over to law enforcement or discarded. Some programs include a policy of calling the victim prior to discarding the kits, and retaining the kit longer if so requested.

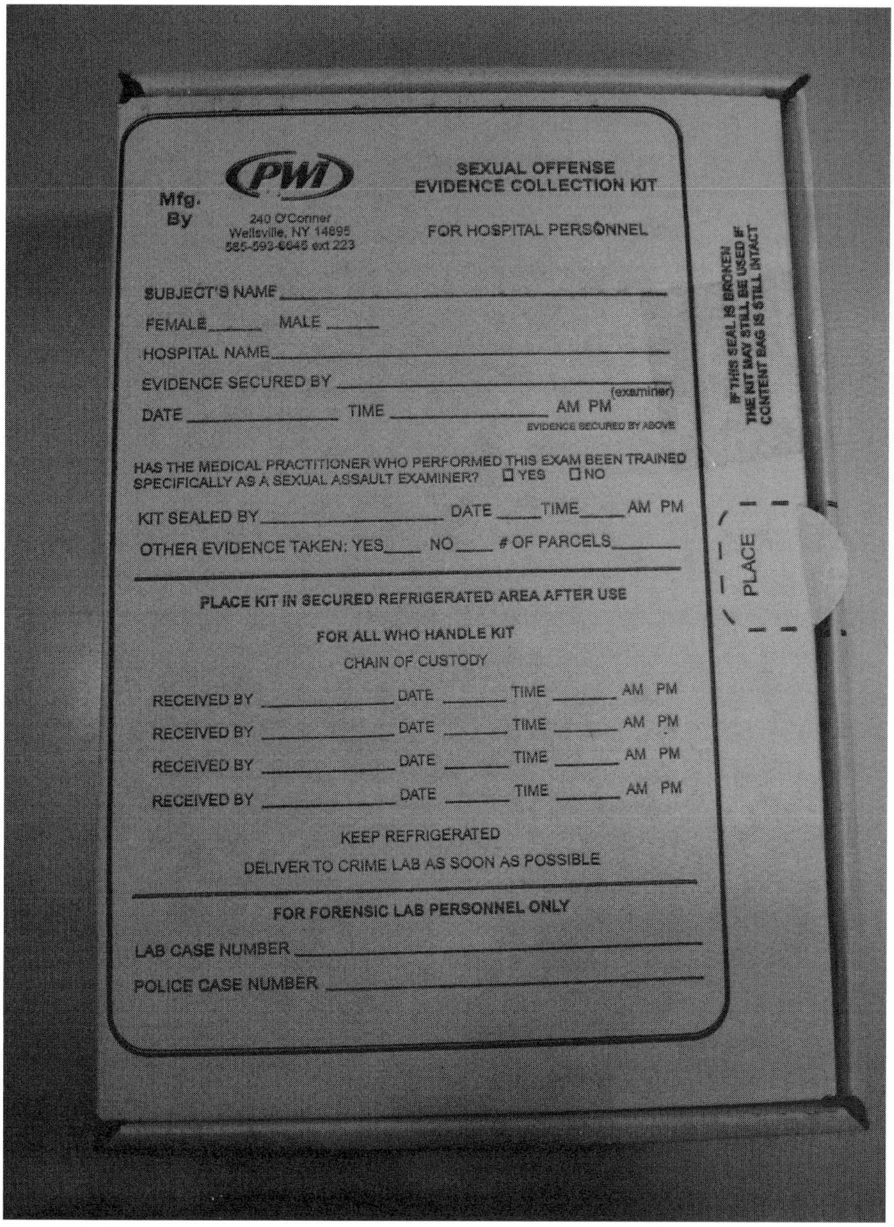

Figure 3.2   New York State Sexual Assault Evidence Collection Kit (SAEK).

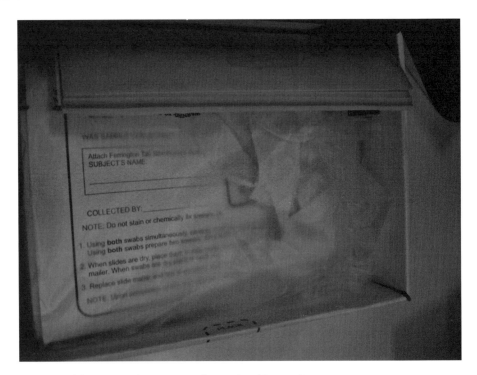

Figure 3.3   Contents of the New York State Sexual Assault Evidence Kit.

The drug-facilitated sexual assault kit

Where these are available they will contain the following items:

1. Urine cup
2. 2 grey-top blood tubes
3. Paperwork to document the symptoms of DFSA

This material is also taken from a sealed kit and resealed when completed. These kits also must be stored and require refrigeration to prevent degradation of the samples.

Sexual assault forensic examiner programs

These programs exist all across the country. They come in a variety of incarnations and go by a variety of acronyms including SAFE, SANE, and SART. SANE programs utilize nurses (Sexual Assault Nurse Examiner) and SART (Sexual Assault Response Team) programs are based on response teams that go to where patients are. Some programs exist in self-contained settings, where either EMS or police takes survivors, or where hotline personnel direct them. They may be transferred to these sites from local emergency rooms or doctor's offices. These programs are extremely beneficial

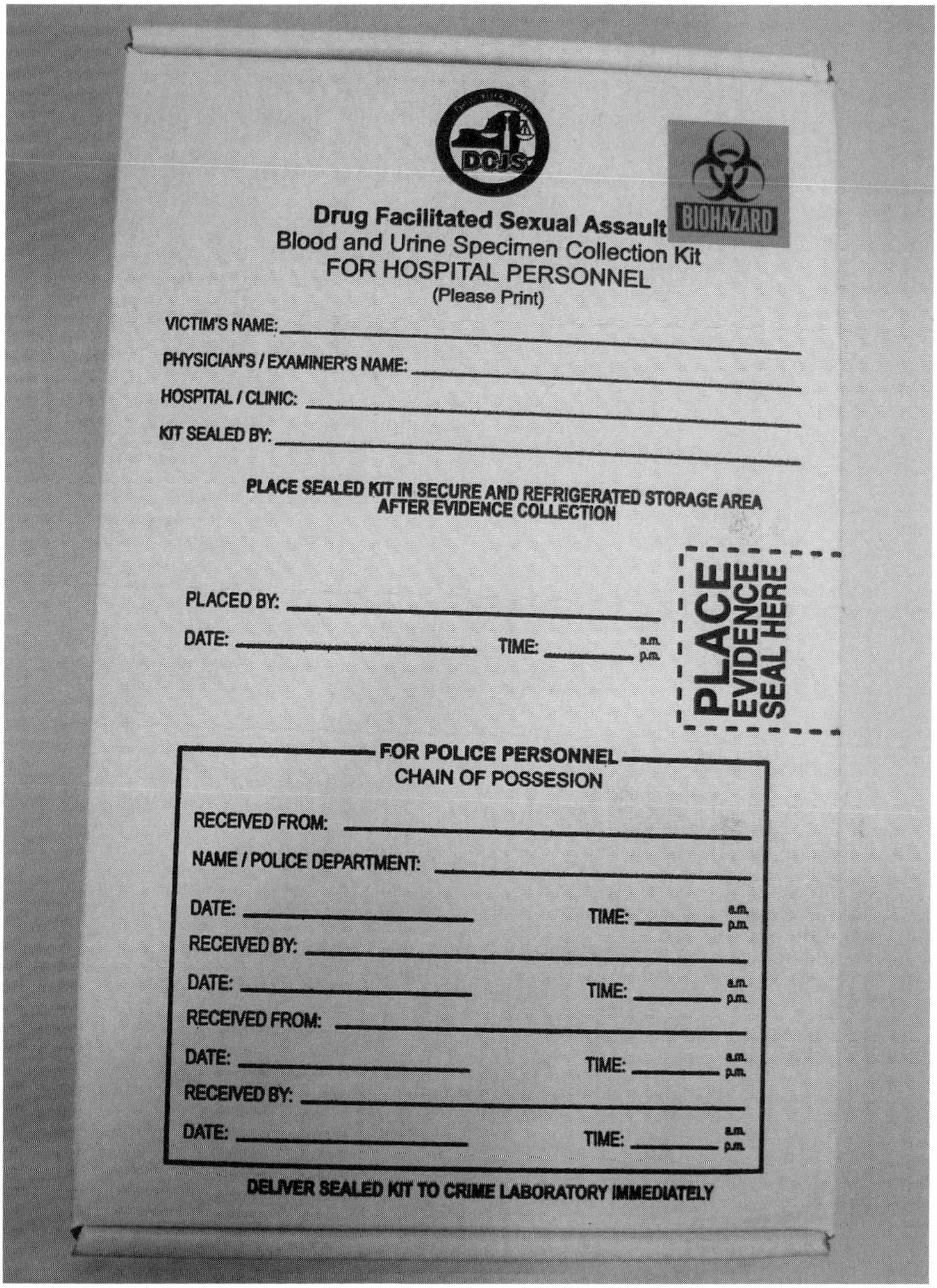

Figure 3.4   New York State Drug-Facilitated Sexual Assault Kit.

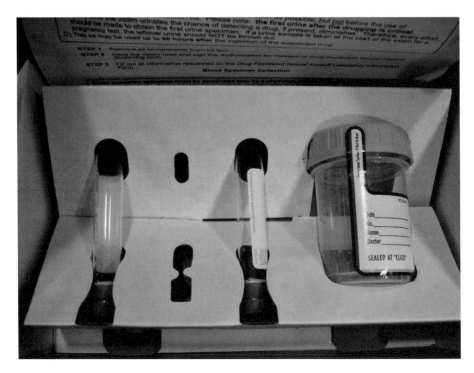

Figure 3.5   Contents of DFSA.

for several reasons. Examiners receive extensive training in evidence collection and their programs provide continuous quality monitoring and improvement, as well as continuing education for the participants. When a patient is seen by one of these examiners, the patient is the only person that the examiner is there to see. There is no time pressure. Often these programs involve more than the examiner – there is often an advocate on-call program, and if affiliated with a rape crisis center, follow-up medical, psychological, and legal care may be included. If your practice or hospital does not have such a program, it would be ideal for you to find out if there is one with which you can become aligned. At the very minimum, know your local rape crisis center's hotline and direct line phone numbers, so they can be a resource for you and your patients. There is some evidence that exams by trained forensic examiners do lead to better DNA acquisition and greater rates of successful prosecution.[2,8]

Examining the patient

After the history, it is time to examine the patient. If the assault occurred within the past 96 hours, you should strongly encourage your patient to have a rape kit collected. Remind her that this does not force her to make a police report, but that it will allow her the opportunity to decide to report later and have the best possibility

Traumagram – Genital

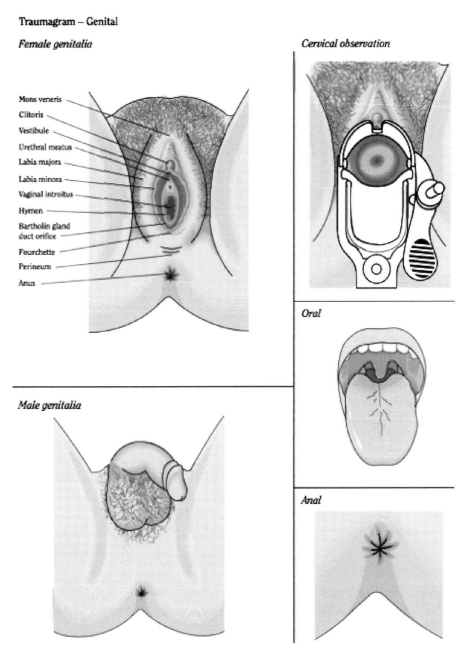

Female genitalia

Mons veneris

Clitoris

Vestibule

Urethral meatus

Labia majora

Labia minora

Vaginal introitus

Hymen

Bartholin gland duct orifice

Fourchette

Perineum

Anus

Cervical observation

Oral

Anal

Male genitalia

Figure 3.6   Genital diagrams with labels. From New York State Protocol for the Acute Care of the Adult Patient Reporting Sexual Assault.

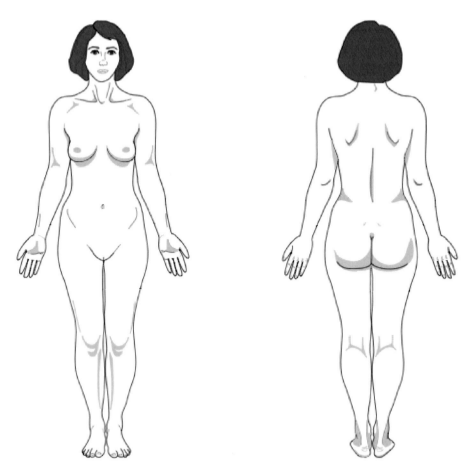

Figure 3.7   Body diagrams. From New York State Protocol for the Acute Care of the Adult Patient Reporting Sexual Assault.

of there being evidence to help her case. You should have already started the kit with the oral samples if your patient has agreed. It is very helpful to victims when you let them know about each of the steps coming up so they are mentally prepared. Also, be sure to continually let the patient know that she is in control of this situation, that you will not do anything she asks you not to do and that she can stop any part of the exam at any time. The order described here will be the routine, but you should be prepared to be flexible, not rule-driven. For example, the perineum and pelvic exam is usually last, but if your patient feels like she needs to urinate urgently, or if she feels she needs to "get that part over with right away," you should conduct these exams first.

The patient's body is a crime scene. Therefore, anything on her body, including debris, marks, secretions, and areas of tenderness are evidence of that crime. As you document your findings, you should be following the principle of "describe it in words, draw it in detail, and take a picture." Please consult the chapter in this book on Forensic Photography for excellent directions on when and how to take these kinds of pictures. Colposcopic photography is a topic only briefly covered in this book, because it requires some expertise and should not be attempted unless the examiner is trained in the use of this tool. However, this is a very worthwhile investment of time, as use of colposcopy greatly increases the likelihood of documenting injuries. While it seems that documented injuries lead to increased conviction rates, the relevance of minor genital injuries and injury patterns in establishing consent is unclear. There have been several cases that have called in to question the validity of this kind of "expert testimony" and at this time researchers are just beginning to approach the question more rigorously.

Initially, the patient should be examined head to toe, with specific attention to areas of her body she reported having soreness or that relate to her account of the assault. In order to accomplish a full exam while minimizing how exposed the victim feels, it can be helpful to give her two patient gowns, one open in the front and one open in the back. If a rape kit is being collected, the examiner should help the patient undress over the appropriate collection paper (either provided within the kit or using a piece of standard exam table paper) while handing her the gowns. After the debris and clothes are collected, the examiner then surveys an area of the victim's body, usually the back first, while allowing her to keep herself covered elsewhere. If a victim reports pain in an area, gently palpate for tenderness. Also palpate any areas where you might expect soreness from the history. For example, if the victim reports that she was choked, but does not have marks on her neck, she may have some tenderness in the area. This is especially true when the victim is being examined immediately after the assault, and bruises have not had time to develop. Police will sometimes re-photograph in 48 hours in order to see more pronounced bruises.

Sometimes clinicians feel uncomfortable examining the breasts, out of concern that the patient will feel further humiliated by this exam. If care is taken to preserve the patient's dignity, this does not have to be the case. The breast area can be a specific target of attack; therefore it is important not to neglect this portion of the exam. Patients may have suction injuries or bite marks, and may have soreness. Examine inside the mouth as well, as forced oral–penile contact can lead to palatal bruising or petechiae. You should also examine the patient using a Wood's lamp, to look for areas of florescence, reflecting possible dried bodily fluids. If a rape kit is to be collected, note these areas and be certain to swab them at the appropriate point in the kit.

If you were not planning to collect a rape kit, the pelvic exam would be appropriate at this time, if the patient is willing.

Collecting the rape kit (*Adapted from the Protocol for the Acute Care of Adult Patients Reporting Sexual Assault*)

Based on the New York State protocol, at this point you would have already per-formed Step 1 (oral swabs and smears) before getting the full history, Step 2 (trace evidence and clothing collection) as the patient undressed and gowned, and Step 3 (underwear collection). It is also reasonable to do the buccal swab (Step 12) early in the exam, as it is not painful or invasive, the patient can easily do it herself, and the specimen needs to dry before the kit can be sealed. The current use of a buccal swab replaces the victim's blood tubes included in older kits. It is very helpful to give the survivor every opportunity to do the steps for herself. This makes the kit less intrusive and gives her both the possibility of feeling more in control and of actively doing something to take care of herself after this tremendous blow to her sense of competence and autonomy. For the sake of reference, a quick review of the above steps will be given, followed by the rest of the steps in order. All envelopes in the kit should be labeled, dated, and signed by the examiner, and "Yes" or "No" marked in the appropriate place to indicate if evidence was collected. Do not leave any questions blank.

Step 1: Oral Swabs and Smears: Two swabs are placed inside the victim's mouth and the mouth and gum pockets are swabbed. The patient can assist with this process. The swabs are smeared together onto the slides and slides and swabs are allowed to dry before being returned to their holders and placed inside the Oral Swabs and Smears envelope. The envelope is then labeled, information filled out, and sealed. To reiterate, this step should be performed as soon as possible, prior to significant history taking. This makes the patient more comfortable and prevents the loss of oral evidence.

Step 2: Trace Evidence and Clothing Collection: This refers to evidence that falls from the patient's clothing or body as she undresses over a large sheet of paper, usually exam table paper. It is then folded and sealed with a label such that the material stays inside. The label should be signed and dated by the examiner. If the patient has not changed clothing since the attack, the clothing should be collected, folded, and placed inside individual paper bags to prevent cross contamination. These bags can then be placed within a larger paper bag, which is then folded over and sealed in the same manner. This does not go inside the kit, but is held or given to law enforcement with the kit. If the clothing is wet, it should be allowed to dry first. If it is not dry, it can be turned over to the police in a plastic bag. However, they must be informed that the clothing is wet so it can be taken out to dry in the crime lab. This is because wet samples will rot and the DNA will degenerate. Additionally, it should be noted if clothing was cut in order to be removed, and the examiner should initial any places where the clothing was cut. Cut lines should avoid any pre-existing tears or stains. Do not overlook the importance of clothing. It is not uncommon for clothing to retain DNA samples from the assailant when none are recoverable from the victim's body. Damage to clothing may also prove useful in establishing the use of force.

If the patient has changed clothes, but the clothing she was wearing at the time of the assault have not yet been cleaned, there is a good chance the clothing may still contain evidence, and law enforcement should be informed.

Step 3: Underwear Collection: The patient's underwear should be collected regardless of whether or not it is the same pair she was wearing. This is because there can be fluid samples on the underwear even at a later time. The underwear is placed in a special paper bag provided in the kit and appropriately labeled and sealed.

Step 4: Debris Collection: Any material found on the patient's body should be removed, placed in the center of the provided paper, which is then folded, and placed inside the envelope. It is critical that the chart contain information regarding what material was collected from where – for example, "leaf debris sticking to patient's back," with a picture drawn on the traumagram, and ideally a photo taken of the material prior to removing it.

Step 5: Dried Secretions and Bite Marks: A Wood's lamp can be used to identify dried secretions, which will fluoresce under the blue light. If secretions or bite marks are identified they are swabbed with two water-moistened swabs together, allowed to dry, placed in the swab box, and sealed in the appropriate envelope. Additionally, if there is matted material in the hair, it would be sampled at this time as well. If multiple sites must be swabbed, additional white envelopes can be used. They should be filled out in the same manner as the ones supplied in the kit, and should never be licked, but taped shut. It may be acceptable to open other kits and use the equivalent envelope in that kit, discarding the rest of the second kit. There should be documentation of how many sites were swabbed. Each sample's label should contain information about where it was obtained, for example, "swab of matted material in pubic hair" or "swab of bite mark from left areola."

Step 6: Fingernail Scrapings: Two wooden sticks and two folded papers are provided. The patient cleans under the fingernails of one hand over one paper, and then places the stick inside the sheet. The paper is folded such that no material is lost and then sealed and labeled left or right. Samples must be taken only from one hand in each paper.

Steps 7 and 9: Pulled Head and Pubic Hairs: These steps are very controversial. They involve the plucking of hairs from the head and pubic area. The hairs must contain the root in order to establish their identity. They must be taken from several sites in the scalp or pubic hair. Many examiners have declined to collect these, citing that this is painful and unnecessary as the victim's hair can be obtained at any time should that become relevant. However, the medical examiner's office in New York has strongly requested that these samples be obtained, pointing out that hair that does not have a root is identified based on its physical characteristics. Therefore, anyone who colors/processes his or her hair may have different hair characteristics over time. Opponents suggest that, at least if the patient is reporting within a short time, the evidence will be analyzed and the person can give the hair standard at a later time, but when the hair is still likely to be the same. This point is well taken with head hair, and often survivors don't find this to be too difficult. The pubic hair is much more painful to pull, and it does seem much less likely to be significantly changed over a fairly short time.

Step 8: Pubic Hair Combing: This step can feel a bit awkward, but the patient can generally do this herself, and it is generally not painful. If the patient has a shaved pubic area this should be noted and still the procedure can basically be followed to allow for any foreign hairs or debris to be collected. A piece of collection paper is placed under her, and she uses the included comb to comb the pubic hairs outwards and downward such that any material that falls out is collected. The comb is then placed inside the paper; the paper is sealed and returned to its envelope.

Step 10: Anal Swabs and Smears: This step is very important, even if the victim denies anal contact. It is best to make collection of swabs from all orifices routine, as the victim may not report the attack she felt to be the most humiliating, and victims may not report or even initially recall everything that happened to her. Of course it should be clear to the patient that she can refuse and/or return to any portion of the exam. This is vital to creating a sense of returned control over her body. Two swabs and slides are provided. The cotton tips can be water moistened and the inside of the anus is swabbed. Perineal secretions should be swabbed in the dried secretions section. It is recommended that the anal swabs be performed before the vaginal swabs to prevent contamination from the vaginal area as well as loss of material from the anal area. If there are any signs of injury or the patient reports pain, an anoscopic exam should be performed at this point.

Step 11: Vaginal/Penile Swabs and Smears: Two sets of paired swabs and slides are included in this step. For vaginal swabs, paired swabs are inserted into the vaginal vault and the area is swabbed; smears are then created with both swabs. The process is then repeated. For penile sampling, the swabs are moistened with water and the penile *shaft* is thoroughly swabbed with both sets of swabs. Do not swab the urethra as would be done for a culture. This is both painful and unnecessary. Secretions from the scrotum or perineum surrounding the penis would be sampled in the dried secretions section.

At this point, the pelvic or genital exam should be performed. Any injuries should be noted, with special attention to the posterior fourchette and the labia minora. Any soreness should be reported in the chart, and significant or otherwise concerning adnexal or cervical motion tenderness should prompt further evaluation such as gynecological consultation, ultrasound, or computed tomography (CT) to rule out internal injuries. Colposcopy can greatly enhance the detection of injuries, to upward of 90 percent from a low of 1 percent. However, the significance of minor injuries with regards to proof of nonconsensual contact is still under debate. Several studies have attempted to delineate patterns of genital injury that are more likely to occur when intercourse is not consensual, but the validity of these findings has been questioned[9,17–19] and the use of colposcopy should not be undertaken unless the clinician is trained in the forensic use of this tool.

Step 12: Buccal Specimen: This step replaces the blood sample in many kits. As stated earlier, it is wise to do this step early in the process, as it also needs to dry. After the patient has cleaned her mouth with water, she can rub the inside of her cheek with the swab. This collects epithelial cells from the patient and allows the determination of her DNA so that it can be distinguished from any other samples obtained. This is also the method that would be used to obtain DNA from a consensual partner.

Completing the Kit: Review the contents to be sure all steps have either been collected or non-collection is noted. Be sure all specimens are dry before sealing them. When all specimens have been placed inside the kit, it is sealed and the information on the outside of the kit is filled out, the kit and any additional packages (i.e., clothing) are turned over to either law enforcement or another designated agent (such as hospital security officers) who brings the kit to a storage facility. Hospitals are required to maintain the kit for a minimum of 30 days. The victim will need to sign either consent to release the evidence or a non-authorization of release, in which case the kit is stored by the facility. At any point until the kit is discarded, the victim can authorize the release of the evidence to the police. She can also request the material (particularly clothing) be returned to her.

Chain of evidence

From the moment the kit is opened, until the time that it is sealed, all contents of the kit must be directly observed by – and in the possession of – the examiner or an assistant who also signs for the kit. This means that the victim, and her family, friends, or advocate must NEVER be left alone with the kit.[2] To do so would raise the possibility of tampering. If the chain of evidence is not absolutely pristine, the kit may not be admissible in court; this would be a tragic waste.

General medical care

After the evidentiary exam is complete, attention can be given to basic medical care including suturing lacerations, abrasion care, and x-rays, if indicated. As a rule, the determination of whether or not to x-ray a patient should be based on clinical indication, not the fact that the patient was assaulted. Numerous negative x-rays will not improve her case, and do expose the patient to radiation. Good clinical judgment combined with the patient's wishes provides the best medical care in this situation and with any other. Tetanus status should have been assessed during the history, and tetanus vaccination should be given if indicated. An anti-emetic should be given to the patient approximately 20 minutes prior to other medications, as the antibiotics and nPEP medications can cause nausea and vomiting.

Laboratory studies

Urine should be collected ideally after the anal/vaginal evidence has been collected. If DFSA is suspected, it is critical that the first urine produced by the patient be collected. It should be routine to save the urine collected for pregnancy testing in case the question of DFSA arises later in the work up. Do not use the clean catch technique to collect urine; if this is needed to determine if a UTI is present, have the patient give a second sample for this evaluation.[2,3]

Blood sample should include baseline CBC, electrolytes, Bun/Creat, LFTs, and hepatitis panel. HIV testing should be done at this time if the mechanisms for counseling and follow-up are in place. Extra blood can be drawn for later testing if a mechanism for this is created.

If blood for DFSA is being drawn, this requires two grey-topped tubes. If there is uncertainty at the time of blood draw, obtain the grey-top tubes – it is preferable to discard tubes rather than require a second venipuncture.

Emergency contraception

Many states mandate that hospitals provide written and verbal information to sexual assault patients regarding emergency contraception, and mandate that the hospitals provide the actual medication on site. As of August 2006, Plan B, a progestin-only oral contraceptive, was made available over the counter for women over 18. This does not generally release hospitals from providing the pills in the ER. This requirement is regardless of the religious affiliation of the hospital, but the Vatican has come out with a position that allows prevention of fertilization for a rape victim, as opposed to the termination or interruption of an existing pregnancy. The only absolute contraindication to the progestin-only pills is current pregnancy. This is because it will not be effective in preventing pregnancy, but if a pregnant patient were to take levenorgestril, there is no evidence it will harm the fetus. The "morning after" pill can be given up to 120 hours after the assault, but is most effective in the first 24 hours.[1,2,13]

Table 3.3 Emergency contraception

Emergency contraception
BEST
1. Plan B – levenorgestril 0.75 mg orally: 1 pill at presentation and one in 12 hours
Alternative
2. Appropriate dose of any oral contraceptive

Prevention of STDs

It seems obvious that any patient who as been subjected to a sexual assault is at risk for developing a sexually transmitted disease such as gonorrhea, chlamydia, or syphilis. Therefore it is considered standard of care to offer prophylaxis against the development of these diseases. There is evidence that currently, women are not being offered these medications.[4] Centers for Disease Control (CDC) guidelines are updated every few years, and addendums are made to reflect current resistance levels. This is easy to check on line at the CDC website.

Of the medications in the above regimen, it should be noted that metronidazole is the least urgent, as it is given to prevent trichomonas and bacterial vaginosis infection, which although unpleasant do not carry significant sequela. It is only important to note this because you must not give metronidazole to anyone with an appreciable alcohol level because of the antabuse-like interaction with alcohol that leads to profound nausea and vomiting, hypotension, headaches, and flushing. If it is taken the patient must be aware that she cannot drink for 48 hours after the dose.

Table 3.4 Medication for STD prophylaxis from *MMWR*. 2006; 55: 1

CDC recommendations for treatment to prevent STD infection in sexual assault victims
1. Ceftriaxone 125 mg IM in a single dose
PLUS
2. Metronidazole 2 g orally in a single dose
PLUS
3. Azithromycin 1 g orally in a single dose
OR
4. Doxycycline 100 mg orally twice a day for 7 days
Do not use floroquinolones, as there is significant resistance in Neiserria gonorrhea.

Post-exposure Hepatitis B and C

Sexual assault also places the patient at risk for contracting Hepatitis B or C. While there is an effective vaccine and immunoglobulin treatment to prevent Hepatitis B infection, Hepatitis C infection cannot be prevented, only screened for. If the patient has been previously infected with, or vaccinated against Hepatitis B and has a known response, it is not necessary to give Hepatitis B vaccine or HBIG. If the patient has not been previously vaccinated or has not completed the series, then the hepatitis vaccination series should be initiated, and HBIG given. Hepatitis B surface antibody (Anti-HBs) titers and Hepatitis C serology, as well as LFTs should be part of the initial battery of tests sent to establish the patient's baseline. Patients receiving the hepatitis vaccination series should have post-vaccination testing done one to two months after their vaccine series is completed.[2]

Post-exposure HIV prophylaxis

Non-occupational exposure HIV post-exposure prophylaxis (nPEP) should be offered to all sexual assault victims unless she explicitly denies "direct contact of the vagina, anus, or mouth with the semen or blood of the perpetrator, with or without physical injury, tissue damage, or presence of blood at the site of the assault."[14] As this often cannot be established with certainty, nPEP should be offered if there was any possibility of this kind of exposure – that is, regardless of whether or not the victim is certain that ejaculation occurred or penile penetration was completed up to 36 hours prior to presentation.[14] Whenever possible, consult with an Infectious Disease (ID) specialist if there is any question. It is also necessary to consult an ID specialist in the case of the victim who is pregnant or breastfeeding, has significant medical problems, or whose assailant is known to be HIV infected. All of these conditions can significantly alter the recommended regimen. If no ID specialist can be reached, the website www.hivguidelines.org provides extensive information and links to further resources. The National Clinicians' Post-Exposure Prophylaxis hotline (1-888-448-4911) is also available 24 hours a day, 7 days a week for clinicians trying to acutely manage these challenging cases.

Ideally the patient should be tested for HIV at the time of initial presentation, as part of a single initial blood draw or by using rapid testing. However, this requires that pre- and post-testing counseling be provided, and if the results are not immediate, a follow-up system for informing patients of their test results must be in place. For this reason many emergency departments do not provide initial HIV testing. With the development of the rapid oral tests, more EDs are creating mechanisms to support this type of point-of-care testing. If immediate testing is not provided, arrangements must be made for testing to occur as soon as possible; ideally from blood already drawn at the time of the initial evaluation. Some hospital labs will perform a "spin and hold" on a serum sample to allow this to be possible. The nPEP should be given even if the patient refuses testing or the results will be delayed. Follow-up testing should be done at 4 weeks, 12 weeks, and 6 months after the assault.[2,14]

Patients should be discharged with enough medication to last until her follow-up appointment; a five-day supply is considered typical.

Completing the encounter

At this point it is important to review everything that has been done with the patient, and find out if she has any questions or issues she still needs addressed. It can be very helpful to have a checklist and pre-printed or computer-based order sets in place to allow practitioners to be consistent and complete in their care of the

Table 3.5 nPEP guidelines from www.hivguidelines.org

Non-occupational PEP recommendations by the CDC
NNRTI-based
Efavirenz + (lamivudine or emtricitabine) + (zidovudine or tenofovir); or Combivir + tenofovir for 28 days (*Do not administer efavirenz to pregnant women*)
PI-based
Lopinavir/ritonavir (Kaletra) + (lamivudine or emtricitabine) + zidovudine (or Combivir) for 28 days

patient.[15] A version of this type of checklist created by the author is included in the quick reference pages. This was designed for use by residents and attendings in an urban emergency department without a SAFE/SANE program.

Patients should have written material on emergency contraception, HIV, and STD prophylaxis, as well as any other care that was rendered. If the kit was not turned over to the police, the patient should be given a contact person with whom she can contact if she wants the kit released at a later time. Be sure the patient has follow-up appointments, medications, and prescriptions. It is especially important that the survivor be given rape crisis center and hotline information. Inquire as to what her plans are for the next few days, and what her social supports are. Respect her decisions if she wants to be alone, but encourage her to use whatever supports she feels comfortable with, and to access the hotline or crisis center early if she is experiencing any distress. Patients sometimes are very calm going through the process of the medical exam and police report, but find that when they are no longer engaged in all that activity, the full force of the events bear down on them.

DNA database

Individuals who commit sexual assault all too often repeat their crime. Every state has some form of database of DNA from persons convicted of a range of crimes, and from rape kits that have yielded DNA. Data from each state is uploaded to a Federal registry called CODIS (Combined DNA Index System). If DNA from a victim matches a known sample in the database, the patient's assailant can be identified. It is also possible that the DNA will match another unidentified DNA sample, linking the crimes and perhaps furthering the process of identifying the perpetrator. Importantly, it is also possible to clear a person as a suspect by demonstrating no match between his DNA and that identified from the victim.[20]

Testifying in court

For SAFE/SANE/SART-trained examiners, testifying in court is not only part of the training, it is one of the main goals of the examiner. This means that the case is being prosecuted, and the examiner now has the opportunity to present his/her findings in a court of law. However, many clinicians dread testifying. It can be difficult to set aside the necessary time for preparation and trial, and clinicians tend to feel anxious about appearing in court, given the hostile legal environment that exists in the United States and are concerned that they will be made to look foolish on the witness stand during cross examination. There are several things that can help you if you feel this way about testifying in court.

1. The more clearly legible your chart is, and the more information it provides, the less likely it is you will actually have to appear in court. It is not uncommon for the prosecutor to use the chart itself, if it is legible and clearly understandable.

2. If you are asked to testify, your chart will be the basis of your testimony. Therefore again, the more legible, clear, and well documented the chart, the less time you will spend on the stand.

3. Remember you are not being sued. You are simply being asked to present your examination findings in court. It may be that you did not find any signs of injury and the prosecution simply wants you to state for the jury that this finding of non-injury is consistent with the possibility of rape. And it is. So you will just be asked to say this.

4. If there are issues to be concerned about regarding your credentials, or other aspects of the case that the defense is expected to focus on, your assistant DA will spend time preparing you. Because of this and the need to be very familiar with the case and your charting, it is well worth the time you put in for preparation. It is in the prosecutor's best interest to have a well-prepared witness; this benefits you by ensuring that you are prepared for any attack made by the defense. Additionally, it is uncommon that a case will hinge on the medical testimony, so attacking your credentials is less likely to be a major focus. If you feel they are not preparing you enough, push for more time, not less.

Resources

Perhaps the best resource for a clinician in need of information for themselves, or for their patient, is the Internet. A simple Google search for "rape crisis center" with a location, will most often yield names, addresses and phone numbers for sites that your patient can utilize. Below are some of the many websites or materials that can be very helpful.

1. Protocol for the Acute Care of Adult Patients Reporting Sexual Assault. New York State Department of Health November 2004. Details the New York State protocol. Includes process descriptions and gives clear rationales behind all of the steps in the process of care, and contains extensive appendices, body diagrams, sample checklists, consent forms, kit instructions, and a great deal more. This is an excellent resource. Accessible on the Web via http://www.health.state.ny.us/professionals/protocols_and_guidelines/sexual_assault/docs/adult_protocol.pdf.

2. Rape Abuse Incest National Network (RAINN). Accessible on the Web at http://www.rainn.org. It provides extensive resource information, national hotline, and political advocacy for survivors.
3. http://ec.princeton.edu/pills/plan-b.html provides detailed patient and professional information about Preven emergency contraception.
4. Frequently updated guideline for HIV prophylaxis can be found at www.hivguidelines.org.
5. The CDC website contains information on a wide range of infectious disease topics, including specific guidelines for STD prevention in sexual assault survivors. http://www.cdc.gov/std/treatment/2006/sexual-assault.htm.
6. New York City Alliance Against Rape: www.nycalliance.org.

Quick Reference Pages

1. If you do not expect to ever collect forensic evidence for a sexually assaulted patient, know where and how you would get a patient of yours to the best possible facility.

2. If you may need to provide acute care to a sexual assault victim, be familiar with the process before treating a patient.

3. If you are frequently providing care to sexual assault victims, consider becoming a trained SAFE/SANE examiner or aligning your facility with a rape crisis center or other SAFE/SANE providers.

4. Make every effort to be sensitive and flexible with a patient who has been sexually assaulted.

5. Be aware of the increased difficulty with the process of care that a patient who is male, lesbian, gay, transgendered, elderly, or disabled may have.

6. Ensure the privacy and dignity of your patient throughout the process of care. Be certain to emphasize this need to your staff as well.

7. Seek opportunities to reinforce to your patient that he/she did not deserve to be assaulted, he/she made the best decisions he/she was able to make, and that it is the assailant, not him/her, who is responsible for what happened.

8. Look for indications early that your patient may have been drugged, and remember that alcohol is the most commonly used "date rape" drug.

9. Encourage your patient to allow an evidence kit to be collected even if he/she does not want to press charges. Evidence collected can be preserved; evidence lost is lost.

10. Be certain your patient has adequate referrals to ensure complete follow-up care for his/her medical and psychological needs.

The following are examples of a checklist and a printed order set that can serve as a guide when clinicians who are not SAFE trained are required to provide care for the sexually assaulted patient.

SEXUAL ASSAULT ACUTE CARE CHECKLIST

Following these steps will ensure the expedient and comprehensive care of sexual assault patients. Some patients may not require all of these interventions, and other patients may require interventions not listed. Examiners must use their clinical judgment in following this outline, including the timeline.

1	Patient identified at triage and brought into gyn room or private area		
2	Contact advocate		
3	Consent patient for care and treatment, including possible photographs and rape kit, or signed refusal of evidence collection. Rape kit if within 96 hours of assault		
4	Draw blood for CBC, Hep Panel, LFTs, possible HIV testing, and any other medically required labs. (At least two speckled tops and a lavender top) SEE DRUG-FACILITATED SEXUAL ASSAULT PROTOCOL IF APPLICABLE		
5	Brief introduction and explanation of procedures, then open kit and obtain ORAL SWABS AND SMEARS (Step #1)		
6	Offer mouthwash, toothbrush, juice, etc. so patient can clean her mouth		
7	History: medical and of the assault, to guide the medical exam		
8	Trace evidence: patient disrobes over exam paper or chuck (Step #2)		
9	Collect clothing, underwear, or diaper – allow to dry if wet (Step #3)		
10	Debris collection: debris from on patient's body (Step #4). Wood's Lamp examination of patient for secretions		
11	Head-to-toe survey for injury/soreness/secretions/bite marks; photographs if deemed useful		
12	Buccal specimen (Step #12 – do *early* as sample must dry)		
13	Swab bite marks and dried secretions (Step #5)		
14	Fingernail scrapings (Step# 6)		
15	Pubic hair combings (Step # 8). PULLED HAIRS ARE NOT REQUIRED (Steps #7 & 9)		
16	Anal swabs and smears (Step #10). DO THIS ROUTINELY		
17	Vaginal/penile swabs and smears (Step #11)		
18	Bimanual exam		
19	Wound care if required		
20	Document all findings in chart in writing and draw on diagrams; photos if appropriate		
21	Urine pregnancy test; SEPARATE URINE FOR DRUG SCREEN if drug-facilitated assault suspected. SEE DFSA PROTOCOL		
22	When all samples are dried and labeled, close and secure kit; DO NOT PUT ANY PAPERWORK INTO THE KIT		
23	Consent or refusal for release to law enforcement		
24	Give anti-emetic medication		
25	HIV prophylaxis (Combivir + Truvada)		
26	STD prophylaxis (GC/Chlam/Trich and HEP B vaccine and HBIG)		
27	Pregnancy prophylaxis		
28	Follow-up care instructions, including Rape Crisis Hotline #		
29	Social services, ID, and GYN referral		
30	Checklist completed, appropriate paperwork to patient, law enforcement, and medical chart		

MD_____   RN_____

Figure 3.8   Example of a checklist, created by the author for use by attendings and residents in a large urban emergency department.

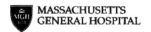

MASSACHUSETTS
GENERAL HOSPITAL

PATIENT IDENTIFICATION AREA

ADULT SEXUAL ASSAULT ORDER SHEET

ALLERGIES: DATE:

TIME	MEDICATION ORDERED	MD SIGNATURE	MEDICATION ADMINISTRATION RECORD	COMMENTS
	STD PROPHYLAXIS: **Gonorrhea:** • Ceftriaxone 250mg IM x 1		Time / Initial / Dose / Site	
	OR if allergic to PCN or cephalosporins and no pharyngeal contact • Spectinomycin 2gm IM x 1		Time / Initial / Dose / Site	
	OR if allergic to PCN or cephalosporins and with pharyngeal contact • Azithromycin 2gm po x 1		Time / Initial / Dose / Site	
	Chlamydia: • Azithromycin 1gm po x 1 (unless already given 2gm Azithromycin for gonorrhea)		Time / Initial / Dose / Site	
	OR if allergic to macrolide antibiotics • Doxycycline 100mg po BID x 7 days		Time / Initial / Dose / Site	
	Trichomoniasis: • Flagyl 2g po x 1		Time / Initial / Dose / Site	
	Hepatitis B: (see comments) • Recombivax 10mcg/1ml IM for age ≥ 20 • For age < 20: age specific dosing		Time / Initial / Dose / Site	Recombivax not needed for patients with known immunity - either had the vaccine or had the disease.
	PREGNANCY PROPHYLAXIS: (see comments) • PLAN B (levonorgestrel) 0.75mg 1 tab now and 1 tab 12 hours later if Hcg is negative.		Time / Initial / Dose / Site	Plan B may be given up to 120 hours after assault.
	OTHER: • Tetanus Toxoid 0.5ml IM x 1 PRN		Time / Initial / Dose / Site	
	• Antiemetic (when giving Azithromycin, Plan B or Flagyl) (specify): _____		Time / Initial / Dose / Site	
	HIV PROPHYLAXIS: (see comments) • HIV PEP med: _____		Time / Initial / Dose / Site	MD should page ID needle stick beeper (36222) for recommendation. Patient must call 617-726-3906 to schedule follow up visit with ID within 2-3 days of ED visit. MD will dispense adequate supply of PEP medication until ID visit.
	• HIV PEP med: _____		Time / Initial / Dose / Site	

TIME	REQUIRED LABS	MD SIGNATURE	RN	COMMENTS
	PREGNANCY TEST: • Urine HCG (HCG serum only when kiosk closed)			
	HEPATITIS SCREEN: • Hepatitis B surface antigen & antibody • Hepatitis C antibody			**NO HOSPITAL TOXICOLOGY SCREEN** (unless medically necessary)
	If starting HIV PEP: (see comments) • CBC with diff, Lytes, Cal, Phos, Mg, LFTS.			**NO HIV TESTING IN THE ED**

INIT.	NURSE'S SIGNATURE	INIT.	NURSE'S SIGNATURE	INIT.	NURSE'S SIGNATURE

White - Medical Record Copy   Yellow - Department Copy   84291 (1/04)

Figure 3.9   Medication Order Sheet used at Mass General. Reproduced from Finkel M. An original, standardized, emergency department sexual assault medication order sheet. *Journal of Emergency Nursing.* 2005; 31: 271.

Table 3.6 nPEP guidelines from www.hivguidelines.org

Non-occupational PEP recommendations by the CDC

NNRTI-based

Efavirenz + (lamivudine or emtricitabine) + (zidovudine or tenofovir); or Combivir + tenofovir for 28 days (*Do not administer efavirenz to pregnant women*)

PI-based

Lopinavir/ritonavir (Kaletra) + (lamivudine or emtricitabine) + zidovudine (or Combivir) for 28 days

For challenging cases, (i.e., pregnant patients, breastfeeding patients, patients sexually assaulted by known HIV patients), consider using the National Clinicians' Post-Exposure Prophylaxis Hotline (1-888-448-4911) to assist in determining the appropriate post-exposure prophylaxis acutely.

References

1. Giardino AP, Datner EM, Asher JB (editors): *Sexual Assault Victimization Across the Lifespan: A Clinical Guide.* Vol 1 & 2. G.W. Medical Publishing, Inc. 2003.
2. Protocol for the Acute Care of Adult Patients Reporting Sexual Assault. New York State Department of Health November 2004. Accessible via: http://www.health.state.ny.us/professionals/protocols_and_guidelines/sexual_assault/docs/adult_protocol.pdf.
3. Ullman S. Psychosocial correlates of PTSD symptom severity in sexual assault survivors. *Journal of Traumatic Stress.* 2007; 20: 821.
4. Amey A. Measuring the quality of medical care for women who experience sexual assault with data from the national hospital ambulatory medical care survey. *Annals of Emergency Medicine.* 2002; 39: 631.
5. Pesola G. Emergency department characteristics of male sexual assault. *Academic Emergency Medicine.* 1999; 6: 792.
6. U.S. Dept of Health and Human Services, Administration for Children & Families, Child Welfare Information Gateway (formerly Nat'l Clearinghouse on Child Abuse & Neglect), 2000. At http://www.childwelfare.gov.
7. Jones H, Powell JL. Old age, vulnerability and sexual violence: Implications for knowledge and practice. *Int Nurs Rev.* 2006; 53: 211–16.
8. Patel M. Management of sexual assault. *Emergency Medicine Clinics of North America.* 2001; 19: 817.
9. McGregor MJ, Du Mont J, Myhr TL. Sexual assault forensic medical examination: is evidence related to successful prosecution? *Ann Emerg Med.* June 2002; 39: 639–47.
10. Straight J. Emergency department care for victims of sexual offense. *American Journal of Health-System Pharmacy.* 2007; 64: 1845.
11. Welch J. Rape and sexual assault. *BMJ.* 2007; 334: 1154.

12. Rovi S. Prophylaxis provided to sexual assault victims seen at U.S. emergency departments. *Journal of the American Medical Women's Association*. 2002; 57: 204.

13. http://ec.princeton.edu/pills/plan-b.html provides detailed patient and professional information about Preven emergency contraception. Accessed 9/07.

14. http://www.hivguidelines.org provides up-to-date post-exposure prophylaxis guidelines. Accessed 9/07.

15. Finkel M. An original, standardized, emergency department sexual assault medication order sheet. *Journal of Emergency Nursing*. 2005; 31: 271.

16. Workowski K. Sexually transmitted diseases treatment guidelines, 2006. *Morbidity and Mortality Weekly Report. Recommendations and Reports*. 2006; 55: 1.

17. Slaugher L, Brown CRV. Colposcopy to establish physical findings in rape victims. *American Journal of Obstetrics and Gynecology*, 1992: 122(1): 83–6.

18. Slaughter L, Brown CRV, Crowley S, Peck R. Patterns of genital injury in female sexual assault victims. *American Journal of Obstetrics and Gynecology*, 1997: 176(3): 609–16.

19. Sachs CJ, Chu LD. Predictors of Genitorectal Injury in Female Victims of Suspected Sexual Assault. *Academic Emergency Medicine*. 2002; 9: 146–51.

20. http://www.dna.gov/uses/solving-crimes/cold_cases/howdatabasesaid/codis. Accessed 9/07.

4

The geriatric patient

Jonathan Glauser, M.D., M.B.A.

Goals and objectives

1. To recognize the patterns of geriatric abuse that exist
2. To learn how to screen and identify geriatric abuse
3. To learn to treat and refer victims of geriatric abuse

Introduction and overview

Elder abuse and neglect has been recognized as a growing problem in the United States. All 50 states have reporting requirements for elder abuse and neglect, although there is no federal policy requiring reporting of elder abuse. Literature suggests that the abusers appear most frequently to be family members and caretakers of the elderly.[1] The responsibility for identifying elder mistreatment often falls on emergency care providers.

There are 45 million people over the age of 60 in the United States, and 3 million over the age of 85. Those over 85 represent the fastest growing segment of the elderly population; it is estimated that the number of persons over the age of 85 will be seven times higher in 2050 than it was in 1980.[2]

Modern reports of elder abuse in the medical literature date from 1975 when the British Medical Journal published a report of "granny battering."[3] In the United States, reports of abuse and neglect in nursing homes in the 1970s led to a systematic study of elder mistreatment by the United States Senate Special Committee on Aging.[4] Since that time, under the auspices of the Department of Health and Human Services, there has been the creation of the National Institute on Elder Abuse. The first federal government measures to address elder abuse came in Title XX of the Social Security Act of 1974, which gave individual states authorization to use Social Service Block Grant funds to protect elderly persons as well as children.[5]

It has been estimated that between one and two million elderly Americans experience some form of mistreatment annually.[6] Other sources cite as many as 2 to

2.5 million cases of elder abuse each year, and that between 1 percent and 10 percent of elders are victims of abuse at some time.[7,8] Reports of abuse have certainly increased with time, with 117,000 reports of elder abuse in 1986 and 293,000 in 1996.[8] Older men and women have similar per capita abuse rates, estimated at a prevalence rate of 32 for every 1,000 adults.[9–11] Factors leading to misdiagnosis and under-reporting include denial by both victim and perpetrator, clinicians' reluctance to report victims, disbelief by medical providers, and clinicians' lack of awareness of warning signs.[12] For these reasons, it has been estimated that only 1 in 14 cases of elder abuse or neglect comes to the attention of authorities.

Elder abuse in family settings has increased in recent years for a number of reasons: the increasing proportion of older adults in the total population, the increase in chronic disabling diseases, progressive dependency, and the increasing involvement of families in caregiving relationships with elders. These trends are likely to continue into the foreseeable future.[13]

It has been shown that elder neglect may be detected in the emergency department by screening protocols.[14] Not only have many emergency departments lacked protocols for elder abuse, but one report stated that many physicians were not even aware of it as an entity.[15] In another study, only 2 percent of all cases reported in the state of Michigan were made by physicians.[16] Hospital protocols have been recommended by the American Medical Association and the American College of Emergency Physicians to aid in the detection and management of elder abuse.[17,18]

It has been found that the risk of death for elder abuse and neglect victims are three times higher than for elderly non-victims.[19] The human cost of abuse and neglect is stark. One report from 1976 noted that 25 percent of elderly patients died within three years of admission, tending to become bewildered, restless, and unable to report their needs soon after admission.[20] As of 2004, the direct medical costs of violent injuries to the elderly were estimated at $5.3 billion.[21]

Definitions

Elder abuse and neglect refers to an act or omission resulting in harm, including death, or threatened harm to the health or welfare of an elderly person. It is often referred to globally as elder mistreatment (EM). The types of abuse of older persons include physical, psychological, sexual, and financial (when the elder's resources have been misappropriated by the caregiver). The 1985 Elder Abuse Prevention, Identification and Treatment Act defines abuse as the "willful infliction of injury, unreasonable confinement, intimidation or cruel punishment with resulting physical harm or pain or mental anguish, or the willful deprivation by a caretaker of

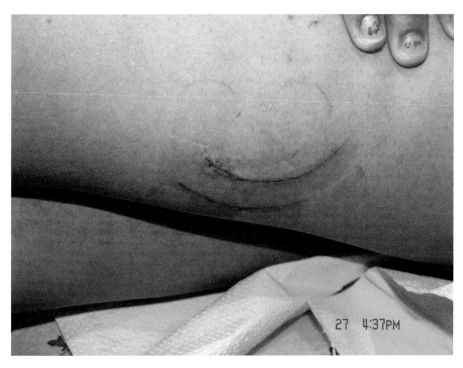

Abrasions: Thirteen-year-three-month-old female child who sustained multiple abrasions and lacerations from thorns during a sexual assault.

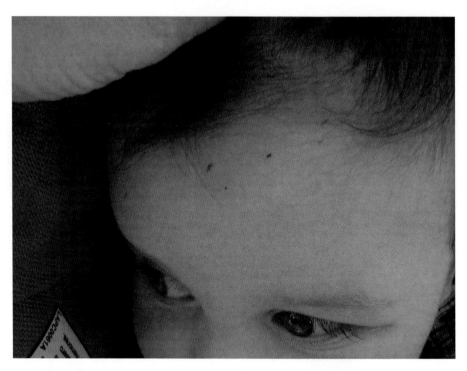

Scratches on the forehead in a six-month-old boy.

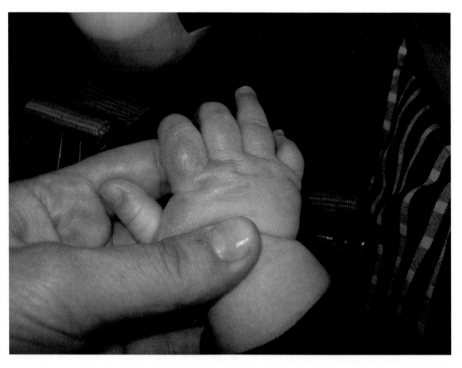

Abuse Mimic: Sucking blister on the index finger of a six-month-old boy.

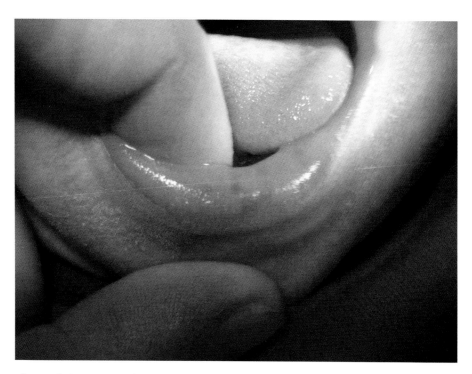

Abuse Mimic: Bruise to the lower lip from vigorous sucking of a pacifier in a six-month-old boy.

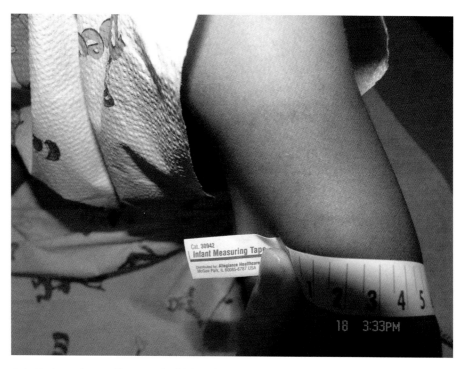

Belt Mark 1: Six-year-five-month old female who disclosed that her father hit her with a belt.

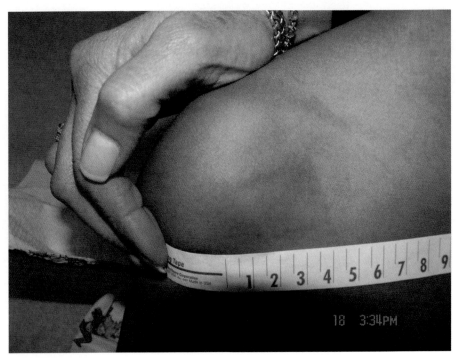

Belt Mark 1: Six-year-five-month-old female who disclosed that her father hit her with a belt.

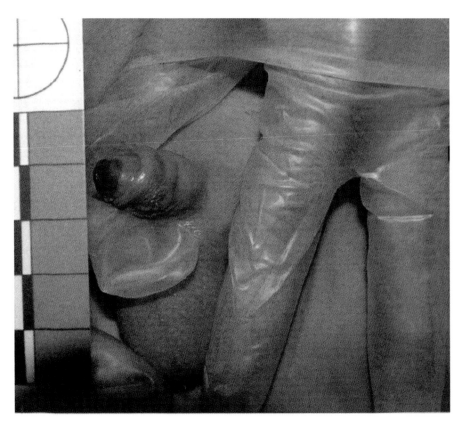

Bruise 2: Ecchymoses and dried blood over the penile tip of a seven-month-old male.

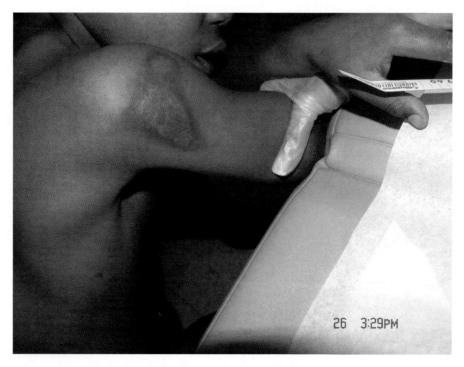

Burn 1: Burn from an unspecified object on the upper right arm of a chronically abused child in foster care.

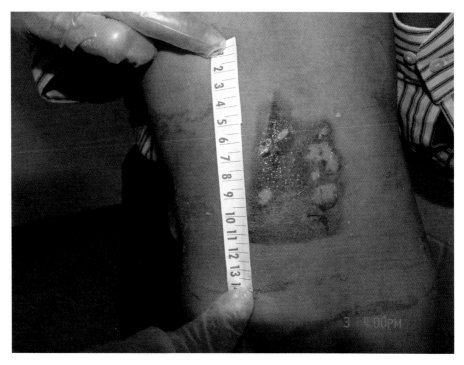

Burn 2: Four-year-old male child who presented to the emergency department with a second-degree burn on his back that was consistent with the pattern of an iron.

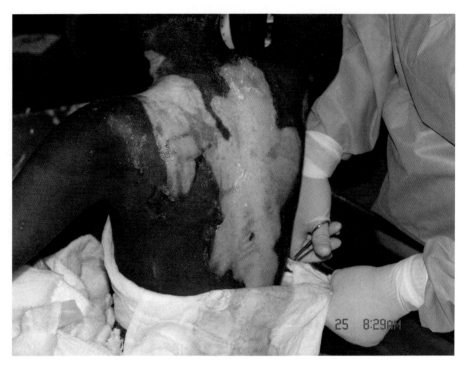

Burn 3: Seven-year-old male child admitted to the burn unit for first- and second-degree burns to 10 percent of his body surface area (back, neck, and torso) which were sustained by a splash burn from boiling water.

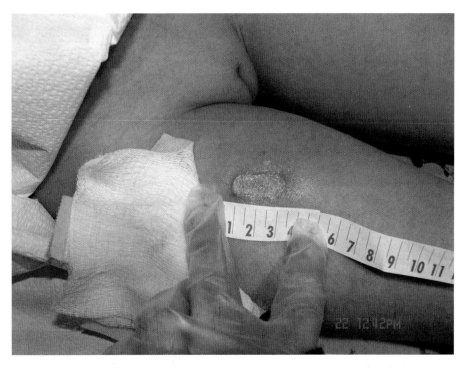

Burn 4: Four-year-old female child with accidental steam burn from steam valve on radiator.

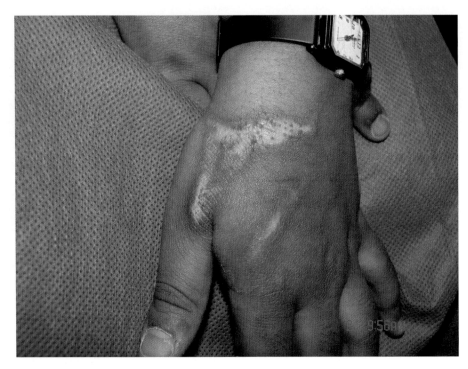

Burn 5: Seven-year-eight-month-old female child who sustained a first-degree burn to the dorsal surface of her left hand while in the care of a babysitter when picking up hot soup from the microwave.

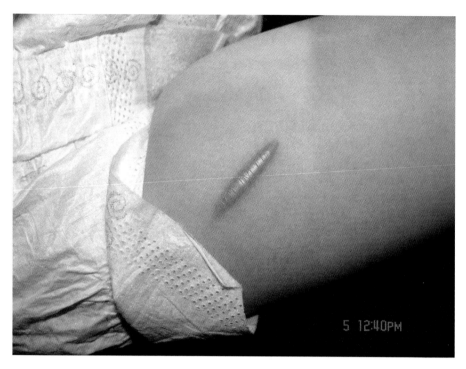

Keloid Scar: One-year-nine-month-old female child with 3cm pink-colored raised keloid scar on the upper outer aspect of the right thigh.

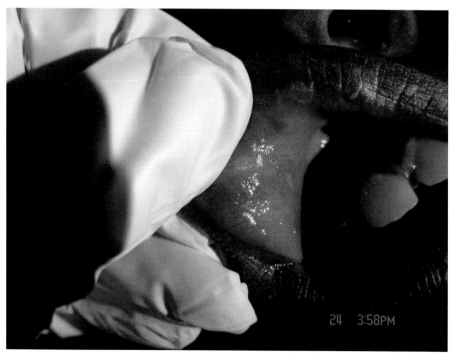

Lip Injury: Seven-year-nine-month-old male child whose biological mother punched him in the mouth with a closed fist.

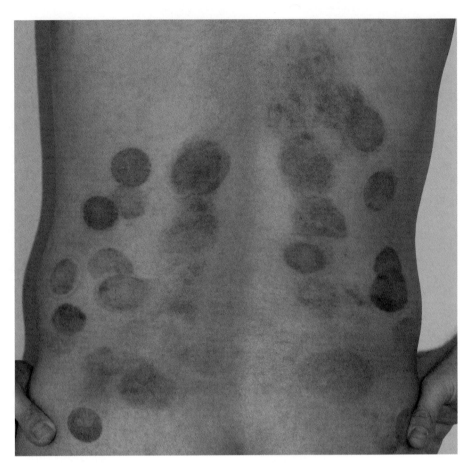

Abuse Mimic: Cupping

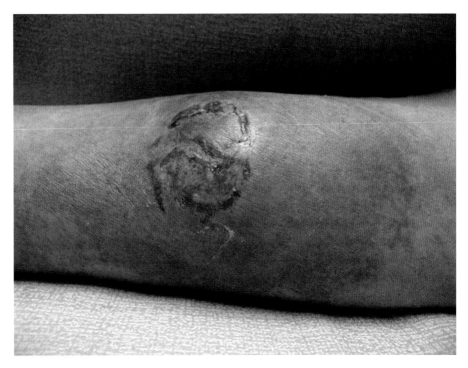

Neutral background.

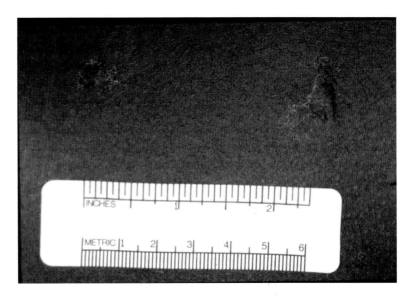

Using a tape measure.

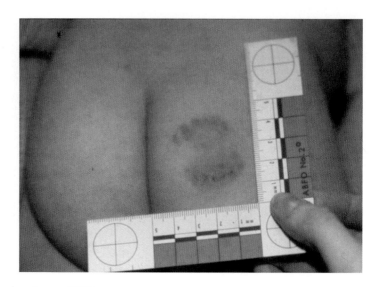

Bite mark, using an ABFO.

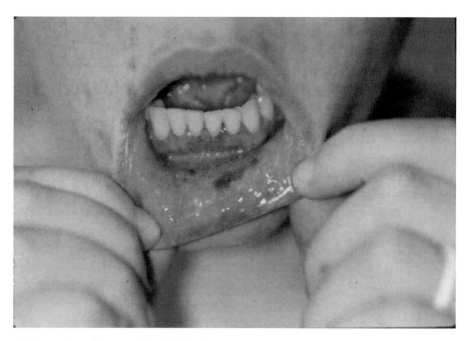

This image is well centered and in focus.

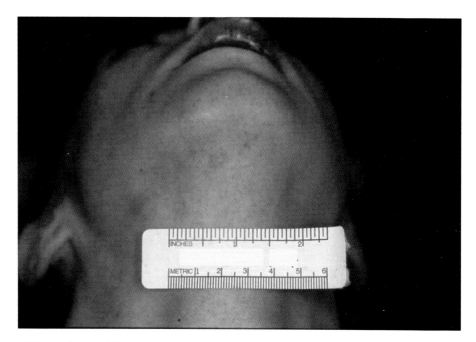

Hidden submental injury.

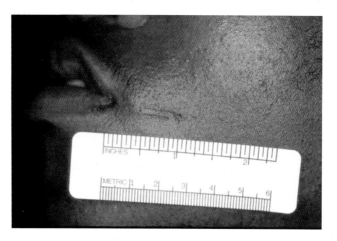

Forensically significant versus medically significant.

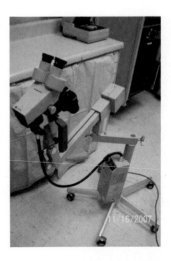

Colposcope with 35mm camera.

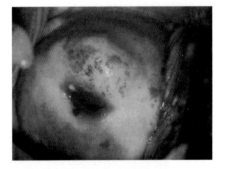

Cervix with petechiae and contusions. Colposcopic photograph courtesy of Bronx SART.

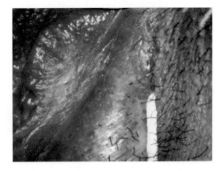

Labia minora abrasion and superficial laceration. Colposcopic photograph courtesy of Bronx SART.

goods or services which are necessary to avoid physical harm, mental anguish, or mental illness."[22]

The American Medical Association in 1987 proposed this definition: "Abuse shall mean an act or omission which results in harm or threatened harm to the health or welfare of an elderly person. Abuse includes the intentional infliction of physical or mental injury; sexual abuse; or withholding of necessary food, clothing, and medical care to meet the physical and mental needs of an elderly person by one having the care, custody, or responsibility of an elderly person."[23]

There are other types of EM: violation of rights, denial of privacy, and denial of participation in decision making.[24] EM may entail more subtle practices, falling under the concept of "undue influence." Undue influence is the substitution of one person's will for the true desires of another. Such influence often entails fraud, duress, threats, or other pressures. Undue influence occurs when one person uses his or her role and power to exploit the trust, dependency, or fear of another to gain psychological control over the weaker person's decision-making, often for financial gain. While dependent and impaired people are especially susceptible, this can happen to people who would be considered otherwise competent.[25]

Elder abuse has been classified into six broad categories:

1. Physical abuse
2. Sexual abuse
3. Financial exploitation
4. Neglect
5. Psychological abuse
6. Violation of rights[24]

These are considered in turn below.

Self-neglect

Separate from the above categories is self-neglect, which encompass behaviors of an elderly person that threaten his/her own safety. These behaviors include failure or unwillingness to provide adequate food, clothing, shelter, medical care, hygiene, or social stimulation for self. By definition, self-neglect excludes situations in which a mentally competent older person who understands the consequences of his/her decisions makes a conscious decision to engage in acts which threaten his/her own health or safety.[27,28] It is the result of an adult's inability due to diminished capacity to perform essential self-care tasks, including the provision of essential food, clothing, shelter, and medical care, as well as the management of financial affairs. A 1997 study indicated that cognitive impairment, poverty, and being of a nonwhite race were independent predictors for self-neglect.[29] A later study indicated that self-neglect contributed to increased mortality. In that report of elderly patients, 40 percent of those in the self-neglect cohort versus 17 percent in the non-investigated cohort died over a 13-year period.[30]

Risk factors

Dependency, either on the part of the victim or of the perpetrator, as well as caregiver stress, are common denominators in abusive situations. Functional impairment leads to dependency and vulnerability of elderly persons, especially those who cannot perform activities of daily living (ADLs). Institutionalization is recognized as a risk factor for neglect and abuse.[11] However, elder abuse occurs most commonly in residential rather than institutional settings.[31] Older persons are most commonly abused by the people with whom they live. Frail, very old (over 75 years) adults who have a diagnosis of depression or dementia, are more likely to be mistreated. Physical or cognitive impairment, alcohol abuse, female sex, and a history of domestic violence are risk factors for elder mistreatment.[32–35] Older adults who require assistance with activities of daily living or have poor social networks have been found to be at higher risk as well.[36] Victims of caregiver neglect are more likely to be widowed, very old, cognitively impaired, and socially isolated. Developmental disabilities, special medical or psychiatric needs, and lack of experience managing finances all place a person at risk, as do patient aggression, verbal outbursts, or embarrassing actions.[10]

The risk to the victim may very well be more related to characteristics of the perpetrator than of the victim. Perpetrators of abuse may be financially dependent on the victim. There may be a family history of violence or substance abuse. Abusers are most often the primary caregiver. Adult children tend to be more inclined to abuse than are spouses, although one survey indicated that 58 percent of domestic elder abuse was by spouses.[11,37] Males abuse more than females.[27] Risk is greater if the caregiver has a financial or emotional dependence on the victim.[37] This dependence may be exacerbated by alcohol or drug abuse, legal or financial difficulties, or psychiatric disease on the part of the caregiver.[10,16] Caregivers may be well-intentioned, but simply overwhelmed by the amount of care required. They may themselves be impaired by mental or physical problems which serve as barriers to the provision of adequate care. A domineering violent or bullying category of provider has been described, prone to financial abuse and neglect, as well as, possibly, sexual abuse.[38] Three characteristics of perpetrators have been identified as risk factors: a history of mental illness and/or substance abuse, excessive dependence on the elder for financial support, and a history of violence within or outside of the family.[39]

Identification of elder abuse

Physical abuse is most easily recognized, although neglect is more common. Psychological and financial abuse may be more easily missed. Difficulty arises when an elderly patient's caregiver seems indifferent or angry toward that person, and is unwilling to cooperate with health care providers. When the abuse is perpetrated within the family network, much effort may be made to conceal it by family members and by the elders themselves.[40]

The history should entail direct and simple questions. Examples of these may include general queries about who handles the patient's finances, who cooks for them, under what circumstances they seek medical care, and whether they feel safe where they live.[41] Specific questions may be posed as to whether the patient has been slapped, struck, kicked, or tied down. The patient, the suspected abuser, and other family members should be interviewed separately without other family staff in the room. The rationale for this is clear: confidentiality is necessary if the interviewer is to ascertain whether the patient has been touched without consent, has had things taken without asking, or is afraid of anyone at home.

Red flags for abuse may include reluctance of the caregiver to leave the patient alone with the health care provider. The caregiver may have sketchy knowledge of the patient's medical conditions. The patient may have missed appointments or exhibited delays in seeking needed care.[42,43]

Clinical presentations may include dehydration, apathy, or depression. The commonest complaints for patients older than age 75 are falls, dehydration, and failure of self-care.[44] Each major category of abuse is considered in turn.

Specific categories of elder abuse

Physical abuse

This is the most recognizable form of abuse: the use of physical force which might result in bodily injury, physical pain, or impairment. It may comprise a wide range of behaviors, including slapping, burning, pushing, striking with objects, any of which are carried out with the intention of causing suffering, pain, or other physical impairment.[45] Neglect was a more common manifestation of mistreatment than frank injury in one review of 36 emergency cases. Dehydration, malnutrition, bed sores, inappropriate clothing, and improper administration of medicines may be indicators of neglect.[35,46] Decubitus ulcers which are untreated or in non-lumbar/sacral areas are suggestive. Elderly patients bruise more easily, and osteoporosis leads to a higher incidence of fractures, so clinical judgment must be used to determine injuries which may not signal abuse.[41] Contusions on the inner arms, inner thighs, palms, soles, scalp, mastoid, or buttocks are worrisome signs of inflicted trauma.[39]

The general appearance should be noted, for hygiene or dirty clothing. The skin mucosa should be examined for dehydration, bruises, decubitus ulcers, lacerations healing by secondary intention, or multiple lesions in various stages of healing. The oral cavity may indicate ecchymosis from forced oral sex, lesions from venereal disease, tooth fractures, or cigarette burns. There may be clustering of bruises or characteristic shape, as from injuries inflicted with a belt or iron. Examination of the head may reveal traumatic alopecia, vitreous hemorrhage, orbital fractures, or retinal detachment. Evidence for occult fracture, immersion burns, or cigarette/cigar burns may be present.[41] Rope or restraint marks on the wrists or ankles may be present.[27]

Sexual abuse

This is broadly defined as nonconsensual sexual contact of any kind with an elderly person. The spectrum of sexual abuse ranges from unwanted touching, indecent exposure, unwanted innuendo to fondling with a non-consenting competent or incompetent person, or rape itself. The patient may complain of genital or anal pain, itching, bruising, bleeding, or may have venereal disease. Torn or stained underwear, with unexplained difficulty walking or sitting, may be present. There may be oral trauma, including fractured teeth.

Financial exploitation

This occurs when family members, caregivers, or friends take control of the elder's resources. Coercion or outright theft may be entailed, with or without the awareness of the victim. Dependent elderly may unwittingly sign over access to savings accounts and other assets when they are in an incapacitated state. An elder's Social Security check may be used by a younger caregiver for his/her own needs. Perpetrators often rely upon the elderly victim for shelter or assets. Theft may be blatant or coerced, with forcible transfer of property, including changing one's will. There may be a discrepancy between the patient's income and living style, or a sudden inability to pay bills, purchase food, or other commodities.[8]

Caregiver neglect

The term "abuse" refers to acts of commission, while "neglect" refers to acts of omission. Neglect may entail failure to meet nutritional and hygienic needs, or to lead as far as manslaughter or suicide.[47] The most common form of elder maltreatment is neglect, broadly defined as the failure of a caregiver to provide basic care to a patient and to provide goods and services necessary to prevent physical harm or emotional discomfort.[48] The refusal or failure to fulfill his/her obligations or duties to an elderly person may include deprivation of food, clothing, hygiene, medical care, shelter, or supervision which a prudent person would consider essential for the well-being of another.[49] Abandonment constitutes the desertion of an elderly person by an individual who is that person's custodian or who has assumed responsibility for providing care to the elder. Desertion of an elder at a hospital, nursing facility, shopping mall, or other public location may occur.

Poor nutrition, poor hygiene, poor skin integrity, contractures, dehydration, fecal impaction, or excoriations may all constitute physical evidence of neglect.[50]

Psychological abuse

This is defined as the infliction of mental anguish, pain, or distress. This may encompass a variety of actions intended to inflict emotional pain or injury, ranging from verbal threats to threats of institutionalization or humiliating statements. Insults, habitual verbal aggression, name calling, and intimidation are all included.[51]

Violation of rights

Examples of this may include denial of privacy or participation in decision-making. Abandonment, as described above, may also be included in this category.

Legal considerations

State laws against elder abuse date from 1973.[35,49] Currently, fifty states and the District of Columbia have passed legislation to establish adult protective service (APS) programs. State APS statutes authorize agencies to investigate cases of elder mistreatment.[52] These laws in general were based upon laws addressing child abuse. Since child abuse laws primarily concerned physical abuse, and children had no money to exploit, older laws tended to be weak on financial exploitation. The remedies offered tend to emphasize removal of the abused person from the setting in which the abuse is occurring.[45,53]

The federal government drafted the first laws regarding elder abuse in 1981 in the US House Select Committee on Aging. Federal definitions of elder abuse were standardized in 1985 with the Elder Abuse Prevention, Identification, and Treatment Act (HR 1674), and addressed further in the 1987 Amendments to the Older Americans Act.[35,45]

Other resources which address the issue of elder abuse include:

1. Criminal Justice Services
2. National Association of State Units on Aging
3. National Center on Elder Abuse
4. National Organization for Victim Assistance
5. National Coalition Against Violence
   (See Resources Section for more details.)

Laws for reporting elder abuse vary from state to state, and physicians should clarify existing law in their own state. Generally, physicians and other reporters are granted immunity when the reporting was done in good faith.[31] Documentation should be clear and legible, as it may become evidence in a court of law.

Obstacles to detection of elder abuse

Victims often have low self-esteem, may blame themselves for the abuse, and do not want to betray their families. They may not want to admit their vulnerabilities, or feel disgraced for having raised a child who would betray him/her in any way.[10,54] They may especially be ashamed to acknowledge his/her own dependency on the abuser – or be loyal to that abuser, and unwilling to press charges against a family member. Abused older adults may be uninformed or misinformed regarding services available.[54] they may harbor a fear of being removed from the home and placed in a nursing institution. This fear may, in fact, be warranted. In a Connecticut study, 60 percent of abused and neglected victims admitted for short-term care remained institutionalized permanently.[55] They may worry about further abuse from a caregiver in retaliation for having divulged information. They may worry about not being believed because the alleged abuser may act differently in public. Many elderly people are isolated and seldom leave the house, resulting in less opportunity for detection of abuse by others. The abuser may control access to others and may stay present during encounters with outsiders to ensure that secrecy is maintained.[56]

There may be differing definitions of abuse by victims from differing cultural backgrounds based on the perception of the intent of the abuser. One example cited was that of a woman who sedated her elderly mother when company came to prevent embarrassment at her mother's senile dementia. That report listed Korean Americans in particular as unwilling to reveal "family shame" to others or to create conflict among their relatives.[57]

Health care visits may be an elderly person's only contact with the outside world. Physicians infrequently report elder abuse, for a variety of reasons. They may not be familiar with reporting laws. They may fear offending patients or their abusers, or are concerned with time limitations in the emergency department. Time limitations may be a pervasive and driving fear in other medical specialties as well. There may be a feeling that requiring physicians to report cases may be patronizing to the victim, who may be perceived as unable to make decisions for himself/herself, especially if he/she is competent.[16] Emergency physicians (EPs) may believe that they do not possess appropriate evaluation skills, or may be uncomfortable asking the caregiver to leave the room during an interview. Some doctors may have the misperception that the law requires them to obtain the patient's permission before reporting.[58]

One recent study attempted to identify specific reasons expressed by primary care physicians for their low compliance with mandatory reporting of elder abuse, which noted: perceptions of decreased physician–patient rapport, worry that mandatory reporting may put abused elders at increased risk, or diminish patient autonomy, and worries regarding patient–clinician confidentiality. Physicians were specifically worried that patients would only report certain things in the strictest confidence, and that the valued relationship between the physician and patient would be compromised by reporting. There were specific concerns that reporting would not remain anonymous, and therefore would hurt a relationship with the patient and his/her family. Physicians tended to worry that the patient's quality of life might decrease in other ways after reporting, as with placement into an unwanted and unsatisfactory care environment. Liability issues were listed as well.[59] Physicians may believe that evidence of elder abuse does not equate to immediate danger for the patient, and therefore, that absolute proof should be required before reporting suspected abuse.[60]

On the other hand, 38 states plus the District of Columbia had laws specifying penalties for failing to report as of 2000. Penalties included reporting to the state's medical licensing authority.[61] A hospital may have no protocols for identifying or addressing elder abuse; one report from 1997 noted that only 31 percent of responding EPs knew of a written protocol for the reporting of elder abuse and neglect.[49] Few medical school curricula as of 1995 had formal training in the detection of elder abuse and neglect and interviewing techniques for potential victims and abusers.[62] Physicians may be reluctant to ask questions about potential abuse because of fear of litigation and possible court appearances.[54,63] For whatever reasons, it is reported that physicians notify the appropriate authorities in only 1 of every 13 cases they identify.[64] One large survey suggested that home care workers were the largest group of reporters (27%), followed by physicians and other health care professionals (18%), and family members (15%).[65] Another review of five years of elder abuse reports in Michigan found that physicians made only 2 percent of the reports. Community members accounted for 41 percent of them, with non-physician health care workers filing 26 percent, and social and mental health workers another 25 percent.[66] All APS laws provide immunity from liability for those who report in good faith. Mandatory reporting laws generally require the reporting of suspected abuse; it is the state agency's job to substantiate the abuse.[58]

Further confounding factors may relate to any underlying medical disorder which the patient may have. Advanced neurologic disease such as multiple sclerosis, amyotrophic lateral sclerosis, or Parkinson's disease may lead to immobilization and severe disability. These individuals are at risk for pressure ulcers, pneumonia, or venous thromboembolism, even with adequate care.[27]

Abuse in long-term facilities

Approximately 5 percent of elderly patients live in long-term institutions. In 1987, Congress enacted legislation that required nursing homes participating in the Medicare and Medicaid programs to comply with certain quality of care requirements. This legislation was included in the Omnibus Budget Reconciliation Act (OBRA), also known as the Nursing Home Reform Act.[53] Every state has a nursing home ombudsman program that responds to reports of neglect or abuse in the nursing home elderly. Physicians may report suspicions of abuse to the state ombudsman or to Adult Protective Services.[41,45]

Abuse in institutional settings may manifest in similar ways to those in residential settings: theft of money or personal property, unsanitary conditions, poor personal hygiene, sexual assault, physical abuse or unexplained injury, bed sores, physical or chemical restraint, or malnutrition and dehydration.[41,47,53]

Elder abuse in nursing homes is well documented. A 1989 study from a random sample of 577 nurses and nursing aides from long-term facilities indicated that 36 percent of respondents had witnessed at least one act of physical abuse in the previous year.[67] A study of 2,400 deaths in Arkansas nursing homes found 50 cases of suspected abuse or neglect, indicating perhaps a larger role for forensic studies in unexplained deaths of older adults in long-term care facilities.[68] Abuse may be related to burnout or personal stress among staff, or to attitudes that residents are childlike and in need of discipline. Primary abusers of nursing home residents were nurse aides and orderlies with no stress training. The Coalition of Advocates for the Rights of the Infirm Elderly (CARIE) has developed an eight-hour program for caregivers working in long-term facilities. The program focuses on recognizing abuse and possible triggers for abuse.[69]

Management and intervention

Patients in immediate danger should be hospitalized, transferred to the care of a friend or reliable family member, or placed in emergency shelters. Suspected abuse should be reported to the appropriate state agency, which can provide a more thorough long-term assessment. Local resources may vary, but may include social work, possible home nursing assistance, safe homes for older battered persons, and calls to the local Adult Protective Services (APS) agency.[47] Admission for a specific medical problem, such as decubitus ulcers or dehydration, may be more acceptable to the patient and the family/caregiver. This may be especially so if the home situation is not easily remedied, as in the case of psychopathology of the abuser with substance abuse or mental illness.

If the patient is not competent to decide for himself/herself, contact with Adult Protective Services should be initiated.[70] Adult Protective Services (APS) is the official state entity charged with promoting advocacy and protecting victims of elder abuse and neglect. All 50 states and the District of Columbia have laws that authorize the provision of APS in elder abuse cases.[71] APS agencies broadly provide access to services that address the social, housing, medical, and legal needs of elderly persons.[72] APS agencies were established by state statutes and may provide immediate evaluation, counseling, and relocation in cases of suspected elder mistreatment. In smaller jurisdictions they are under local law enforcement. They can establish a court-ordered guardianship or conservatorship to arrange shelter, finances, and care. Once a report has been filed to APS, a social worker is assigned to the case and makes a home visit. After conducting an interview and screening the case, the social worker may suggest solutions. Generally the patient and the caregiver should be interviewed separately. The patient's decision-making capacity must be assessed. If an adult is suffering from mental illness or cognitive impairment and represents an immediate risk for hurting himself/herself, emergency removal orders may need to be pursued authorizing temporary involuntary hospital admission. Legal guardianship, also called conservatorship, is the permanent removal of a person's right to make his/her own decisions. This requires judicial oversight and due process for wards and conservatees.[73]

If the patient is competent, his/her wishes must be honored, even if those wishes do not appear to be in the patient's best self-interest. Ultimately, team members recruited to manage elder abuse and neglect cases may include physicians, nurses, social workers, APS caseworkers, law enforcement personnel, prosecutors, clergy, and representatives from financial institutions.[72] In non-emergency cases, APS workers usually have between 30 and 60 days to complete an investigation and determine the validity of an allegation.

In 16 states, every citizen is a mandatory reporter for elder abuse, with reporting laws generally applying to professionals who interact with vulnerable populations. Failure to report is a punishable offense in 42 states, and good faith reporters are immune from civil and criminal lawsuits.[74] Protective services must keep the identity of the reporter confidential.

Two studies found that, by being referred to APS, elderly persons were more likely to be institutionalized.[75,76] With increasing demand for APS, there may be pressure to solve difficult problems through nursing home placement,[77] although the irony of using a system intended to protect the health and independence of the vulnerable elderly population by institutionalizing them has not been lost on at least one author.[54]

On occasion, medical case management teams are convened to provide consultation and support to hospital staff, to assist in the multidisciplinary evaluation of suspected abuse, and to develop treatment plans. Team members generally are composed of a physician, nurses, and social workers.[78] They may make house calls. Services provided may include physical and occupational therapy, nutritional

Table 4.1 Resources for elder abuse

Whom to contact	Services they provide
Clinical Justice Services American Association of Retired Persons 601 E. St., NW Washington, DC 20049 202-434-2222	Self-instruction training program, pamphlets, and brochures on elder abuse prevention
National Association of State Units on Aging* National Center on Elder Abuse 1201 15th St. NW, Suite 350 Washington, DC 20005-2842 202-898-2586 www.elderabusecenter.org	Individual services, help for state and local programs, provider training. Provides information and resources, including phone numbers for reporting elder mistreatment and laws in individual states
Administration on Aging U.S. Health and Human Services 200 Independence Avenue SW Washington, DC 20201 www.aoa.gov	Administration of grants Listing of community resource centers and foundations Information on legislation, Older Americans Act
National Organization for Victim Assistance 510 King St., Suite 424 Alexandria, VA 22314 1-800-TRY-NOVA or 703-535-6682 www.try.nova.org	Referrals, resources in every state
National Coalition Against Domestic Violence* P.O. Box 18749 Denver, CO 80218 303-83-1852/104 ncadv.org	Training and education on domestic violence, publications, and programs
Local resources *Adult Protective Services *Police *State elder abuse hotlines Toll free (Available 24 hours) (Consult local directory)	Protection
National Domestic Violence Hotline: Toll- free 800-799-SAFE; TTY 800-787-3224 (Hearing-impaired line)	Intervention Cannot take reports Confidential – Available 24 hours
Long-term Care Ombudsman Resource Center www.ltcombudsman.org	Provides background information on support, technical assistance
National Council on the Aging 409 Third Street SW, Suite 200 Washington, DC 20024 800-424-9046 www.noa.org	Addresses many aging issues through various programs
American Bar Association 750 N Lake Shore Drive Chicago, Illinois 60611 312-988-5000 Commission on Law and Aging www.abanet.org/aging	Provides information on laws pertinent to elders; has contact information by state and other law-related services for legal assistance providers. Provides mandatory reporting requirements for each state

* These organizations also have research or advocacy functions.

improvement, or treatment of disease states. Legal intervention teams have been utilized as well. Their purpose may be to address financial management, probate and guardianships, or other legal and housing issues. Civil courts can issue protective orders, create guardianships, order assets to be frozen, adjudicate lawsuits, and issue emergency removal orders.[72] In extreme cases, Fatality Review Teams have been convened to review deaths of older persons. These teams require participation by the medical examiner.[79] A variety of agencies exist which offer information, research services, and advice regarding abuse and neglect of the elderly (see Table 4.1).[43,72,80,81]

In some cases of unintentional neglect, education of the caregiver may be the only intervention necessary. Options for support to decrease the stress and anxiety that preceded the abuse may include home health aides, respite services, day programs, or accessible transportation to unburden the caregiver.[10] Ultimately, the goal of treatment is not to punish the victim or the abuser, but to stop the abuse. When mistreatment results from the caregiver being overburdened, intervention may be welcomed by all parties. Options for the caregiver in less acute situations include periodic respite care, support groups, home health services, adult day care, and church activities or pastoral visitations.[31]

Conclusions

Elder abuse patients have substantial interactions with emergency departments. Geriatric abuse as a health care issue is a relatively recent phenomenon and still evolving. Millions of elderly persons experience progressive dependency, social isolation, poorly rated self-health and psychological decline. Physicians are well situated for detecting and reporting suspected cases, although many barriers exist on the individual level. These visits frequently require hospital admission.

References

1. Hardin E, Khan-Hudson A. Elder abuse – "society's dilemma." *J Nat Med Assoc*. 2004; 97(1): 91–4.
2. The Program Resources Department, the American Association of Retired Persons, and the Administration on Aging. *A Profile of Older Americans 1993*. Washington, DC: U.S. Department of Health and Human Services.
3. Burston GR. Granny battering. *BMJ*. 1975; 3: 592–3.
4. U.S. House Select Committee on Aging and U.S. House Science and Technology Subcommittee on Domestic, International, Scientific Planning Analysis and Cooperation Domestic Violence 1978, Washington DC: U.S. Government Printing Office.
5. Protecting America's Seniors: A History of Elder Abuse and Neglect from the United States Senate, Special Committee on Aging 2002.

6. Shields LB, Hunsaker DM, Hunsaker JC. Abuse and neglect: a ten-year review of mortality and morbidity in our elders in a large metropolitan area. *J Forensic Sci*. 2004; 49(1): 122–7.

7. Lachs M, Berkman L, Fulmer T, Horwitz R. A prospective community-based pilot study of risk factors for the investigation of elder mistreatment. *J Am Geriatr Soc*. 1994; 42: 169–73.

8. Cohen M, Halevi-Levin S, Gagin R, Friedman G. Development of a screening tool for identifying elderly people at risk of abuse by their caregivers. *J Aging Health*. 2006; 18: 660–85.

9. Tartara T, Kuzmeskus L. Elder abuse in domestic settings. Elder Abuse Information Series, No. 1, Washington, DC, National Committee on Elder Abuse (NCEA), 1996–1997.

10. Kleinschmidt KC. Elder abuse: A review. *Ann Emerg Med*. 1997; 30(4): 463–72.

11. Pillemer K, Finkelhor D. The prevalence of elder abuse: a random sample survey. *Gerontologist*. 1988; 28: 51–7.

12. Levine JM. Elder neglect and abuse. A primer for primary care physicians. *Geriatrics*. 2003; 58(10): 37–44.

13. Schiamberg LB, Gans D. Elder abuse by adult children: an applied ecological framework for understanding contextual risk factors and the integrational character of quality of life. *Int Jour Aging and Hum Develop*. 2000; 50(4): 329–59.

14. Fulmer T, Pavesa G, Abraham I, et al. Elder neglect assessment in the emergency department. *J Emerg Nurs*. 2000; 26(5): 436–43.

15. Cammer Paris BE. Violence against elderly people. *Mt Sinai J Med*. 1996; 63: 97–100.

16. Homer AC, Gilleard C. Abuse of elderly people by their caregivers. *Br Med J*. 1992; 301: 1359–62.

17. American Medical Association: AMA Diagnostic and Treatment Guidelines on Elder Abuse and Neglect, Chicago, American Medical Association 1992.

18. Policy Statement: American College of Emergency Physicians: Management of elder abuse and neglect. *Ann Emerg Med*. 1998; 31: 149–50.

19. American Medical Association White Paper on Elderly Health Report of the Council on Scientific Affairs. *Arch Intern Med*. 1990; 150: 2459–72.

20. Baker A. Slow euthanasia – or "she will be better off in a hospital." *BMJ*. 1976; 2: 571–2.

21. Mouton CP, Rodabough RJ, Rovi SLD. Prevalence and 3 year incidence of abuse among postmenopausal women. *Am J Public Health*. 2004; 94: 605–12.

22. U.S. House of Representatives HR 1674. The Elder Abuse Prevention, Identification, and Treatment Act. 1985.

23. Council on Scientific Affairs. Elder abuse and neglect. *JAMA*. 1987; 257: 966–71.

24. Wieland D. Abuse of older persons: an overview. *Holistic Nurs Pract*. 2000; 14(4): 40–50.

25. Quinn MJ. Undue influence and elder abuse: recognition and intervention strategies. *Geriatric Nurs*. 2002; 23(1): 11–16.

26. Greenberg EM. Violence and the older adult: the role of the acute care nurse practitioner. *Crit Care Nurs Quarterly*. 1996; 19(2): 76–84.

27. Gorbien MJ, Eisenstein AR. Elder abuse and neglect: An overview. *Clin in Geriatr Med*. 2005; 21: 279–92.

28. Tatara T. Understanding the nature and scope of domestic elder abuse with the use of state aggregate data: summaries of the key findings of a national survey of state APS and aging agencies. *J Elder Abuse Negl*. 1993; 5: 35–57.

29. Lachs MS, Williams C, O'Brien S. Older adults: an 11-year longitudinal study of adult protective service use. *Arch Intern Med*. 1996; 156: 449–53.

30. Lachs MS, Williams CS, O'Brien S. The mortality of elder mistreatment. *JAMA*. 1998; 280: 428–32.

31. Marshall CE, Benton D, Brazier JM. Elder abuse: using clinical tools to identify clues of mistreatment. *Geriatrics*. 2000; 55(2): 42–53.

32. Swagerty DL, Takahashi PY, Evans JM. Elder mistreatment. *Am Fam Phys*. 1999; 59(10): 2804–8.

33. Wierucka D, Goodridge D. Vulnerable in a safe place: institutional elder abuse. *Can J Nurs Admin*. 1996; 9(3): 82–104.

34. Comijs H. Elder abuse in the community: Prevalence and consequences. *J Am Geriatr Soc*. 1998; 46: 885–8.

35. Jones JS. Elder abuse and neglect: responding to a national problem. *Ann Emerg Med*. 1994; 23: 845–8.

36. Fulmer T. Elder mistreatment. *Ann Rev Nurs Research*. 2002; 20: 369–95.

37. Pillimer K, Suitor JJ. Violence and violent feelings: what causes them among family caregivers? *J Gerontol*. 1992; 47: S165–S172.

38. Ramsey-Klawsnik H. Elder-abuse offenders: a typology. *Generations*. 2000; 2: 17–22.

39. Collins KA. Elder mistreatment: A review. *Arch Pathol Lab Med*. 2006; 130: 1290–6.

40. Kosberg J. Hidden problem of elder abuse: Clues and strategies for health care workers. In F Safford & G.I. Krel (Eds.) *Gerontology for Health Professionals, a Practice Guide*, Washington D.C. NASW Press: 130–47.

41. Lachs M, Pillemer K. Abuse and neglect of elderly persons. *N Engl J Med*. 1995; 332: 437–43.

42. Kruger RM, Moon CH. Can you spot the signs of elder mistreatment? *Postgrad Med*. 1999; 106: 169–83.

43. Ahmad M, Lachs MS. Elder abuse and neglect: What physicians can and should do. *Cleve Cl J Med*. 2002; 69: 801–8.

44. Lowenstein SR, Crescenzi CA, Kern DC, et al. Care of the elderly in the emergency department. *Ann Emerg Med*. 1986; 15: 528–35.

45. Clarke ME, Pierson W. Management of elder abuse in the emergency department. *Emerg Med Clin N Am*. 1999; 17(3): 631–44.

46. Jones J, Dougherty J, Schelble D, Cunningham W. Emergency department protocol for the diagnosis and evaluation of geriatric abuse. *Ann Emerg Med*. 1988; 17: 1006–15.

47. Lynch SH. Elder abuse: what to look for, how to intervene. *AJN*. 1997; 97(1): 27–33.

48. Levine JM. Elder neglect and abuse: a primer for primary care physicians. *Geriatrics*. 2003; 58: 37–44.

49. Conlin M. Silent suffering: A case study of elder abuse and neglect. *J Am Geriatr Soc*. 1995; 43: 1303–08.

50. Fulmer T, Ashley J. Clinical indicators of elder neglect. *Appl Nurs Res*. 1989; 2: 161–7.

51. Kruger RM, Moon CH. Can you spot the elder mistreatment? *Postgrad Med*. 1999; 106(2): 169–78.

52. Capezuti E, Brush BL, Lawson WT. Reporting elder mistreatment. *J Geront Nurs*. 1997; 23(7): 24–32.

53. Stiegel LA. Recommended Guidelines for State Courts Handling Cases Involving Elder Abuse. *American Bar Association*. 1995.

54. Dong XQ. Medical implications of elder abuse and neglect. *Clin Ger Med*. 2005; 21(2): 293–313.

55. Faulkner LR. Mandating the reporting of suspected cases of elder abuse: an inappropriate, ineffective and ageist response to the abuse of older adults. *Fam Law Q*. 1982; 16: 69–91.

56. Cammer Paris BE. Violence against elderly people. *Mt Sinai J Med*. 1996; 63: 97–100.

57. Moone A, Williams O. Perceptions of elder abuse and help-seeking patterns among African-American, Caucasian-American, and Korean-American elderly women. *The Gerontologist*. 1993; 33: 386–95.

58. Wei GS, Herbers JE. Reporting elder abuse: A medical, legal, and ethical overview. *JAMWA*. 2004; 59: 248–54.

59. Rodriguez MA, Wallace SP, Woolf NH, Mangione CM. Mandatory reporting of elder abuse: Between a rock and a hard place. *Ann Fam Med*. 2006; 4: 403–09.

60. Cohn F, Salmon ME, Stobo JD, eds. *Confronting Chronic Neglect: The Education and Training on Family Violence*. Washington, DC: National Academy Press, 2002.

61. Welfel EF, Danzinger PR, Santoro S. Mandated reporting of abuse/maltreatment of older adults: A primer for counselors. *J Couns Dev*. 2000; 78: 284–92.

62. Hazzard W. Elder abuse: definitions and implications for medical education. *Acad Med*. 1995; 70: 979–81.

63. Clark-Daniels CL, et al. Abuse and neglect of the elderly: Are emergency department personnel aware of mandatory reporting laws? *Ann Emerg Med*. 1990; 19: 970–7.

64. Conlin M. Silent suffering: A case study of elder abuse and neglect. *J Am Geriatr Soc*. 1998; 46: 885–8.

65. Tatara T. *Suggested State Guidelines for Gathering and Reporting Domestic Elder Abuse Statistics for Compiling National Data*, 1990. Washington, DC: National Aging Resource Center on Elder Abuse.

66. Rosenblatt DE, Cho KH, Durance PW. Reporting mistreatment of elder adults: the role of physicians. *J Am Geriatr Soc*. 1996; 44: 65–70.

67. Pillemer K, Moore DW. Abuse of patients in nursing homes: findings from a survey of staff. *Gerontologist*. 1989; 29: 314–20.

68. Ortmann C, Fechner G, Bajanowski T. Fatal neglect of the elderly. *Int J Legal Med*. 2001; 114: 191–3.

69. Administration on Aging. Department of Health and Human Services. *AGING*. 1996; 367: 1–136.

70. Subcommittee on Health and Long-Term Care of the Select Committee on Aging, House of Representatives: *Elder Abuse: A Decade of Shame and Inaction*. Washington, DC. U.S. Government Printing Office, 1992.

71. National Center on Elder Abuse. Elder Abuse Law Background Information. At www.elderabusecenter.org/default.cfm/?p=backgrounder.cfm.

72. Dyer CB, Heisler CJ, Hill CA, Kim LC. Community approaches to elder abuse. *Clin Geriatr Med*. 2005; 21(2): 429–47.

73. Keith PM, Wacker RR. It's hard to guard the aged: role strain of male and female guardians. *J Gerontol Social Work*. 1993; 21: 41–58.

74. A response to the abuse of vulnerable adults: the 2000 survey of state adult protective services. Available at: www.elderabusecenter.org/pdf/research/apsreport030703.pdf.

75. Blenkner M. A research and demonstration of protective services. *Soc Casework*. 1971; 52: 483–97.

76. Lachs MS, Williams CS, O'Brien S. Adult Protective Service use and nursing home placement. *Gerontologist*. 2002; 42: 734–9.

77. Wolf RS, Pillemer K. *Helping Elderly Victims: The Reality of Elder Abuse*. New York: Columbia University Press, 1989.

78. Matlaw JR, Spence DM. The hospital elder assessment team: a protocol for suspected cases of elder abuse and neglect. *JEAN*. 1994; 6: 23–7.

79. Nerenberg L. Multidisciplinary elder abuse prevention teams: a new generation. Available at: www.elderabusecenter.org/default.cfm.

80. Aravanis SC, Adelman RD, Breckman R. Diagnostic and treatment guidelines on elder abuse and neglect. *Arch Fam Med*. 1993; 2: 371–88.

81. Jones JS, Veenstra TR, Seamon JP. Elder mistreatment: national survey of emergency physicians. *Ann Emerg Med*. 1997; 30: 473–9.

5

Mentally ill or cognitively impaired patients

Stephanie Cooper, M.D.

Goals and objectives

1. To understand the increased risk of abuse that faces mentally ill and intellectually disabled (ID) people
2. To learn to identify, manage, and refer patients who are mentally ill or intellectually disabled who have been abused

Abuse of mentally ill and intellectually disabled people

Overview

Mentally ill and intellectually disabled people are among the vulnerable populations more likely to be victimized and abused. Obstacles to reporting abuse within these disenfranchised groups have made this problem more difficult to chronicle, treat, and prevent. This chapter will provide an overview of the prevalence of abuse, the types of abuse, and strategies for better reporting and preventing abuse within the psychosocially vulnerable cohorts of mentally ill and intellectually disabled patients.

Abuse is a public health issue. Maltreatment can lead to physical trauma, emotional trauma, and even death. Mentally ill patients are prone to worsening of their psychiatric condition after being abused. Intellectually disabled patients may suffer worsening of their primary disability, or, they may develop secondary disabilities resulting from the victimization. In both populations, physical, sexual, and emotional abuse aggravates the pre-existing condition, requiring additional health interventions and both medical and psychological assistance.

Abuse of the intellectually disabled

Definition of intellectually disabled

Intellectually disabled (ID) people are defined as individuals who have unique needs with regards to information processing. Intellectual disability can be congenital or acquired through accident or disease. The disability can affect memory, learning, speaking, problem solving, and other cognitive skills. Definitions of intellectual disability vary widely, and can include such terms as mental retardation, developmental disability, cognitive disability, and developmental disability with intellectual limitations. The term "developmental disability" can be used interchangeably with "intellectual disability," but the former implies a wider spectrum of disability.[1] Frequently, impairments in intellectual ability are coincident with physical and psychological impairments. A person is considered intellectually disabled if cognitive function is impaired enough to limit performing activities of daily living.

Types of abuse

Due to their backdrop of disability, abuse of people with cognitive impairment occurs in a myriad of ways, including unique forms of maltreatment that leverage the individual's lack of adaptive capacity. In addition to physical abuse (hitting, pushing, kicking, etc.) and sexual abuse, intellectually disabled people may suffer abuse by behaviors that constrain their adaptive devices, such as turning off an electric communication device, or disabling an electric wheelchair.[2] Neglect of this population may include withholding food, failing to provide adequate shelter, refusing assistance with necessary activities such as personal hygiene and toileting, or failing to provide medical care. Because many people with intellectual disabilities do not have control over their own finances, they may be subject to financial abuse such as absconding with checks, or charging unnecessary fees. Caregivers, functioning as interventional gatekeepers, can restrict the individual's access to services ranging from transportation to health care. In addition to caregiver abuse, peer abuse is an important modality of victimization in this population. Intimate partner violence among people with intellectual disability is poorly understood, though several studies indicate this is a common problem among people with mild to moderate intellectual deficit.[3]

Connection between violence and disability

The high rates of abuse experienced by people with intellectual disabilities result partly from the fact that violence causes disabilities and partly from society's response to disabilities, which increases the risk of violence. Abuse in infancy, such as shaken baby syndrome, can result in intellectual disability. In addition, extreme violence experienced by pregnant women can lead to reduced uterine blood flow and possible neurohormonal effects on the fetus.[4] People with disabilities are at increased risk of experiencing abuse, as their disability may impair escaping from danger (such as not being able to use a telephone to call for help). Also, disability is linked to poverty, which may predispose the individual to environments where violence is common.

Prevalence of abuse among people with ID

It is widely believed that people with disabilities are much more likely to be maltreated than people without disabilities. However, gathering incidence and prevalence data has been difficult due to limitations on reporting. As a result, less than 20 studies between 1994 and present chronicled prevalence of abuse within adult populations with intellectual disabilities.[5] Baseline estimates reveal that people with disabilities are two to five times more likely to experience abuse than those without disability.[6] Powers and colleagues found a prevalence of physical abuse of approximately 67 percent among women with both physical and intellectual disabilities.[7]

Sexual abuse in intellectual disability

Approximately 20 percent of U.S. females and 5 to 10 percent of U.S. males are sexually abused annually; people with intellectual and developmental disability are at higher risk than the baseline population. Adults with intellectual disability are 1.4 times more likely to have been sexually abused than their non-disabled cohort.[8] One expert in the field estimates that 15,000 to 19,000 people with developmental disabilities are raped each year in the U.S.[9] Prevalence estimates of sexual abuse vary widely, ranging from a recent study/literature review citing a prevalence of 25 to 53 percent,[10] to an older study quoting a 90 percent prevalence of sexual abuse among people with developmental disabilities.[11] Among patients with ID referred for sex education, the prevalence of sexual abuse was 61 percent for women and 25 percent for men.[12]

Abuse of children with intellectual disabilities

Children with intellectual disabilities are four to ten times more likely to suffer abuse than children without disability.[13] Approximately one in three children with ID will be sexually abused before the age of 18.[14] Abuse of this population occurs whether children are living in the community or in congregate care settings. Children living in the community with cognitive impairment were more likely to be victims of violence compared to a same-aged control cohort.[15] Lifetime prevalence estimates of abuse for children and adolescents with intellectual disability ranged from 11 to 28 percent.[16,17]

Sullivan and Knutson examined a hospital sample and found that the incidence of maltreatment was 1.7 times greater than children without disabilities. Furthermore, disability contributed to the abuse in 47 percent of cases, and in 37 percent, child protection services (CPS) professionals felt that the abuse resulted in a disability. Both the severity and duration of sexual and physical abuse was greater among children with multiple disabilities. The most common disabilities among the abused children were behavior disorders, speech disorders, mental retardation, and hearing impairments.[18] Estimates of abuse were even higher in another study which found that 88 percent of inpatient ID children were exposed to physical, psychological, and sexual abuse. An astonishing 66 percent had been the victims of violence.[19]

The Law Commission of Canada investigated institutional abuse of children with intellectual disabilities, and reported, "The fact that physical and sexual abuse was common in many institutions intended to protect, nurture and educate young people reflects a tragic breach of trust by those who were abusers. It is an indictment of the supervisory processes in place at those institutions. And it is a damning commentary on the casual attitude that we took towards the children we placed in residential facilities."[20]

Why people with ID are at increased risk for abuse

People with intellectual disability can be considered more prone to abuse for a variety of cultural and behavioral reasons. Culturally, they may be isolated and socially vulnerable in addition to cognitive and potentially physical vulnerabilities. To function within the context of requiring care from others, people with ID may have learned compliant behavior as a survival skill. Limited social interactions, low self-esteem, and limited assertiveness skills contribute to an inability to defend oneself.[21] In addition, people with cognitive deficits may lack the ability to speak, or have limited communication skills such that they cannot voice dissent.

Risk factors correlative with sexual abuse include powerlessness, communication deficits, impaired judgment, family isolation, and living arrangements that increase vulnerability – all of which are common in the ID population. In many cases, adults with ID were not knowledgeable about sexual relationships. Frequently, they were unable to distinguish abusive from consenting sexual encounters. Per researchers McCabe and Cummins, only 3 percent of adults in their sample were able to answer the question "what is sexual abuse?"[22]

Reporting issues

Another reason why people with intellectual disabilities are more prone to maltreatment involves the inherent limitations of reporting abuse within this population. Establishing that an abuse incident has occurred requires evidence and documentation. In many cases, intellectually disabled people may not understand the legal ramifications of being abused. They may be unaware that the treatment they are experiencing is what others in society would deem "abuse." People with ID may not know that they could or should report abuse, how to discuss the events, or which authorities to contact. Assuming that people with cognitive limitations gain access to the appropriate authorities, they may lack the capacity to communicate in a fashion that chronicles the abuse. (In cases of severe ID, people may only be able to provide sounds or gestures to signal their needs.) In essence, to document an incident of abuse, social services and law enforcement may require information that cognitively disabled people are unable to provide.[23] Due to reporting limitations in this population, it is estimated that only 3 percent of sexual abuse of people with developmental disabilities will ever be reported.[24] Underreporting limits abuse prevention, as offenders remain unprosecuted, and victims remain untreated.

Reporting abuse is also obfuscated by cultural factors. People with intellectual disabilities often depend on the caregiving of others. If caregivers are both nurturers and abusers, victims may be unwilling to report maltreatment due to fear of losing the positive aspects of the relationship. Additionally, many people with intellectual disability dwell in group homes; social isolation and lack of alternative living scenarios may encourage their silence.

Caregiver abuse

Abuse by the primary caregiver is common among people with intellectual disability. Among adults living in the community and receiving assistance in their homes, one study revealed that 30 percent underwent verbal, physical, or financial abuse.[25] Powers and colleagues discovered even higher rates of abuse among women who used personal assistance services. Forty percent had been emotionally abused, 35 percent financially abused, 19.5 percent had been neglected, 14 percent physically abused, and 11 percent sexually abused by their caregivers. Additionally, these women reported both physical and sexual abuse from people who had not been their personal assistants.[26]

Sequelae of abuse

Abuse, though underreported in this population, is not silent in its sequelae. Increased incidence of psychiatric and behavioral disturbance is associated with sexual abuse among people with cognitive disabilities.[27] After-effects of abuse also include higher rates of anxiety and depression. One study, comparing sequelae of abuse among developmentally disabled and non-disabled cohorts, found that both the experience and its aftermath may be more deleterious among the ID group. Significantly higher rates of depression, anxiety, sexual maladjustment, and even dual psychiatric diagnosis were found in victims of sexual exploitation with intellectual disability relative to controls.[28]

Psychological ramifications of abuse can trigger self-injurious behavior. Cognitively impaired people may self-injure to deal with stress or anger, re-enact the abuse, or attempt to communicate the maltreatment.[29] Direct physical sequelae of abuse can exacerbate existing symptoms or ability to adapt. For instance, a hand injury sustained by a person who depends on his/her hands for communication (signing or using adaptive technology) can significantly worsen the disability.

Recognition of abuse

For abuse to be prevented and treated, both caregivers and health care practitioners must recognize the signs and symptoms. Since caregivers are familiar with the individual's unique form of communication, they are first-line agents in detecting behavior changes. Caregivers are thus critical in translating patterns that could signal the occurrence of maltreatment.[30] Also, caregivers may be the only witness to the patient's physical stigmata of abuse.

The health care practitioner should be aware that physical and sexual abuse is a frequent occurrence in the intellectually disabled community. The provider should therefore be sure to look for physical signs of abuse such as abrasions, contusions, genital discomfort, STDs, and unexpected pregnancy.[31] By maintaining professional attitudes and a culture of support, providers will help patients and caregivers share their stories.

Reducing risk of abuse

Prevention of abuse within the intellectually disabled community begins with increasing awareness. Health educators can disseminate information to health care professionals as well as disability service providers. Training for law enforcement and legal personnel may facilitate reporting and obtaining testimony. Additionally, changing overarching societal attitudes (such as devaluation of people with disabilities) and rewriting myths (such as the erroneous notion that cognitively impaired people don't feel pain), which contribute to abuse of this vulnerable population, is crucial to lessening its frequency.[32]

Education and awareness programs for people with intellectual disabilities may also reduce risk of abuse. Interventions that promote assertiveness, choice-making, body integrity, personal rights, and self-defense help reshape compliant behaviors.[33,34] Some disability professionals argue that increasing awareness of sexuality via sex education classes is key to prevention.[35]

Service organizations must carefully screen providers and exclude high-risk individuals and offenders. These organizations should provide environments that are physically and emotionally safe.

Treatment of abuse

Historically, there has been debate about whether people with ID could benefit from therapy to deal with abuse. Many current researchers stress that therapy is useful if not mandatory to lessen the psychological impact of maltreatment. Finding a clinician proficient in disability, sexuality, and abuse, however, can be difficult.[36] Several studies have shown that support groups for victims of abuse have reduced trauma and depression. One such support group for sexually abused people with ID also included an educational support group for the victim's caregivers.[37]

Interdisciplinary therapy, repetition, role-playing, and a strong support network were crucial to therapeutic improvement.

Special population: cognitive impairment in the elderly

Adults who undergo progressive decline in cognitive function the hallmark of Alzheimer's disease – are particularly at risk for abuse. Prevalence of abuse among elders with dementia ranges from 5 to 12 percent.[38] Abuse may be reciprocal in this population, as the cognitively impaired elderly are likely to bite, kick, push, or hit their primary caregivers. Up to 33 percent of caregivers reported physical abuse directed toward them at least once during the course of caregiving.[39] Surveys of caregivers showed that 6 to 12 percent admitted to engaging in violent behavior toward the patient in their care.[40] Risk factors for caregiver violence included helping individuals with more significant functional impairments, and working longer hours. As our society ages, abuse among the cognitively impaired elderly will become a growing concern.

Abuse of the mentally ill

Definition of mentally ill

Mental illnesses are typified by alterations in mood, thought, and behavior associated with significant distress and impaired functioning over an extended time-period. The terms schizophrenia, mood disorder (including bipolar disorder and major depression), and personality disorder are various types of mental illness. Symptoms can range from mild to severe. Mental illnesses affect all cultures, races, and socioeconomic groups, and have a significant public health impact. In the United States, an estimated 26 percent of Americans over age 18 suffer a diagnosable mental disorder yearly, although only about 6 percent suffer a serious mental illness (SMI).[41] A person is considered seriously mentally ill when his/her psychological disposition precludes him/her from consistently managing the tasks of daily life.

Types of abuse

In addition to physical and sexual abuse, the limited coping skills of people with serious mental illness create opportunity for other types of abuse. Explosive behavior traits mixed with impoverished, dangerous living environments can ignite physical abuse. Mentally ill people are the victims of physical violence at a rate far exceeding the baseline population.

Neglect is another troubling form of abuse that strikes this vulnerable cohort. Many severely mentally ill people are homeless, or reside in group homes. In either scenario, they are frequently without access to reliable food and water, a reasonably thermoregulated environment, safety from physical assault, and means to navigate the social service and mental health system.

Connection between violence and mental illness

Mental illness is thought to result from a complex interplay of biological, genetic, environmental, and neurohormonal factors. While there is a definite genetic underpinning, experiences such as trauma and chronic stress can lead to long-term changes in brain function. Multiple studies have shown that a history of severe physical and/or sexual trauma in childhood correlates with mental illness in adulthood.[42–45] In turn, additional abuse can aggravate existing mental illness, exacerbating the reciprocal interaction between biology and lived experience.[46]

Prevalence of physical and sexual abuse among people with SMI

Although historically, people with mental illness have been considered perpetrators of abuse, recent research shows that they are far more likely to be victims of violence. Teplin and colleagues found that the rate of violent crime against seriously mentally ill people residing in the community was more than 11 times the rate in the general population.[47] Specifically, people with serious mental illnesses were eight times more likely to be robbed, 15 times more likely to be assaulted, and 23 times more likely to be raped compared to people in the general population. Personal theft – theft of property from one's person – was dramatically increased among people with serious mental illness. In the general population, personal theft occurs at a rate of 0.2 percent compared to a rate of 21 percent among the mentally ill – 140 times more frequently. Extrapolating these findings to the U.S. population indicates that nearly 3 million people with severe mental illness are victims of one or more violent crimes each year.[48]

A study among outpatients with schizophrenia and schizoaffective disorder examined the likelihood of being crime perpetrators versus crime victims. After three years of monitoring, 22 percent of subjects had been charged with a crime, while 38 percent had been crime victims. For seriously mentally ill people in this study, the likelihood of being a victim of violent crime was 14 times the likelihood of being arrested for committing one.[49]

Violence and physical abuse also occur at the hands of intimate contacts. Cascardi and colleagues (1996) studied victimization of recently admitted mentally ill inpatients by family members or intimate partners. Sixty-three percent with an intimate partner reported physical abuse within the past year, including being punched, hit, choked, or threatened with a weapon. Of the inpatients who lived with relatives, 46 percent had been physically abused by family members within the last year.[50,51]

Abuse among episodically homeless women with severe mental illness was so common as to be "normative" for this population. Goodman and colleagues surveyed urban women diagnosed with schizophrenia, schizoaffective disorder, bipolar disorder, borderline personality disorder, or unspecified psychosis. Of 99 women surveyed, 97 percent had experienced abuse. Specifically, 87 percent of the women reported childhood physical abuse and 65 percent reported childhood sexual abuse. As adults, 87 percent of the women had been physically abused, and 76 percent had been sexually abused. Both strangers and intimate partners perpetrated adulthood sexual and physical assault. For this cohort of episodically homeless women with SMI, no differences in abuse were found among ethnicity, education, or diagnosis. In many cases, abuse was a recurrent and recent event. Within a month of the interview, 28 percent of study participants had been sexually or physically abused. The authors of this study concluded that "rape and physical battery" were "inextricably woven" into the fabric of these women's lives.[52]

Prevalence of neglect among people with mental illness

In 1965, the U.S. government passed the Community Mental Health Centers Act, which initiated the release of schizophrenic patients from institutions into the community. Inadequate social and financial support, as well as lack of social and psychiatric care services, rendered many of these people homeless. As a result, an estimated 20 to 40 percent of homeless people in the United States have serious mental illness.[53]

Many states dealt with the largess of homeless, deinstitutionalized mentally ill people by encouraging group homes. Recent publicity of the maltreatment and neglect within these facilities, however, has spawned widespread investigation. In 2002, the *New York Times* reviewed deaths of people with SMI living in group homes in New York City and revealed a total of 946 deaths between 1995 and 2001. These deaths included 126 persons in their 20s, 30s, and 40s, as well as fourteen suicides and several preventable deaths such as appendicitis. Conditions of the group homes were described as "vermin-ridden" and filthy, with staff occasionally "threatening residents."[54]

Special populations and abuse: prisoners

According to the Human Rights Watch organization, there are currently three times more mentally ill people in prison than in mental health hospitals.[55] By another estimate, over a million inmates in the American prison system suffer from mental illness – one in every six prisoners.[56] While incarcerated, people with SMI may suffer abuse from guards or other prisoners at disproportionately high rates. Recent research on prisoners in the Mid-Atlantic States reveals that mentally ill inmates are sexually victimized at higher rates (1 in 12) than their non-mentally ill counterparts (1 in 33). Among prisoners with serious mental illness, the incidence of sexual victimization was three times higher among female inmates compared to males, and higher among non-whites compared to whites, regardless of gender.[57]

Why people with SMI are at risk for abuse

People with serious mental illness are more prone to abuse for a variety of cultural, psychological, and environmental reasons. On a cultural level, the bias that mentally ill people provoke violence may be used as a justification to victimize them.[58] Perhaps due to media focus on crazed killers and random acts of violence, the public overestimates the association between mental illness, violence, and their own personal risk.

Psychological disability increases personal vulnerability. Symptoms of mental illness such as impaired sense of reality, disorganized thinking, poor impulse control, and difficulty problem solving diminish the individual's ability to both perceive risk and protect oneself from threat.[59] When provoked, a prior history of abuse may predispose the mentally ill to lashing out or behaving violently; limited problem solving may lead to explosive behavior rather than containment.

Furthermore, many people with SMI live in high-risk environments. Without social or financial resources, they may be marginalized to impoverished and dangerous neighborhoods. Poverty, homelessness, substance use, poor support networks – all common in severe mental illness – correlate with abuse.[60]

Reporting issues

Reporting abuse is difficult in any population, but among people with SMI, is limited by many factors. In cases of neglect by family members or group homes, there may be no third-party witness to the abuse. When complaints are lodged with oversight agencies (such as group home violations) corrective action may be slow or nonexistent.

Authorities may doubt the reliability of mentally ill people's testimony. Among people who experience visual and auditory hallucinations, can report of abuse be valid? Goodman and colleagues (1999) claim that self-reports of trauma among seriously mentally ill people can be considered reliable.[61]

Additionally, several studies indicate that people with SMI may underreport physical and sexual abuse. Despite the prevalence of family member and intimate partner violence, the majority of victims did not consider their maltreatment to be abuse.[62] Consequently, physical abuse was only documented on 25 percent of these patient's charts. In one study, 33 percent of male patients had experienced childhood sexual abuse, but few of them labeled it as such.[63] In essence, despite relatively high rates of abuse, perceived vulnerability is quite low.[64]

Sequelae of abuse

Abuse can trigger a negative feedback cycle among people with serious mental illness. Physical or sexual abuse can exacerbate psychiatric disorders, creating further psychosocial dysfunction. Higher levels of anxiety, hallucination, delusion, and thought disorder were found in patients who had experienced abuse as both children and adults.[65,66] Consequent behavior patterns – decreased cognitive function, increased substance abuse, and frayed social interactions – then contribute to further abuse. This negative cycle has led to the conclusion that victimization increases the likelihood of repeat victimization.[67,68]

People with serious mental illness living in a context of repeated trauma do not become desensitized. Rather, psychiatric symptoms in multiply traumatized women worsened relative to the intensity of new abuse. Not surprisingly, the more frequent, recent, and varied the abuse, the worse damage to self-esteem, trust, and intimacy.[6]

Post-traumatic stress disorder (PTSD) is a common response to physical and sexual abuse. Symptoms associated with PTSD include avoidance, overrarousal, and re-experiencing the trauma in the absence of real-time threat. PTSD is common but underreported among people with severe mental illness. One study found that 43 percent of mentally ill people exhibited PTSD, but only 2 percent of these had PTSD documented in their charts.[70]

Seriously mentally ill people may respond to abuse by engaging in high-risk and self-harming behaviors. The epitome of self-harm – suicide – has been linked to recent sexual and physical abuse among the mentally ill. Astonishingly, males who had been sexually or physically abused within the last 30 days were significantly more likely to attempt suicide.[71] In addition, risky sexual behavior and increased seroprevalence of HIV has been linked to a history of physical and sexual abuse.[72,73] Victimization also correlates with homelessness, decreased quality of life[74], and increased utilization of mental health and hospital resources.

Recognition of abuse

The prevalence of criminal victimization as well as physical and sexual abuse in this vulnerable population should encourage mental health professionals and medical care providers to screen for signs and symptoms. Providers should ask specific and deliberate questions, understanding that many people with SMI may not label certain behaviors (slapping, pushing, unwanted genital contact) as "abuse." Providers should recognize that when people with severe mental illness experience abuse, it may significantly exacerbate their psychological problems. For instance, when emergency medicine providers treat SMI patients for assault, they should recognize that the patient might benefit from a psychiatric consult to deal with the psychological ramifications of the physical abuse.

For patients presenting with worsening psychological symptoms, providers should consider abuse as a potential cause. The temporal link between suicide attempts and recent abuse underscores the importance of investigating possible abuse in all patients with serious mental illness.

Documenting the abuse is key to raising awareness and improving services for victims. Providers who work with this vulnerable population must recognize their role in elucidating a history of abuse, and their responsibility to document physical and psychological signs and symptoms. Failure to address abuse histories may confirm patients' belief in the need to deny the reality of these traumatic experiences.[75]

Reducing risk of abuse

A multifactorial approach should be used to reduce risk of abuse among people with serious mental illness. To begin with, society should be educated that people with SMI are more often the victims than the perpetrators of abuse. With increased awareness, the public may exhibit more compassion for the mentally ill, and less tolerance of their victimization.

Reducing risk of abuse on an individual level relies on minimizing modifiable risk factors. Substance use correlates with physical and sexual abuse and criminal victimization in populations with and without mental illness. Treating substance abuse will decrease personal vulnerability and possibly reduce the risk of revictimization.[76] Criminal victimization in this population is linked to a complex interplay of residential instability/homelessness, poverty, and substance abuse. Providing stable, physically safe environments are crucial to developing a sense of personal control.[77]

People with SMI can minimize vulnerability by learning specific skill sets that emphasize conflict management and personal protection. Outreach should target high-risk groups within the mentally ill community, such as the homeless, substance abusers, and those with a significant history of childhood sexual abuse.

In addition, risk-reduction can be enhanced by partnership with law enforcement. Police officers often function as "streetcorner psychologists."[78] Their role as protective resources should be highlighted, and they should be trained to understand the social context of constant threat experienced by many people with mental illness. Armed with this awareness, police may be more likely to document, investigate, and prosecute abuse of the mentally ill.

Conclusion

Mentally ill and intellectually disabled people are among the vulnerable populations more likely to be victimized and abused. Obstacles to reporting abuse have precluded documentation, thus limiting awareness and the ability to provide support and treatment for victims. Abuse of mentally ill and intellectually disabled people leads to worsening of their respective disabilities. Furthermore, victimization has been shown to lead to repeat victimization. For society to help quash this cycle of abuse, further investigation of this important public health problem is necessary. Ideally, increased understanding of the prevalence and circumstances of abuse will lead to abuse prevention in these psychosocially disenfranchised populations.

References

1. Public Health Agency of Canada. Family Violence and People with Intellectual Disabilities. National Clearinghouse on Family Violence. Accessed online 10/2/07 at http://www.phac-aspc.gc.ca/ncfv-cnivf/familyviolence/html/fvintellectu_e.html.

2. Nosek MA. Women with disabilities and the delivery of empowerment medicine. *Arch Phys Med Rehabil*. 1997 Dec; 78(12 Suppl 5): S1–2.

3. Public Health Agency of Canada.

4. Public Health Agency of Canada.

5. Horner-Johnson W, Drum C. Prevalence of maltreatment of people with intellectual disabilities: A review of recently published research. *Mental Retardation and Developmental Disabilities Research Reviews*. 2006; 12: 57–69.

6. Sobsey D. *Violence and Abuse in the Lives of People with Disabilities: The End of Silent Acceptance?* Baltimore: Paul H. Brookes Publishing Co, 1994.

7. Powers LE, Curry MA, Oschwald M, et al. Barriers and strategies in addressing abuse: A survey of disabled women's experiences. *J Rehabil*. 2002; 68: 4–13.

8. Powers LE, et al. (2002).

9. Sobsey D. (1994).

10. Horner-Johnson W, et al. (2006).

11. Valenti-Hein D, Schwartz L. *The Sexual Abuse Interview for Those with Developmental Disabilities*. James Stanfield Company. Santa Barbara, CA, 1995. Valenti Hein and Schwartz as reported in the *ARC*.

12. McCarthy M, Thompson D. A prevalence study of sexual abuse of adults with intellectual disabilities referred for sex education. *Journal of Applied Research in Intellectual Disabilities*. 1997; 10(2): 105–24.

13. Horner-Johnson W, et al. (2006).

14. Perlman N, Ericson K. Issues related to sexual abuse of persons with developmental disabilities: An overview. *Journal on Developmental Disabilities*. May 1992; 1(1): 19–23.

15. Svetaz MV, Ireland M, Blum R. Adolescents with learning disabilities: Risk and protective factors associated with emotional well-being – Findings from the National Longitudinal Study of Adolescent Health. *Adolesc Health*. 2000; 27: 340–8.

16. Sullivan PM, Knutson JF. The association between child maltreatment and disabilities in a hospital-based epidemiological study. *Child Abuse Negl*. 1998; 22: 271–88.

17. Verdugo MA, Bermejo BG, Fuertes J. The maltreatment of intellectually handicapped children and adolescents. *Child Abuse Negl*. 1995; 19: 205–15.

18. Sullivan PM, Knutson JF. (1998).

19. Ebeling H, Nurkkala H. Children and adolescents with developmental disorders and violence. *J Circumpolar Health*. 2002; 61(suppl 2): 51–60.

20. Law Commission of Canada.

21. Muccigrosso, L. Sexual abuse prevention strategies and programs for persons with developmental disabilities. *Sexuality and Disability*. Fall 1991; 9(3): 261–71.

22. McCabe MP, Cummins RA. The sexual knowledge, experience, feelings and needs of people with mild intellectual disability. *Educ Train Ment Retard Dev Disabil*. 1996; 31: 13–21.

23. Baladerian N. Sexual abuse of people with developmental disabilities. *Sexuality and Disability*. 1991; 9(4): 323–35.

24. Valenti-Hein D, Schwartz L. (1995).

25. Oktay JS, Tompkins CJ. Personal assistance providers' mistreatment of disabled adults. *Health Social Work*. Aug 2004; 29(3): 177–87.

26. Powers LE, et al. (2002).

27. Sequera H, Howlin P, Hollins S. Psychological disturbance associated with sexual abuse in people with learning disabilities: Case-control study. *British Journal of Psychiatry*. 2003; 183(5): 451–6.

28. Matich-Maroney J. Sexual exploitation and its aftereffects in developmentally disabled adults. Dissertation Abstracts International Section A: Humanities and Social Sciences. Vol 57(8-A), Feb 1997, pp. 3681.

29. Burke L, Bedard C. Self-injury considered in association with sexual victimization in individuals with a developmental handicap. *Canadian Journal of Human Sexuality*. Fall 1994; 3(3): 253–62.

30. Burke L, Bedard C, Ludwig S. Dealing with sexual abuse of adults with a developmental disability who also have impaired communication: Supportive procedures for detection, disclosure and follow-up. *Canadian Journal of Human Sexuality*. Spr 1998; 7(1): 79–91.

31. Sobsey D. (1994).

32. Sobsey D. (1994).

33. Sobsey D, Mansell S. The prevention of sexual abuse of people with developmental disabilities. *Developmental Disabilities Bulletin*. 1990; 18(2): 51–66.

34. Muccigrosso L. (1991).

35. Peckham N, Howlett S, Corbett A. Evaluating a survivor's group pilot for women with significant intellectual disabilities who have been sexually abused. *Journal of Applied Research in Intellectual Disabilities*. Jul 2007; 20(4): 308–22.

36. Baladerian N. (1991).

37. Peckham N, et al. (2007).

38. Coyne, A. The relationship between dementia and elder abuse. *Geriatric Times*. July/Aug 2001; 2(4). Available online at http://www.cmellc.com/geriatric times/g010715.html.

39. Coyne A. (2001).

40. Pillemer K, Suitor J. Violence and violent feelings: what causes them among family caregivers? *J Gerontol*. 1992; 47(4): S165–S172.

41. Kessler R, Chiu W, Demler O, Walters E. Prevalence, severity, and comorbidity of twelve-month DSM-IV disorders in the National Comorbidity Survey Replication (NCS-R). *Archives of General Psychiatry*. 2005 Jun; 62(6): 617–27.

42. Lysaker PH, Buck KD, LaRocco VA. Clinical and psychosocial significance of trauma history in the treatment of schizophrenia. *J Psychosoc Nurs Ment Health Serv*. Aug 2007; 45(8): 44–51.

43. Shevlin M, Houston J, Dorahy M, and Adamson G. Cumulative traumas and psychosis: an analysis of the National Comorbidity Survey and the British Psychiatric Morbidity Survey. *Schizophr Bull*. June 22, 2007; 193–9.

44. Read J, Agar K, Argyle N, Aderhold V. Sexual and physical abuse during childhood and adulthood as predictors of hallucinations, delusions and thought disorder. *Psychology and Psychotherapy: Theory, Research and Practice*. 2003; 76(Pt.1):1–22.

45. Goodman LA, Fallot RD. HIV risk behavior in poor urban women with serious mental disorders: association with childhood physical and sexual abuse. *Am J Orthopsychiatry*. 1998 Jan; 68(1): 73–83.

46. Public Health Agency of Canada. A report on Mental Illnesses in Canada. http://www.phac-aspc.gc.ca/publicat/miic-mmac/chap_1_e.html

47. Teplin LA, McClelland GM, Abram KM, Weiner DA. Crime victimization in adults with severe mental illness: comparison with the National Crime Victimization Survey. *Arch Gen Psychiatry*. 2005; 62: 911–21.

48. Teplin LA, et al. (2005).

49. Brekke JS, Prindle C, Bae SW, Long JD. Risks for individuals with schizophrenia who are living in the community. *Psychiatr Serv*. 2001; 52: 1358–66.

50. Cascardi M, Mueser KT, DeGiralomo J, et al. Physical aggression against psychiatric inpatients by family members and partners. *Psychiatr Serv*. 1996; 47: 531–3.

51. Stuart, H. Violence and mental illness: an overview. *World Psychiatry*. 2003 June; 2(2): 121–4.

52. Goodman LA, Dutton MA, Harris M. Episodically homeless women with serious mental illness: Prevalence of physical and sexual assault. *Amer J Orthopsychiat*. 1995; 65(4): 468–79.

53. Hockberger R, Richards J. Thought disorders. In Rosen's *Emergency Medicine*. St. Louis MO, 2002. p 1541.

54. Levy, C. For mentally ill, death and misery. In *The New York Times*. April 28, 2002. Available online at http://query.nytimes.com/gst/fullpage.html?res=9407EEDB113EF93BA15757COA9649C8B63.

55. Human Rights Watch. United States: Mentally Ill Mistreated. Accessed online at http://hrw.org/english/docs/2003/10/22/usdom6472.htm. 10/1/2007.

56. Kinsler P, Saxman A. Traumatized offenders: don't look now, but your jail's also your mental health center. *J Trauma Dissociation*. 2007; 8(2): 81–95.

57. Wolff N, Blitz C, Jing S. Rates of sexual victimization in prison for inmates with and without mental disorders. *Psychiatr Serv*. August 2007; 58:1087–94.

58. Stuart H. (2003).

59. Teplin LA, et al. (2005).

60. Teplin LA, et al. (2005).

61. Goodman LA, Thompson KM, Weinfurt K, Corl S, Acher P, Mueser KT, Roserberg SD. Reliability of reports of violent victimization and posttraumatic stress disorder among men and women with serious mental illness. *J Trauma Stress*. 1999 Oct; 12(4): 587–99.

62. Cascardi M, et al. (1996).

63. Ladd B, Moore E. Prevalence and denial of sexual abuse in a male psychiatric inpatient population. *J Trauma Stress*. 2005 Aug; 18(4): 323–30.

64. Hiday VA, Swartz MS, Swanson JW, Borum R, Wagner HR. Criminal victimization of persons with severe mental illness. *Psychiatr Serv*. 1999; 50: 62–8.

65. Read J, Agar K, Argyle N, Aderhold V. Sexual and physical abuse during childhood and adulthood as predictors of hallucinations, delusions and thought disorder. *Psychology and Psychotherapy: Theory, Research and Practice*. March 2003; 76(1): 1–22.

66. Lysaker PH, Buck KD, LaRocco VA. Clinical and psychosocial significance of trauma history in the treatment of schizophrenia. *J Psychosoc Nurs Ment Health Serv*. 2007 Aug; 45(8): 44–51.

67. Lam JA, Rosenheck R. The effect of victimization on clinical outcomes of homeless persons with serious mental illness. *Psychiatr Serv*. 1998; 49: 678–83.

68. Teplin LA, et al. (2005).

69. Goodman LA, Dutton MA. (1996).

70. Mueser KT, Goodman LB, Trumbetta SL, et al. Trauma and posttraumatic stress disorder in severe mental illness. *Journal of Consulting and Clinical Psychology*. 1998; 66: 493–9.

71. Tiet QQ, Finney JW, Moos RH. Recent sexual abuse, physical abuse, and suicide attempts among male veterans seeking psychiatric treatment. *Psychiatr Serv*. 2006 Jan; 57(1): 107–13.

72. Devieux JG, Malow R, Lerner BG, Dyer JG, Baptista L, Lucenko B, Kalichman S. Triple jeopardy for HIV: substance using severely mentally ill adults. *J Prev Interv Community*. 2007; 33(1–2): 5–18.

73. Goodman LA, Rosenberg SD, Mueser KT, Drake RE. Physical and sexual assault history in women with serious mental illness: prevalence, correlates, treatment, and future research directions. *Schizophr Bull*. 1997; 23(4): 685–96.

74. Lam JA, Rosenheck R. (1998).

75. Goodman LA, Dutton MA. (1995).

76. Teplin LA, et al. (2005).

77. Goodman LA, Dutton MA. (1995).

78. Teplin LA. Criminalizing mental disorder: the comparative arrest rate of the mentally ill. *Am Psychol*. 1984; 39: 794–803.

Mental illness references

Brekke JS, Prindle C, Bae SW, Long JD. Risks for individuals with schizophrenia who are living in the community. *Psychiatr Serv*. 2001; 52: 1358–66.

Cascardi M, Mueser KT, DeGiralomo J, et al. Physical aggression against psychiatric inpatients by family members and partners. *Psychiatr Serv*. 1996; 47: 531–3.

Devieux JG, Malow R, Lerner BG, Dyer JG, Baptista L, Lucenko B, Kalichman S. Triple jeopardy for HIV: substance using severely mentally ill adults. *J Prev Interv Community*. 2007; 33(1–2): 5–18.

Eisenberg L. Violence and the mentally ill: victims, not perpetrators. *Arch Gen Psychiatry*. 2005; 62: 825–6.

Friedman SH, Loue S. Incidence and prevalence of intimate partner violence by and against women with severe mental illness. *J Womens Health (Larchmt)*. 2007 May; 16(4): 471–80.

Goodman LA, Fallot RD. HIV risk behavior in poor urban women with serious mental disorders: association with childhood physical and sexual abuse. *Am J Orthopsychiatry*. 1998 Jan; 68(1): 73–83.

Goodman LA, Rosenberg SD, Mueser KT, Drake RE. Physical and sexual assault history in women with serious mental illness: prevalence, correlates, treatment, and future research directions. *Schizophr Bull*. 1997; 23(4): 685–96.

Goodman LA, Thompson KM, Weinfurt K, Corl S, Acher P, Mueser KT, Roserberg SD. Reliability of reports of violent victimization and posttraumatic stress disorder among men and women with serious mental illness. *J Trauma Stress*. 1999 Oct; 12(4): 587–99.

Goodman LA, Dutton MA. The relationship between victimization and cognitive schemata among episodically homeless, seriously mentally ill women. *Violence Vict*. 1996 Summer; 11(2): 159–74.

Goodman LA, Dutton MA, Harris M. Episodically homeless women with serious mental illness: Prevalence of physical and sexual assault. *Amer J Orthopsychiat*. 1995; 65(4): 468–79.

Ladd DD, Moore E. Prevalence and denial of sexual abuse in a male psychiatric inpatient population. *J Trauma Stress*. 2005 Aug; 18(4): 323–30.

Lam JA, Rosenheck R. The effect of victimization on clinical outcomes of homeless persons with serious mental illness. *Psychiatr Serv*. 1998; 49: 678–83.

Levy, C. For mentally ill, death and misery. In *The New York Times*. April 28, 2002. Available online at http://query.nytimes.com/gst/fullpage.html?res=9407EEDB113EF93BA15757 COA9649C8B63.

Lysaker PH, Buck KD, LaRocco VA. Clinical and psychosocial significance of trauma history in the treatment of schizophrenia. *J Psychosoc Nurs Ment Health Serv*. 2007 Aug; 45(8): 44–51.

Hiday VA, Swartz MS, Swanson JW, Borum R, Wagner HR. Criminal victimization of persons with severe mental illness. *Psychiatr Serv*. 1999; 50: 62–8.

Kessler RC, Chiu WT, Demler O, Walters EE. Prevalence, severity, and comorbidity of twelve-month DSM-IV disorders in the National Comorbidity Survey Replication (NCS-R). *Archives of General Psychiatry*. 2005 June; 62(6): 617–27.

Kinsler P, Saxman A. Traumatized offenders: don't look now, but your jail's also your mental health center. *J Trauma Dissociation*. 2007; 8(2): 81–95.

Mueser KT, Goodman LB, Trumbetta SL, et al. Trauma and posttraumatic stress disorder in severe mental illness. *Journal of Consulting and Clinical Psychology*. 1998; 66: 493–9.

Public Health Agency of Canada. A report on mental illnesses in Canada. http://www.phac-aspc.gc.ca/publicat/miic-mmac/chap_1_e.html.

Stuart H. Violence and mental illness: an overview. *World Psychiatry*. 2003 June; 2(2): 121–4.

Shevlin M, Houston J, Dorahy M, and Adamson G. Cumulative traumas and psychosis: an analysis of the National Comorbidity Survey and the British Psychiatric Morbidity Survey. *Schizophr Bull*. June 22, 2007.

Teplin LA, McClelland GM, Abram KM, Weiner DA. Crime victimization in adults with severe mental illness: comparison with the National Crime Victimization Survey. *Arch Gen Psychiatry*. 2005; 62: 911–21.

Teplin LA. Criminalizing mental disorder: the comparative arrest rate of the mentally ill. *Am Psychol*. 1984; 39: 794–803.

Tiet QQ, Finney JW, Moos RH. Recent sexual abuse, physical abuse, and suicide attempts among male veterans seeking psychiatric treatment. *Psychiatr Serv*. 2006 Jan; 57(1): 107–13.

Marley JA, Buila S. Crimes against people with mental illness: types, perpetrators, and influencing factors. *Soc Work*. 2001; 46: 115–24.

Read J, Agar K, Argyle N, Aderhold V. Sexual and physical abuse during childhood and adulthood as predictors of hallucinations, delusions and thought disorder. *Psychology and Psychotherapy: Theory, Research and Practice*. March 2003; 76(1): 1–22.

Silver E. Mental disorder and violent victimization: the mediating role of involvement in conflicted social relationships. *Criminol*. 2002; 40: 191–212.

Wolff N, Blitz C, Jing S. Rates of sexual victimization in prison for inmates with and without mental disorders. *Psychiatr Serv*. Aug 2007; 58: 1087–1094.

Intellectual disability references

Baladerian N. Sexual abuse of people with developmental disabilities. *Sexuality and Disability*. 1991; 9(4): 323–35.

Burke L, Bedard C. Self-injury considered in association with sexual victimization in individuals with a developmental handicap. *Canadian Journal of Human Sexuality*. Fall 1994; 3(3): 253–62.

Burke L, Bedard C, Ludwig S. Dealing with sexual abuse of adults with a developmental disability who also have impaired communication: Supportive procedures for detection, disclosure and follow-up. *Canadian Journal of Human Sexuality*. Spr 1998; 7(1): 79–91.

Coyne A. The relationship between dementia and elder abuse. *Geriatric Times*. July/Aug 2001; 2(4). Available online at http://www.cmellc.com/geriatric times/g010715.html.

Ebeling H, Nurkkala H. Children and adolescents with developmental disorders and violence. *J Circumpolar Health*. 2002; 61(suppl2): 51–60.

Family Violence and People with Intellectual Disabilities. National Clearinghouse on Family Violence. Public Health Agency of Canada.

Horner-Johnson W, Drum C. Prevalence of maltreatment of people with intellectual disabilities: A review of recently published research. *Mental Retardation and Developmental Disabilities Research Reviews*. 2006; 12: 57–69.

Levy H, Packman W. Sexual abuse prevention for individuals with mental retardation: Considerations for genetic counselors. *J Genet Counsel*. 2004; 13: 189–205.

Matich-Maroney J. Sexual exploitation and its aftereffects in developmentally disabled adults. *Dissertation Abstracts International Section A: Humanities and Social Sciences*. Feb 1997; 57(8-A): 3681.

McCabe MP, Cummins RA. The sexual knowledge, experience, feelings and needs of people with mild intellectual disability. *Educ Train Ment Retard Dev Disabil*. 1996; 31: 13–21.

McCarthy M, Thompson D. A prevalence study of sexual abuse of adults with intellectual disabilities referred for sex education. *Journal of Applied Research in Intellectual Disabilities*. 1997; 10(2): 105–24.

Muccigrosso, L. Sexual abuse prevention strategies and programs for persons with developmental disabilities. *Sexuality and Disability*. Fall 1991; 9(3): 261–71.

Nosek MA. Women with disabilities and the delivery of empowerment medicine. *Arch Phys Med Rehabil*. 1997 Dec; 78(12 Suppl 5): S1–2.

Oktay JS, Tompkins CJ. Personal assistance providers' mistreatment of disabled adults. *Health Social Work*. Aug 2004; 29(3): 177–87.

Peckham N, Howlett S, Corbett A. 2007. Evaluating a survivor's group pilot for women with significant intellectual disabilities who have been sexually abused. *Journal of Applied Research in Intellectual Disabilities*. Jul 2007; 20(4): 308–22.

People with Mental Retardation and Sexual Abuse. www.people1.org/articles/article_sex_abuse.htm from the ARC accessed 10/1/2007.

Perlman N, Ericson K. Issues related to sexual abuse of persons with developmental disabilities: An overview. *Journal on Developmental Disabilities*. May 1992; 1(1): 19–23.

Pillemer K, Suitor J. Violence and violent feelings: what causes them among family caregivers? *J Gerontol*. 1992; 47(4): S165–S172.

Powers LE, Curry MA, Oschwald M, et al. Barriers and strategies in addressing abuse: A survey of disabled women's experiences *J Rehabil*. 2002; 68: 4–13.

Sequera H, Howlin P, Hollins S. Psychological disturbance associated with sexual abuse in people with learning disabilities: case-control study. *British Journal of Psychiatry*. Nov 2003; 183(5): 451–6.

Sobsey D. (1994) *Violence and Abuse in the Lives of People with Disabilities: The End of Silent Acceptance?* Baltimore: Paul H. Brookes Publishing Co.

Sobsey D, Mansell S. The prevention of sexual abuse of people with developmental disabilities. *Developmental Disabilities Bulletin*. 1990; 18(2): 51–66.

Talbot TJ, Langdon PE. A revised sexual knowledge assessment tool for people with intellectual disabilities: is sexual knowledge related to sexual offending behavior? *Journal of Intellectual Disability Research*. 2006; 50(7): 523–31.

Valenti-Hein D, Schwartz L. (1995). *The Sexual Abuse Interview for Those With Developmental Disabilities*. James Stanfield Company. Santa Barbara, CA.

6

Immigrants and ethnic minority populations

Indrani Sheridan, M.D., F.A.C.E.P., F.A.A.E.M.

Goals and objectives

1. To better appreciate the role that culture plays in abuse situations
2. To learn about how a minority patient may perceive the practitioner investigating abuse in order to overcome this potential barrier
3. To understand how the use of a cultural translator may facilitate the practitioner investigating a potentially abusive situation

Introduction

There is culture-based bias in Medicine. Despite our best efforts and intentions, physician–patient miscommunication and misjudgment abound whenever there is a difference in the cultural background of the people.[1–5] Unfortunately, many studies demonstrate that patients belonging to an ethnic minority receive unequal treatment and experience poorer outcomes in their medical treatment.[6–8] Most startling is that this inequity occurs independent of income, insurance, severity of illness, co-morbidities, or any other factors that one might guess could potentially impact care.[9–12]

Simply put, belonging to an ethnic minority group puts patients at increased risk of misdiagnosis, inadequate treatment, poor preventative care, and a greater occurrence of complications.[13,14] Unequal treatment for ethnic minorities and immigrants is well documented in many areas of care, including pain control, treatment of coronary artery disease, and screening for malignancies.[15–17] Of equal, if not greater concern, is the fact that misperceptions and unequal treatment of immigrants and ethnic minorities also occur in the area of abuse.[18–21]

Immigration data show that there are currently about 30 million residents in the United States who are foreign-born. The annual immigration rate is greater than 10 percent.[22,23] The U.S. Department of Commerce predicts that in 50 years, 60 percent of the population in this country will be attributable to immigration and the direct descendants of immigrants.[24]

While the focus of medical training is to prepare doctors to treat organic and functional disease, traditionally very little attention is paid to cultural factors despite the pervasive influence that culture has on presentation, expression, and natural history of disease and injury. In addition, non-verbal communication is often misinterpreted by both the sender and recipient when there is a cross-cultural interaction, particularly when the interaction is highly emotionally charged or reaches into sensitive areas for the interacting cultures. Interpreting these non-verbal cues is an art that is almost completely ignored in medical education, but one that is increasingly necessary as we deal with more and more people from the non-dominant culture. Even when the medical practitioner is not from the dominant culture, most often, the basis of the training that he/she received comes from a White, Western, heterosexual male perspective. This undoubtedly influences interactions with patients on multiple conscious and subconscious levels.

Immigrants, ethnic minorities, and the dominant culture

An immigrant is a person who moves from one country to another country. Most commonly, the cultural background of an immigrant is not the same as the predominant culture in the country to which he/she has moved. This makes immigrants a cultural minority. Within a country, immigrants and ethnic minority populations may overlap. Their members differ technically in definition, yet their issues are largely the same. There are certain characteristic difficulties that are unique to either immigrant or ethnic minority populations, but for the purpose of this chapter, it is useful to consider the terms as interchangeable, and principles discussed as being applicable to both groups.

Distinguishing between minority and dominant cultures is important for delivering the best possible level of care. As noted above, the roots and assumptions of medical training are deeply embedded in the dominant culture and often practitioners may be unaware of how this affects their treatment of patients. Particularly for immigrant and ethnic minority communities, at the very minimum, recognizing that there are cultural differences is the first step toward providing culturally competent care.

Does abuse occur more commonly in ethnic minority populations?

Multiple studies describe the epidemiology of physical abuse, such as domestic violence, sexual assault, child abuse, and the medical and social problems associated with substance abuse.[25–27] Data exists regarding the incidence of abuse among the five main ethnic populations who live in the United States: White Caucasian, African-American, Hispanic, Native American Indian, and Asian.[28–30] However, the occurrence of abuse in immigrant populations has not been as well documented except for studies of very specific, country-related populations, for example in Somali refugees, Haitian, Puerto Rican, and others. Even these studies, however, do not distinguish between ethnic groups coming from the same country.[31,32]

While there are definite trends seen within each minority group, indicating that certain patterns of abuse occur more frequently in sub-populations of cultures, these trends disappear or become secondary to social and environmental factors, education level, and economic status when these are statistically controlled for.[33–35] It appears that the latter factors, particularly poverty, have a more significant impact on the incidence and nature of abuse than does the ethnic group under consideration.[36–38] To express this in another way, within a particular stratum of society, all members share the same risk for occurrence of abuse, independent of culture, and that risk increases as income and education levels decrease.

Reported cases: Just the tip of the iceberg

Apart from the complex reasons that abuse is underreported in general, there are very real problems with both the identification and handling of abuse that are unique to ethnic minority patients. It is impossible to accurately quantify the number of unreported cases. When talking with patients, friends, members of the wider community, and people who may sometimes become involved with abuse cases via a circuitous route (e.g., teachers, coaches, clergy, loan or probation officers), it becomes clear that not only is abuse under-reported, but even when the victim wants to speak up, it is sometimes "swept under the rug," not talked about, not acknowledged, ignored, or downplayed. Worse still, the victim of abuse can be seen to somehow share responsibility for what happened to him/her, made to feel guilty, ashamed, or unworthy.[37–39] The direct and indirect consequences of reporting versus not reporting can make the situation much worse for a victim socially, psychologically, physically, and emotionally. Layering cultural, ethnic, and nationality factors over this multiplies this complexity several-fold.

Some immigrants may be working or living illegally in the United States, or they may believe that they have broken a law (e.g., by failure to pay a fine) and are afraid of being arrested if they provide details about themselves. In many countries, contact with legal authorities is strongly associated with discrimination or oppression. Immigrants may be distrustful or fearful of any encounter that takes place through official channels or involves the police. As a result, they often isolate themselves from the very same services and organizations that could potentially help them.[40,41]

It is important to concede that sometimes immigrants do experience discrimination at the hands of the protective services. When this occurs, the resultant mistrust of police, schools, legal, and social service providers is extremely hard to dispel in these communities. Immigrant women, in particular, are often threatened by their spouses or domestic partners of the consequences they will suffer if they ask for help. Children may be told that the policeman will take them away if they do not behave, hence deepening the distrust for all protective services.

In some cultures it may be considered disrespectful to criticize one's spouse, in-laws, older sibling, or relative, and so reporting abusive behavior becomes problematic for the victim. The victim may be ostracized from the family or social group, lose support, be ridiculed, isolated, or even have the abusive situation escalate.[42,43] In Western, particularly American society, the values of individual freedom, rights, and happiness are paramount. However, many other cultures place the highest value on responsibility to the family, community, or group, as well as respect, steadfastness, and courage. Victims are expected to suffer in silence, try to make the situation better, stay in the abusive situation for the good of the home or the wider family, and avoid scandal or public revelation of a problem that may taint the family's reputation. Additionally, immigrant women often suffer both linguistic and cultural isolation making it almost impossible for them to seek assistance.

Unfortunately, there is sometimes a lack of reporting on the victim's part because the victim believes that nothing can be done to help them. A victim may have witnessed others living through the same form of abuse, (e.g., siblings, a friend, or other women in the community), and know someone who either tolerated the abuse and fared well or badly, or complained and fared very badly as a result. This feeling of helplessness is common among victims of abuse at all levels and is often associated with a feeling of unworthiness of help.

Circumstances like these are hard to change. For the medical profession, changing a deep-rooted cultural norm should not be the goal. A realization on the part of the practitioner that these influences exist goes a long way toward earlier detection or recognition of abuse, more sensitive handling of victims, and a greater understanding of how to work within the given circumstance to best protect the victim.

Hidden barriers to appropriate care

As stated above, minorities of all kinds (both recent immigrants and those who have been here for more than ten years) often receive unequal care. Of note, they frequently bring additional factors to bear during the patient–physician encounter. Such factors make it less likely that medical personnel will be able to detect abuse or handle it within the appropriate culture-specific perspective. The descriptions that follow will examine some of these factors in the hope that through understanding, we can better assist these patients.

Factors that represent barriers to care may include: language discordance, immigration status, legal status, preconceived ideas about a particular group (on both the therapist's and the patient's part), "blind spots" in one's own thinking, lack of knowledge and understanding of common cultural practices, patient's ability to access required care, and as alluded to above, cultural taboos about being a victim, about reporting abuse, or turning in the abuser. There are probably many other factors that we can only begin to suspect or comprehend from the outside. Such factors may make it difficult for a patient to come forward to seek care, and therefore unlikely that physicians would detect abuse situations in such patients.

Dealing with the health care system can be challenging for anyone and particularly for immigrants in the face of language difficulties, inability to pay, lack of familiarity with the resources available to them, and the myriad stressors that can accompany living and working in a new country.[36,44,45] Cultural norms that place the male as head of the household and the spokesperson for all of his dependents make it difficult for battered women and children to speak of the abuse or even to speak of routine illnesses, especially when these topics are of a sensitive nature.

There are often taboos regarding speaking about various subject matters, such as sex, violence, drug use, drinking, family matters, or certain conditions like mental illness. In some cultures, marital rape is not considered rape as it is in the United States context. Developmentally disabled patients may be considered to be the responsibility of the family and hidden from the community. Immigrants may recognize that their practices would be "unacceptable" to the dominant culture and unwilling to disclose these.

At the other extreme are situations where established medical conditions may be ignored because of a cultural belief that this is a good thing, a blessing, or the sufferer is one of the "chosen." An example of this is the Hmong, who sometimes view epilepsy as communication with the higher spirits, and so will not seek medical attention for a child who has recurrent or prolonged seizures. Cultures that are more fatalistic (e.g., Islamic, Latin American), may believe that it is God's will that the patient has these symptoms, that the well-being of the patient is in the hands of God, and that certain interventions are not welcome.

Some ethnic minorities may have an inability to effectively describe or express what is happening to them. This can occur because of naiveté, youth, lack of exposure or education, or skewed expectations and definitions of what is acceptable or normal in a relationship. This can also happen because the interpreter doesn't know the idioms, is too young (e.g., when children are used as interpreters), or the subject matter is too delicate for the person to mention.

Understanding these variables is a daunting task for someone from outside of that culture, because so often, the person is unaware himself/herself of what is happening or find it hard to explain to an "outsider" why this is important to his/her culture.

They may even find it too obvious to require explanation, so both the victim and the health care provider are not aware that key information is missing when trying to understand their patient's needs.

Education is one method of changing behavior. There is no easy substitute for familiarity with the common cultural practices and rituals in which our patients might engage, that could lead either to harm or the appearance of harm.[46] The physician also runs the risk of failure to stop the harmful practice or habit if the patient is under the impression that the physician does not fully understand what is going on or why, and so pays no attention to the advice given. Additional examples of culturally based beliefs that can represent large or small obstacles to communication and patient care are given in Table 6.1.

Whose definition is used? Considering context when suspecting abuse

Understanding the roots or intention of cultural practices is of paramount importance. Without such understanding, one may identify an action as having an intent to abuse or cause harm, when the real purpose is to protect or heal. In some cases, it is possible that there is intent to cause harm, and we may correctly identify abuse and manage the case appropriately. In other cases, injury is a result of complications arising from action or treatment that is intended to relieve symptoms, cure a problem or produce a desirable effect. What constitutes this "desirable effect" is highly culture and time specific.

An example of an intended healing action that could cause harm is a burn that is caused by moxibustion, the process of burning a dried herb, usually mugwort, directly on the skin in order to increase the circulation of "qi" or vital energy within the body. Herbal remedies have always been around, and either by misapplication, overdose, poisoning, or simply because they may not work, findings of abuse may result following their use. Families may try herbal remedies for a long period before consulting with a Western practitioner, at which point, the patient may be beyond the point of regaining full health. These issues also apply to recognized over-the-counter medications used in modern Western society, sometimes leading to poisoning, malnutrition, coagulopathies, bone disorders, and various other maladies.

An example of the second situation, where serious complications and harm can result from the direct and intended effect of treatment, is that of blood-letting. This was a very common practice in the Middle Ages, in order to release bad humors that were present in the body and reestablish a balance of energy. In modern times the cutting of someone in this fashion would prompt allegations of assault. Yet blood-letting was accepted and widely recognized enough to be described as a standard of care.

Table 6.1 Examples of culturally based taboos that can represent large or small obstacles to communication and/or patient care

- Some Arabic men will not let a male physician examine their wife, or do pelvic or rectal examinations.
- Across many cultures, there are various prohibitions about using pork-, beef-, chicken-, horse-, eggs-, or embryo-derived medications (many vaccines, endocrine medications, blood products, and prostheses are derived this way).
- Sikh men are required to grow their hair, and keep it covered in a turban, away from the eyes of anyone other than their spouse.
- Some Islamic women are required to keep their face, head, and the rest of their body fully covered.
- Among the Chinese, it is bad luck to speak of death or dying, and doing so, even for discussing prognosis or for informed consent purposes, may offend, or elicit fear and uneasiness.
- In some East Indian and other Southeast Asian cultures, touching the head or the feet has strong religious, social, or moral meanings and implications, as does direct eye contact.
- There are widespread religious practices involving any death that occurs during certain days of the week, times of the day, or seasons of the year, with a large impact on how the remains are handled by the ED, possibilities for post-mortem, removal of the body, etc.
- Diverse cultures use beads, bracelets, strings, anklets, and amulets to ward off evil. Touching or removing these can incite fear and non-cooperation in patients.
- Vietnamese patients view the physician as an expert. Therefore, diagnosis should be arrived at with limited examination, laboratory data, or other diagnostic tests. If a physician probes a great deal into symptoms he/she may be viewed as incompetent because he/she was not able to arrive at a diagnosis easily or immediately.
- South Asian Hmong parents believe it is bad luck to admire a baby excessively because "spirits" may hear the praise and come to take the baby away. Thus simple praise aimed at putting parents at ease may have the opposite effect.

Many cultures throughout the world engage in practices which may be considered mutilation elsewhere or in a different time. Examples of these include various forms of body piercing, swaddling, binding the skull to mold it to a specific shape, scarification or genital alterations as a right of passage into adulthood, or for example, circumcision for religious or prophylactic health reasons. The latter is viewed in the United States as a beneficial health care practice. Most of the other actions above would be perceived negatively, but they are unlikely to be viewed as abuse by members of the predominant U.S. culture. Female genital mutilation, however, is now considered a human rights violation despite the fact that many immigrant cultures still continue the practice.

Sometimes physical harm can result from cultural practices that are not in themselves abusive. For example, acupuncture can produce infection, and has even been known to cause a pneumothorax. In an effort to be true to their religious beliefs, a Jehovah's Witness may refuse blood transfusion for his/her child resulting in clear and imminent danger to that child. It is therefore important to keep context in mind when we suspect or diagnose or manage abuse. See Table 6.2 for additional examples of alternative medical practices that may lead to a suspicion of abuse.

However safe or unsafe alternative practices might be, it is important to remember that the laws that exist in America today strive to preserve each individual's right to uphold their religious or cultural beliefs and practices as far as possible. Many of the ethnic minority practices are firmly based in written religious beliefs and are defensible in the minds of the people who live by them. Figure 6.1(a–e) illustrates graphically how the beliefs or opinions of various people can vary regarding a particular practice.

Corporal punishment

The issue of corporal punishment is perhaps the most difficult of all. The reader may refer to Fontes (2005) and Straus (2001) for further in-depth reading on this complex issue. There are wide variations both between and within different cultures, as to what is acceptable when punishing wrong behavior in children. To complicate matters further, the definition of abuse spans more than simply applying physical force. Humiliating or threatening a child can certainly be considered abuse, and while even in extreme cases where verbal, emotional, or psychological abuse is clear, what is not at all clear is how we are supposed to handle this situation within our roles as patient advocates and protectors of victims of abuse. Immigrant women who do suffer from verbal, psychological, and emotional abuse are often told by their families, religious advisors, and communities to accept the abuse and be "good wives" or daughters.

There are many factors that lower the threshold for the occurrence of child abuse. While a full discussion of these factors is beyond the scope of this chapter the topic is covered in the child abuse chapter. With regard to the immigrant population there are additional reasons that the potential for abuse may be greater. The most obvious is that parents have very broad discretion in how they discipline their children and the child's behaviors that trigger an occasion for discipline varies enormously from one culture to another. This aspect will be explored in more detail later in this chapter.

Other issues that are more germane to immigrants than the general population are the higher incidence of single-parent families, paternal unemployment,

Table 6.2 Examples of alternative medical practices that may or may not lead to a suspicion of abuse

---

- Hypnosis, aromatherapy, meditation, homeopathy, yoga, and allied physical disciplines.
- Acupuncture: Originating in China more than 2,000 years ago, acupuncture involves stimulation of anatomical points on the body by penetrating the skin with thin, solid, metallic needles that are manipulated by the hands or by electrical stimulation. Imbalance leads to blockage in the flow of "qi" (vital energy) along pathways known as "meridians." It is believed that there are 12 main meridians and 8 secondary meridians and that there are more than 2,000 acupuncture points on the human body that connect with them. Acupuncture restores the delicate balance of two opposing and inseparable forces: yin and yang.
- Cupping: application of a heated cup to the skin, which creates a vacuum as it cools, which may cause the appearance of ecchymoses in the skin. The purpose of cupping is to open the five "meridians" through which healing energy or "qi" can flow to the vital organs.
- Moxibustion: the process of burning a dried herb (usually Mugwort) directly on the skin, or above specific acupuncture points, also to increase the circulation of "qi."
- Ayurvedic medicine: a holistic system of healing that evolved among the Brahmin sages of ancient India some 3000 to 5000 years ago. It focuses on establishing and maintaining balance of the life energies through the use of herbal remedies and various exercises.
- Coining / Cao Gio: Vietnamese, Cambodians, and the people of Laos practice rubbing the skin with a coin to alleviate various common symptoms of illness by releasing excess "wind" or energy considered responsible for illness. The back, neck, head, shoulder, and chest are common sites of application. This procedure often generates skin eruptions in a pine tree pattern with 2 long vertical marks along either side of the spine and several lines paralleling the ribs. Although mimicking the lesions of trauma, it is not a harmful procedure, and no complications are known.
- A few cultures in the Caribbean actively practice Voodoo, with attendant prohibitions and prescriptions involving talismans, amulets, concoctions to drink or apply topically, with attendant resistance to having any of these removed or interfered with during patient care. Many of their rituals involve animals or animal products, with attendant risks of exposure to zoonoses.
- Latino remedies: herbal teas and abdominal massage with oils, or administration of oral substances containing lead, such as greta and azarcon for "Empacho" (blocked intestine); having the child wear an azabache, or seed-like charm, on a necklace or bracelet is believed to protect against "Mal de ojo" (evil eye). "Mollera caida" (fallen fontanelle) is believed to result when an infant pulls away from the breast too quickly, or when a bottle is pulled away from the infant too quickly. Folk remedies to "realign the fontanelle" include sucking on the fontanelle, pushing up against the soft palate, or even hanging the infant over a basin of hot water and tapping the feet.

---

harmless physical finding
e.g. coining

intent was to cause harm ⟷ no intent to cause harm

harmful physical finding
e.g. death

harmless physical finding

intent was to cause harm ⟷ no intent to cause harm

harmful physical finding

harmless physical finding

intent was to cause harm ⟷ no intent to cause harm

harmful physical finding

Figure 6.1a–e   Whose definition of abuse do we use?

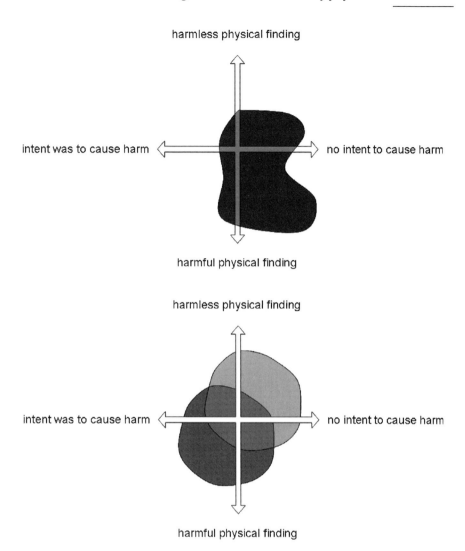

harmless physical finding

intent was to cause harm

no intent to cause harm

harmful physical finding

harmless physical finding

intent was to cause harm

no intent to cause harm

harmful physical finding

Figure 6.1a–e   (*continued*)

poverty, having multiple jobs with little time to spend with children, or very little time for recreational activities as a family, social isolation, prejudice, inadequate housing, and lack of a strong social network to support the family in times of stress.[43,47]

Fontes makes the point that cultural minorities who engage in physical abuse fall into four major categories. These categories are important because they can be used to guide intervention and preventive measures.

The first category consists of people who are excellent parents in every other way, who have high ideals for their children and are very supportive, but their authoritarian style of discipline is "heavy-handed." These parents require restructuring in their discipline practices by providing alternative ways to handle disobedience or disruptive behavior in their children.

The second category consists of religious groups who believe in the value of severe corporal punishment or other child rearing practices that society considers dangerous. Interventions with this group are particularly difficult, most often ineffective, and limited in scope by the nature of their belief system. Laws exist in the United States to protect and uphold religious freedom, and it becomes difficult to design a clear algorithm for the evaluation of potential abuse and subsequent intervention. A constructive way of dealing with these situations stems from the observation that every culture has norms that raise the risk of abuse for children as well as values that have the potential to protect children from abuse. The most effective interventions use this method to leverage change by appealing to the values that are in line with the hoped-for outcome.

The third group represents those caretakers who are struggling with extreme poverty, mental illness, substance abuse, or other severe stressors, who cannot effectively handle parenting issues without resorting to violence or abuse. In these cases, restructuring or addressing the environmental issues is an essential part of addressing the abuse. Without attention to these details, educational interventions are likely to be minimally effective or longstanding.[49]

The fourth group comprises parents who punish their children in cruel or malicious ways that would be considered abusive in any culture.

There is another facet to consider in understanding the immigrant parent being investigated for abuse by a Western practitioner. Many common child rearing practices in America may be seen as cruel or abusive by other cultures. It is hard for immigrants to process the suggestion that they may be subjecting their child, spouse, or elderly parent to abuse when they perceive their health care provider is guilty of similar activities. Examples of Western practices that might be seen as abusive: sending children to bed without supper to punish disobedience, giving them "timeout" standing in the corner, forbidding play outdoors, withholding lunch money, taking away toys, leaving children to sleep alone, allowing babies to cry themselves to sleep. The idea that a sitter or preschool teacher functions as the primary caretaker while the parents work is considered neglectful or uncaring by certain cultures. These cultures place children and their needs at the very center of societal structure. Western parents are often perceived as lacking warmth and ineffective in raising their own children. Certain behaviors, such as temper tantrums reinforce this view by other cultures. A health care provider from the dominant Anglo-American culture may lack credibility in dispensing advice in such circumstances.

Ultimately, familiarity with cultural norms may help us to distinguish between punishment techniques that are typical for that ethnic group from those that are unusual and might warrant suspicion of abuse.[48] There are no easy answers to this sensitive issue, except possibly universal prohibition of any kind of physical discipline and substituting alternative, more acceptable methods to accomplish the same goal.

Language barriers

By law, language interpreters should be made available to all patients seeking medical services.[50] In reality, this is not the norm, particularly in smaller towns and rural areas. Few hospitals have interpreters on hand at all times (although some staff may speak other languages). Some hospitals have a pool of interpreters from which to draw but these are often not "on call" and available to the emergency medicine department in a timely enough manner. Very few hospitals are able to find and provide interpreters for the less commonly taught languages and even when the language can be interpreted, the culture may not be. For example, there is a distinct difference in culture and language between Puerto Rican and Honduran Spanish and between Christians and Muslim Arabs. Certain software solutions such as those produced by companies such as MedBridge (http://www.inocom.com), attempt to bridge the gap in time between when the patients first present and when a live translator can be produced. As these programs develop in depth and sophistication, the thrust is to incorporate as much culturally based information as possible into its function, applying well-known cultural norms and standards to better facilitate communication between doctors and patients.

Some victims may prefer an ethnically different therapist. They perceive someone outside their community as being more objective and able to maintain confidentiality.[51] However, others feel that only a person of their ethnic background can understand the issues involved and know what to do. Setting up the right blend of patient and therapist is not always within our control, but it is important to get an optimal match if at all possible.

There is no doubt that the involvement of a trained interpreter is an essential part of the cross-cultural clinical encounter for therapeutic reasons. Studies have also noted marked increase in satisfaction on the part of patients, even to the extent of relief of symptoms without the administration of medication.[19,52]

Legal requirements

It is very important to understand the state and federal laws pertaining to reporting abuse or suspected abuse. While there may be slight variations locally, the laws and regulations concerning reporting are clear and consistent. However, the manner in which the physician and her/his team interpret or apply these laws, particularly when dealing with immigrant patients or their families, can sometimes be problematic.

Title VI of the 1964 Civil Rights Act and additional federal legislation signed by President Clinton in 2001 confirm the rights of peoples with limited English proficiency to various kinds of services including health care.[53] These services must include informing immigrants of their rights and the right to an interpreter.[37] On the other side of the matter, all 50 states have statutes regarding reporting requirements for suspected abuse and neglect. In the case of child abuse, all health workers are required to report suspected cases. Problems arise when the need for interpretation of both language and culture is combined with suspected abuse and the health team is not prepared to deal with all of these tangled aspects. Other chapters in this text speak more specifically to the legal aspects of reporting abuse. We will focus here on the areas where intercultural communication and cultural competence become key to treating the patient, the family, and the situation.

The case of illegal immigrants

Immigrants are often suspicious if not fearful of authority in all its guises. They may have come to the United States from countries where the law and police are not to be trusted. They may have suffered abuse themselves at the hands of presumed or actual authorities in their original countries. It becomes particularly difficult to treat suspected cases of abuse when the person or his/her family members are illegal. Patients may have been warned or threatened by the abuser, family members, or even their community that they will either be deported, their partners deported, or their children removed from their care if they seek health care for reasons of abuse. The abuser may hide or destroy important documents or refuse to sign papers. For these reasons, federal law has been specifically modified to protect battered and abused women and their children.[41]

For women who are married to U.S. citizens or lawful permanent residents, new federal laws provide some protection. Modifications to both immigration laws and the passage of the Violence Against Women Act in 1994 provide various forms of legal relief and services to both immigrant men and women victims of domestic violence.[54] These are bolstered, in most states, with additional support that allows the battered patient to access services (e.g., shelters, financial support) and legal means to prevent deportation. The state courts do not determine immigration issues but rather focus on enhancing the safety of the battered patient.[54] Equally as important to the battered patient is that state and local law enforcement officials are not required to contact the Immigration and Naturalization Service (INS), and are more interested in protecting the safety and health of the battered patient. Communicating this notion of safety and safeguards to the patient is of utmost importance in promoting trust and full disclosure of whatever has led up to the abuse situation.

For illegal immigrants, there are few legal remedies or recourse. They do face the possibility of deportation. Nevertheless, most health care providers and local law enforcement officials are more interested in getting the patient's medical needs addressed as a priority.

Working toward equality for immigrants and cultural minorities

Based on research the following policy recommendations are suggested[41,55,56]:

There needs to be improved research on immigrants and ethnic minority populations. Specifically, more information is needed on prevalence and incidence of partner violence, nature and characteristics of abuse, contributing factors, and culturally appropriate education concerning partner violence. "Culturally competent" shelters and counseling services should be established. Finally, the factors that contribute to partner violence among ethnic minorities, such as poverty and lack of educational and economic opportunities must be addressed. For the physician, educational efforts must begin in medical school and be an integral part of the continuing medical education process, so that as new information is obtained, and population characteristics shift, every physician is able to adjust their knowledge base and practice appropriately. Providing ready access to cultural data must be made a priority, especially for those who work in the emergency setting, or who see large populations of immigrants or ethnic minorities in their everyday practice.

Effecting change: Working toward cultural competence

Increased physician awareness and behavior modification can potentially lead to greater recognition of abuse, and avoidance of the potential to suspect abuse because of a misunderstanding of certain cultural norms. Ideally, as we learn more about the cultural norms of various ethnic minorities, we will become better in the role of recognition and treatment, with appropriate referrals and follow-up care. Identification of medical, social, emotional, and economic complicating factors can help us to deal more effectively with victims of abuse, to minimize the chance of recurrence.[46]

It is important that the therapist is aware of culturally appropriate interventions that may be used with ethnic minorities when appropriate.[49] Culturally sensitive practice is described as awareness that race, social class, ethnic group membership, and cultural background must be taken into consideration in understanding the client's lifestyle and value system. Support groups can reduce the level of isolation and provide valuable resources to the victim in the event of community ostracism. Emergency physicians and teams should be aware of such types of support services if these are available for ethnic minorities and immigrants.

Conclusion

When working with people from different cultural groups it is easy to assume that behaviors that run contrary to our expectations are culturally based. Social factors beyond income and education are also very important. These include factors such as illiteracy, immigration experiences, religion, social stressors, and social support networks. As practitioners, we need to be sensitive to the cultural traditions that are different from Euro-American norms, and exercise caution in concluding that everything that appears to be abusive, is in fact abuse. It is also equally important for us to be able to recognize the potential for harm occurring in a patient as a result of practices common to his/her particular ethnic background. There also may be systemic variables that play a significant role in determining behavior. These can be macro-systemic, that is, based on historical and cultural practices or micro-systemic, that is, that stem from the family structure.[57] The immigrant/ethnic minority patient that presents to the Emergency Department is embedded in a system made more complicated by the factors outlined above.

While it is not practical to learn everything there is to know about all of the ethnic minorities that present to our Emergency Departments, it is mandatory to be familiar with the central beliefs, customs, and habits of the people who come most often to us for treatment.[46,58] Any intervention that is culturally sensitive must be user-friendly. The client must feel welcome, respected, understood, not blamed or shamed, and the logistics of complying with the intervention must be practical and attainable for the persons involved in order for it to be effective.[37,40,59,60] In our well-meaning attempt to serve and protect all of our patients from harm, it is also necessary to respect their cultural boundaries, be uncritical of their practices, and to work in tandem with them to help them safely navigate through our complex health care system.[61] Table 6.3 suggests some examples of useful questions to keep in mind during the cross-cultural medical interview. In light of our power to effect dramatic change in the lives of our patients, we have a compelling obligation to examine our personal assumptions about race and ethnicity, and to match our medical knowledge with familiarity with the cultural norms and practices of our patients. As a matter of social justice and in order to provide the best possible medical care, we owe them no less than this.

Table 6.3 Cross-cultural interview questions*

What do you call this illness?

What do you think has caused this illness?

Why do you think this illness started when it did?

What problems do you think this illness causes? How does it work?

How severe is this illness?

How long do you think it will last?

What kind of treatment do you think is needed?

What are the most important results you hope for with treatment?

What do you fear most about the illness?

*Kleinman A, Eisenberg L, Good, B. Culture, illness, and care: clinical lessons from anthropologic and cross-cultural research. *Annals of Internal Medicine*. February 1978; 88: 251–8.

References

1. Abreu JM. Conscious and nonconscious African American stereotypes: impact on first impression and diagnostic ratings by therapist. *Journal of Consulting and Clinical Psychology*. June 1999; 67(3): 387–93.

2. James TL, Feldman J, Mehta SD. Physician variability in history taking when evaluating patients presenting with chest pain in the emergency department. *Academic Emergency Medicine*. February 2006; 13(2): 147–52.

3. Lane WG, Rubin DM, Monteith R, Christian CW. Racial differences in the evaluation of pediatric fractures for physical abuse. *Journal of the American Medical Association*. October 2, 2002; 288: 1603–09.

4. McKinlay JB, Potter DA, Feldman HA. Non-medical influences on medical decision-making. *Social Science & Medicine*. March 1996; 42: 769–76.

5. Van Ryn M, Burke J. The effect of patient race and socioeconomic status on physician's perceptions of patients. *Social Science & Medicine*. 2000; 50: 813–28.

6. Finucane TE, Carrese JA. Racial bias in presentation or cases. *Journal of General Internal Medicine*. March–April 1990; 5: 120–1.

7. Kleinman A, Eisenberg L, Good B. Culture, illness, and care: Clinical lessons from anthropologic and cross-cultural research. *Annals of Internal Medicine*. February 1978; 88: 251–8.

8. Smedley BD, Stith AY, Nelson AR. *Unequal Treatment: Confronting Racial and Ethnic Disparities in Health Care*. Institute of Medicine. Washington, DC: The National Academies Press, 2003.

9. Daumit GL, Powe NR. Factors influencing access to cardiovascular procedures in patients with chronic kidney disease: race, sex, and insurance. *Seminars in Nephrology*. July 2001; 21: 367–76.

10. Epstein AM, Ayanian JZ, Keogh JH, et al. Racial disparities in access to renal transplantation – clinically appropriate or due to underuse or overuse? *The New England Journal of Medicine*. November 23, 2000; 343(21): 1537–44.

11. Gornick ME, Eggers PW, Reilly TW, et al. Effects of race and income on mortality and use of services among Medicare beneficiaries. *The New England Journal of Medicine*. September 12, 1996; 335(11): 791–9.
12. Roetzheim RG, Pal N, Tennant C, et al. Effects of health insurance and race on early detection of cancer. *Journal of the National Cancer Institute*. 1999; 91(16): 1409–15.
13. Cone DC, Richardson LD, Todd KH, Betancourt JR, Lowe RA. Health care disparities in emergency medicine. *Academic Emergency Medicine*. November 2003; 10(11): 1176–83.
14. Johnson PA, Lee TH, Cook EF, Rouan GW, Goldman L. Effect of race on the presentation and management of patients with acute chest pain. *Annals of Internal Medicine*. April 15, 1993; 118(8): 593–601.
15. Todd KH, Lee T, Hoffman JR. The effect of ethnicity on physician estimates of pain severity in patients with isolated extremity trauma. *The Journal of the American Medical Association*. March 1994; 271: 925–8.
16. Todd KH. Pain assessment and ethnicity. *Annals of Emergency Medicine*. April 1996; 27: 421–3.
17. Todd KH, Deaton C, D'Adamo AP, Goe L. Ethnicity and analgesic practice. *Annals of Emergency Medicine*. January 2000; 35(1): 11–6.
18. Ayanian JZ, Udvarhelyi IS, Gatsonis CA, Pashos CL, Epstein AM. Racial differences in the use of revascularization procedures after coronary angiography. *The Journal of the American Medical Association*. May 26, 1993; 269(20): 2642–6.
19. Kressin NR, Petersen LA. Racial differences in the use of invasive cardiovascular procedures: review of the literature and prescription for future research. *Annals of Internal Medicine*. September 4, 2001; 135(5): 352–66.
20. Miner J, Biros MH, Trainor A, Hubbard D, Beltram M. Patient and physician perceptions as risk factors for Oligoanalgesia: A prospective observational study of the relief of pain in the emergency department. *Academic Emergency Medicine*. February 2006; 13(2): 140–6.
21. Nazroo JY. The structuring of ethnic inequalities in health: economic position, racial discrimination, and racism. *American Journal of Public Health*. February 2003; 93(2): 277–84.
22. Schmidley AD. (2001). Profile of the foreign-born population in the United States: 2000. 2001 Current Population Reports, Series P23-206. Washington, DC: U.S. Census Bureau.
23. U.S. Census Bureau (2004). Annual Estimates of the Population by Sex, Race and Hispanic or Latino Origin for the United States: April 1, 2000 to July 1, 2003 (NC-EST2003-03). Available on: http://www.census.gov/main/www/cen2000.html. Accessed April 26, 2007.
24. U.S. Bureau of the Census, U.S. Department of Commerce (1996). Population projections of the United States by age, sex, race, and Hispanic origin: 1995 to 2050. Current Population Report, 25-1130.
25. O'Keefe M. Racial/ethnic differences among battered women and their children. *Journal of Child and Family Studies*. 1994; 3(3): 283–305.
26. Richie BE, Kanuha V. (1993) Battered women of color in public health care systems: racism, sexism, and violence. In *Wings of Gauze: Women of Color and the Experience of Health and Illness*, ed. B. Blair & S. E. Cayleff. Detroit, MI: Wayne State University Press, pp. 288–99.

27. West CM. Partner Violence in Ethnic Minority Families. Family Research Laboratory, University of New Hampshire. Available on: http://www.agnr.umd.edu/nnfr/research/pv/pv_ch7.html. Accessed January 29, 2007.

28. Bachman R. (1993). *Death and Violence on the Reservation: Homicide, Family Violence, and Suicide in American Indian Populations.* Westport, CT: Auburn House.

29. Buchwald D, Tomita S, Hartman S, Furman R, Dudden M, Manson SM. Physical abuse of urban Native Americans. *Journal of General Internal Medicine.* August 2000; 15(8): 562–4.

30. Suitor JJ, Pillemer K, Straus MA. Marital violence in a life course perspective. In *Physical Violence in American Families: Risk Factors and Adaptations to Violence in 8,145 Families*, ed. M. A. Straus & R. J. Gelles. New Brunswick, NJ, 1990: Transaction, pp. 305–19.

31. Abraham M. (2000). *Speaking the Unspeakable: Marital Violence among South Asian Immigrants in the United States.* New Brunswick, New Jersey: Rutgers University Press.

32. McFarlane J, Wiist W, Watson M. Characteristics of sexual abuse against pregnant Hispanic women by their male intimates. *Journal of Women's Health.* August 1998; 7(6): 739–45.

33. Asbury J. Violence in families of color in the United States. In *Family violence: Prevention and Treatment*, ed. R. L. Hampton, T. P. Gullota, G. R. Adams, E. H. Potter, & R. P. Weissberg. Newbury Park, CA: Sage, 1993, pp. 159–78.

34. Brice-Baker JR. Domestic violence in African-American and African-Caribbean families. *Journal of Social Distress and the Homeless.* 1994; 3(1): 23–38.

35. Caetano R, Schafer J, Cunradi CB. Alcohol-related intimate partner violence among White, Black and Hispanic couples in the United States. *Alcohol Research & Health.* 2001; 25(1): 58–65.

36. Cazenave NA, Straus MA. Race, class, network embeddedness and family violence: a search for potent support systems. In *Physical Violence in American families*, ed. M. A. Straus & R. J. Gelles. New Brunswick, NJ, 1990: Transaction, pp. 321–40.

37. Fontes LA. *Child Abuse and Culture: Working with Diverse Families.* New York: Guilford, 2005.

38. Futa KT, Hsu E, Hansen DJ. Child sexual abuse in Asian American families: an examination of cultural factors that influence prevalence, identification, and treatment. *Clinical Psychology: Science and Practice.* 2001; 8(2): 189–209.

39. Kanuha V. Sexual assault in Southeast Asian communities: issues in intervention. *Response to Victimization of Women and Children.* 1987; 10(3): 4–6.

40. Fontes LA. Child discipline and physical abuse in immigrant Latino families: reducing violence and misunderstanding. *Journal of Counseling and Development.* 2002; 80: 31–40.

41. Franco FE. Unconditional safety for conditional immigrant women. *Berkeley Women's Law Journal.* 1996; 11: 99–141.

42. Feiring C, Coates DL, Taska LS. Ethnic status, stigmatization, support, and symptom development following sexual abuse. *Journal of Interpersonal Violence.* 2001; 16(12): 1307–29.

43. Fontes LA. Disclosures of sexual abuse by Puerto-Rican children: oppression and cultural barriers. *Journal of Child Sexual Abuse.* 1993; 2(1): 21–35.

44. Kanuha V. Women of color in battering relationships. In *Women of color: Integrating ethnic and gender identities in psychotherapy*, ed. L. Comas-Diaz & B. Greene. New York: Guilford Press, 1994, pp. 428–54.

45. Zayas LH. Childrearing, social stress, and child abuse: clinical considerations with Hispanic families. *Journal of Social Distress and the Homeless*. 1992; 1(3–4): 291–309.

46. Sheridan I. Treating the world without leaving your ED: opportunities to deliver culturally competent care. *Academic Emergency Medicine*. August 2006; 13(8): 896–903.

47. Johnson D. Stress, depression, substance abuse, and racism. *American Indian and Alaska Native Mental Health Research*. 1994; 6(1): 29–33.

48. Fontes LA. *Sexual Abuse in Nine North American Cultures: Treatment and Prevention*. California: Sage, 1995.

49. Garbarino J, Ebata A. The significance of ethnic and cultural differences in child maltreatment. *Journal of Marriage and the Family*. 1983; 45(4): 773–83.

50. U.S. Department of Health and Human Services, Office of Civil Rights (1998). Guidance Memorandum on Prohibition against National Origin Discrimination: Persons with limited English proficiency. Washington, DC. Available at http://www.hhs.gov/ocr/lep. Accessed Feb 24, 2007.

51. Cooper-Patrick L, Gallo JJ, Gonzales JJ, et al. Race, gender, and partnership in the patient–physician relationship. *The Journal of the American Medical Association*. August 11,1999; 282(6): 583–9.

52. Baker DW, Hayes R, Fortier JP. Interpreter use and satisfaction with interpersonal aspects of care for Spanish-speaking patients. *Med Care*. October 1998; 36: 1461–70.

53. Title VI of the Civil Rights Act of 1964. Policy Guidance on the Prohibition Against National Origin Discrimination as it Affects Persons with Limited English Proficiency, 65 Federal Register 52,762 (August 30, 2000). Available at: www.hhs.gov/ocr/lep/guide.html. Accessed February 10, 2006.

54. Weissman DM. Addressing domestic violence in immigrant communities. *Popular Government*. 2000; 65: 13–18.

55. Jasinski JL. *Structural inequalities, family and cultural factors, and spousal violence among Anglo and Hispanic Americans*. Doctoral Dissertation, University of New Hampshire, Durham. 1996.

56. Williams OJ. Domestic partner abuse treatment programs and cultural competence: the results of a national survey. *Violence and Victims*. 1994; 9(3): 287–296.

57. Yick AG. Feminist theory and status inconsistency theory: application to domestic violence in Chinese immigrant families. *Violence Against Women*. 2001; 7: 545–62.

58. Terao SY, Borrego J, Urquiza AJ. A reporting and response model for culture and child maltreatment. *Child Maltreatment*. May 2001; 6(2): 158–68.

59. Walker LEA. *Abused Women and Survivor Therapy*. Washington, DC: American Psychological Association. 1994.

60. Williams EE, Ellison F. Culturally informed social work practice with American Indian clients: guidelines for non-Indian social workers. *Social Work*. 1996; 41(2): 147–51.

61. Brach C, Fraser I. Can cultural competency reduce racial and ethnic health disparities? A review and conceptual model. *Medical Care Research and Review*. 2000; 57(Suppl. 1): 181–217.

62. Behl LE, Crouch JL, May PF, Valente AL, Conyngham HA. Ethnicity in child maltreatment research: a content analysis. *Child Maltreatment*. 2001; 6(2): 143–7.

63. Boudewyn AC, Liem JH. Childhood sexual abuse as a precursor to depression and self-destructive behavior in adulthood. *Journal of Traumatic Stress*. July 1995; 8(3): 445–59.

64. Field CA, Caetano R. Longitudinal model predicting partner violence among white, black, and Hispanic couples in the United States. *Alcoholism: Clinical and Experimental Research*. 2003; 27(9): 1451–8.

65. Field C, Caetano R. Ethnic differences in intimate partner violence in the U.S. general population. The role of alcohol use and socioeconomic status. *Trauma, Violence, & Abuse*. 2004; 5(4): 303–17.

66. Straus MA, Donnelly DA. *Beating the Devil Out of Them: Corporal Punishment in American Families and its Effect on Children*, 2nd edn. New York: Lexington Books, 2001.

67. Weinick RM, Zuvekas SH, Cohen JW. Racial and ethnic differences in access to and use of health care services, 1977 to 1996. *Medical Care Research and Review*. 2000; 57(suppl. 1): 36–54.

Quick Reference Pages

Many cultural practices fall into one or another of the categories above, somewhere along a continuum of intent to harm and no intent to harm on one axis, and on another axis, actions that produce physical findings on examination on one end of the spectrum, to those that produce no physical evidence whatsoever, on the other. Very few practices that are unique to a particular culture (as opposed to fairly universal or ubiquitous) consist of a single point along one or another of these axes, or on the plane. The drawings below attempt to illustrate how one behavior, custom, or action may result in a blend of intention and result, leaning more or less prominently into one or more quadrant. Various examples are proposed, illustrating the complexity of the "real-life" situations that clinicians face in trying to decide whether or not an action represents an occurrence of abuse.

To make matters even more complicated, various participants may view the same action as being represented on completely different or partially overlapping parts of the diagram. For example, the "accused" may have one view of his/her action, the "victim" another, and the physician a third. In this scenario, another physician, for example, may have yet a fourth opinion that differs entirely from the other three! Whose definition of abuse is correct? Is there a universally accepted method for determining this answer? Unfortunately, even in purely clinical terms there is not.

Examples may include:

Body piercing (earrings in children), tattoos, ritual scarification, circumcision, hair removal, exposing children intentionally to someone who is sick so that they may develop immunity (e.g., to chickenpox)

Examples may include:

Physical abuse as punishment (beatings, non-accidental burns, chaining someone to the bed or floor, locking a child in a basement without access to sunlight), sexual assault, domestic violence or marital rape

Examples may include:

Exposing someone to second-hand smoke, thereby increasing his/her risk of cancer, reactive airway disease, or other toxicities; not using adequate sunscreen on a child or disabled person leading to severe sunburn; inadequate supervision around a swimming pool, a park, a public street, or in the home around potentially toxic or high accident-prone areas; inadequate nutrition because of religious, social, or other reasons leading to vitamin deficiencies, growth retardation, or disease; child rearing practices that may put children at risk of harm, for example, diluting formula with too much water to save money, swaddling, re-using disposable items

Examples may include:

The classic example of this situation is corporal punishment. There are often as many opinions as to what is acceptable as there are people involved. Often, as explained before, there is no universally accepted set of rules or guidelines for determining what is appropriate, within the "grey areas," even though in most cases, the extreme ends of the spectrum are easier to define. In this climate of uncertainty there is an ongoing effort to at least design a practical algorithm which a clinician may use in determining when to activate the ancillary services related to abuse. In the previous diagram, the different colors may represent the interpretation of a single behavior by two different people, for example, a parent and the physician treating the child.

7

Care of victims of torture

Moira Davenport, M.D.

Goals and objectives

1. To learn what types of torture exist and screen patients who are potential survivors of torture
2. To understand the acute and chronic effects of torture on patients
3. To learn how to treat, document, and refer survivors of torture

'Medicine and torture both hold a topographical affinity for each other in the sense that both reside and 'colonise' the private space of the sentient body of a human being: one to save a life and the other to destroy it.'

– Merlau-Ponty[1] (Vinar, 2005)

The recent atrocities at Abu Ghraib have once again focused attention on victims of torture. Photographs from this prison site vividly illustrate the immediate physical damage sustained by victims of torture; however, these pictures do not fully illustrate the extensive long-term medical and psychological injuries sustained by these individuals. Furthermore, most victims of torture do not present in such a dramatic fashion. The United Nations (UN) High Commission of Refugees estimates that worldwide there were 9.7 million victims of torture in 2004 and Amnesty International estimates that 104 countries still practice some form of torture today.[2,3] As victims of torture often flee their homeland after the abuse, physicians worldwide should be familiar with the medical needs of torture victims. This chapter will familiarize physicians with the current definitions of torture and types of torture used today as well as common medical and psychological concerns of these individuals.

Following the Nuremberg trials, the United Nations has played a key role in defining torture and in delineating means to prevent its practice worldwide. The Office of the High Commission for Human Rights defines torture as "every act conducted intentionally which causes severe pain or suffering, whether physical or mental, in order to obtain confession or information from somebody or a third person punishing him for an act he or a third person has committed or is suspected of having committed, or intimidating or coercing him or a third person, or for any reason based on discrimination of any kind, when such pain or suffering is inflicted by or at the instigation of or with the consent or acquiescence of a public official or other person acting in an official capacity." It does not include the pain or suffering arising from, inherent in, or incidental to lawful sanctions.[4]

The United Nations High Commission for Refugees (UNHCR) defines refugee as any person who has 'a well-founded fear of being persecuted for reasons of race, religion, nationality, membership of a particular social group or political opinion, is outside the country of his nationality and is unable, or owing to such fear, is unwilling to avail himself of the protection of that country; or who, not having a nationality and being outside the country of his former habitual residence as a result of such events is unable, or owing to such fear, is unwilling to return to it.'[4]

The UNHCR also states that 'No State Party shall expel, return ("refouler") or extradite a person to another State where there are substantial grounds for believing that he would be in danger of being subjected to torture.'[4]

The UN recommends guidelines for investigating claims of torture which may be helpful for the medical practitioner evaluating a potential victim of torture:

1. Clarification of the facts. Establishment and acknowledgement of individual and State responsibility for victims and their families.
2. Identification of measures needed to prevent recurrence.
3. Facilitation of prosecution and/or, as appropriate, disciplinary sanctions for those indicated by the investigation as being responsible. Demonstration of the need for full reparation and redress from the State, including fair and adequate financial compensation plus provision of the means for medical care and rehabilitation.
4. The investigative authority shall have the power and obligation to obtain all the information necessary to the inquiry. They shall also have the authority to oblige all those acting in an official capacity allegedly involved in torture or ill-treatment to appear and testify. The same shall apply to all witnesses.
5. Alleged victims of torture or ill-treatment, witnesses, those conducting the investigation and their families shall be protected from violence, threats of violence or any other form of intimidation that may arise pursuant to the investigation. Persons potentially implicated in torture or ill-treatment shall be removed from any position of control or power, whether direct or indirect, over complainants, witnesses and their families, as well as those conducting the investigation.
6. Alleged victims of torture or ill-treatment and their legal representatives shall be informed of, and have access to, any hearing, as well as to all information relevant to the investigation, and shall be entitled to present other evidence.
7. Medical experts involved in the investigation of torture or ill-treatment shall behave at all times in conformity with the highest ethical standards and, in

particular, shall obtain informed consent before any examination is undertaken. The examination must conform to established standards of medical practice. In particular, examinations shall be conducted in private under the control of the medical expert and outside the presence of security agents and other government officials.[5]

The difference between a refugee and an asylum seeker

The UN defines refugees as 'any individual outside of the country of nationality who is unable or unwilling to return because of persecution or a well-founded fear of persecution on account of race, religion, nationality, membership in a particular social group, or political opinion.' Those granted asylum are afforded country-specific political protections; however, not all refugees apply for asylum. An asylum seeker usually has more legal protections and options until asylum has been granted or denied than a refugee who has not applied for asylum.

Based on the UN guidelines, each country has its own policies on victims of torture/asylum seekers/refugee health. An interesting side note to the above guidelines is that although 'a state may have an obligation not to deport, but the question remains as to what extent it is then responsible to take measures allowing the individual to exist and subsist.'[6]

The United States has a long history of banning torture starting with the Constitution; the 5th Amendment ('the prohibition against self-incrimination was adopted specifically to prohibit the use of torture to extract confessions') and the 8th Amendment ('prohibiting cruel and unusual punishment') are clearly written to protect against torture.[7] This theme has been repeated, both through state criminal laws banning assault and battery, and Congress ratifying both the Torture Victim Protection Act (1991) and the International Convention against Torture and Other Cruel, Inhuman or Degrading Treatment or Punishment (1994).[7]

As a medical practitioner, it is helpful to know that most victims of torture do undergo a rudimentary medical screening in their country of residence before being allowed to immigrate to the 'safe' country. This is done primarily to rule out infectious diseases, such as tuberculosis, leprosy, and HIV.[8] Based on the victim's country of origin, permission to travel may be granted once treated for any active infection. Extent of screening varies from country to country based on national resources and on the political situation.

Current requirements for the medical evaluation of torture victims in the European Union

The European Union (EU) states that 'member states shall ensure that applicants receive the necessary health care, which shall include at least emergency care and essential treatment of illness.[9] Norredam evaluated trends in EU countries, which received 282,480 applications for asylum in 2004.[2] They found that all EU countries require some form of medical screening of asylum seekers. This was variability in methodology including systemic screening (Nordic countries) and screening only at reception centers (Austria, France, Spain, and Britain). The specific government agencies responsible for screening also varied, with federal governments controlling some programs and state governments controlling others.

Screening for specific conditions varied widely, with no country requiring both physical and mental screening. Only 77 percent of countries actually required a physical examination as part of the screening program and 61 percent required psychological testing as part of the screening program. Considering that one in six asylum seekers has a severe physical problem and two-thirds have experienced psychological problems, it is likely that large numbers of asylum seekers are not receiving the care they need under the current screening guidelines. It may be helpful in evaluating these patients to remember that their prior medical screening may have neglected their mental health or physical health issues.

Medical care for torture victims in Australia and New Zealand

Australia and New Zealand have similar deficits in evaluating the health care of torture victims. All immigrants to Australia are first evaluated by the Department of Immigration, Multicultural, and Indigenous Affairs (DIMIA) and then by the Refugee Review Tribunal (RRT). This two-tiered system is designed to be non-adversarial yet still determine if the applicant faces a real chance of persecution. The process also accepts that 'an individual can have a well founded fear of persecution even though the possibility of the persecution occurring is well below 50 percent.'[10] However, even with these guidelines, there is 'no requirement for decision makers to seek expert psychological evidence even in situations where applicants present with complex trauma histories.' In fact, there are no specific parameters that must be met in the medical care afforded to refugees in Australia.[10,11]

Financial concerns of providing health care to asylum seekers

Controversy exists in that several countries limit access to health care for certain subpopulations of asylum seekers. Among EU countries, the most common limitation applied is that asylum seekers are only eligible for emergency medical care. Other nations limit the health care available to pregnant women and to children. Torture victims may also have limited access to immigration opportunities and to health care based on their medical conditions. This is particularly evident with HIV+ individuals. In 1996 the UNHCR met with representatives of the Australian and New Zealand governments to discuss the issue of providing care to refugees and the potentially devastating financial costs of meeting all their health care needs, 'if issues of public health became linked in the minds of the public with refugee resettlement, there would be an adverse reaction which could have devastating consequences on resettlement itself' and that the countries 'can't afford to become the world's infirmary.'[12] These discussions contributed to the development of the UNHCR developing a quota system to determine the number of refugees a country could safely accept and assimilate each year.[12]

Types of torture

It may be helpful in evaluating a potential victim to understand the types of torture used and the injury patterns associated with them.

Several classes of torture are used around the world. Several varieties of direct torture are commonly practiced. Burning, administration of electrical shocks, and physical mutilation (particularly of the genitals) often lead to deformities easily detected on physical examination. Electrical shocks may be delivered in one of two ways. The first is via direct application of electrode to the victim's body (picana) and the other is done by strapping the victim into a metal chair or bed and running the current through the furniture/body circuit (parilla). Physical findings may vary based on the type of application used.

Other forms of direct torture such as beating (with objects or via punching), binding, blunt head trauma, kicking, or prolonged suspension may produce temporary evidence of trauma such as abrasions and ecchymoses. The object used to beat victims of torture varies between countries. Bamboo or other wood sticks are commonly used in Africa, while the lathi (a long, pointed wooden stick) is the preferred weapon in Bangladesh. Rifle butts are another commonly used object, as are the fists of the abuser.[13] These methods of abuse also illustrate the importance of diagnostic adjuncts, such as radiographic imaging, to the physical examination. Although visible evidence of trauma may have resolved, healing fractures in a pattern consistent with the report of abuse may help to confirm a victim's history. Binding, another form of direct trauma, may produce long-term soft tissue damage, particularly at involved joints.

Water is another popular medium used in torture. The most basic method of water torture involves withholding water from the victim, leading to severe dehydration. Victims are often submerged in large bodies of water; this water is often polluted with human excrement, human bodies, and other pollutants. Lastly, 'water torture' involves pouring water, often hot and/or polluted, into the victim's nose and/or mouth, creating the sensation of choking or drowning (this method has also been called water boarding).

Psychological torture includes threats (against self or against family members), witnessing the torture of others (especially family members), mock execution, and near drowning.

Sensory deprivation is a form of psychological torture, and includes blindfolding and isolation.

Some methods of torture combine physical and psychological components. Exposure is an example of this combined form of torture, which may include exposure to the elements, bodily fluids, or inhumane/unsanitary conditions. More extreme examples of exposure include forced prolonged standing and repeated activities outside of the realm of normal function. The former Soviet Union was known to practice 'elephant.' Victims would have a gas mask placed over their faces and then gradually had the oxygen content decreased, creating the sensation of suffocation. Lastly, withholding is another torture method. By withholding food, water, sleep, warmth, or medications, perpetrators of torture are able to combine physical and psychological methods of abuse.[14]

Torture methods employed vary between countries. Several Middle Eastern countries have been found to favor Palestinian hanging over traditional hanging. In the Palestinian method victims are suspended with the shoulders internally rotated and behind the back as opposed to a more traditional method of suspending a victim with the shoulders in a position of maximum forward elevation/abduction. While both methods have been found to result in significant long-term shoulder morbidity in survivors, the Palestinian method results in a higher rate of shoulder dislocation. In early 2000, Turkish officials discovered the cadavers of several political prisoners found to have been tortured via the 'hogtie' method. This uncommon form of binding ties both the victim's hands and feet behind the back, effectively leaving the victim in a ball like position and thus unable to resist subsequent attacks. The hogtie method ultimately leads to death via positional asphyxia.[15] The chicken kebab method of torture is also seen in some Eastern European countries. In this method the victim's knees and elbows are flexed to 90°. The victim is then hung by his knees and placed in a ball like position by binding the wrists with the band resting on the anterior tibia at the ankle joint.[16] Victims of the kebab method of torture are subjected to compression injuries and the consequences of neurovascular compromise.

Ghotna is commonly practiced in India. In this method a long pole is placed across the legs of the victim; the torturer then stands on the pole, often for an extended period of time.[17] Ghotna can result in a variety of musculoskeletal complications, including rhabdomyolysis, nerve damage, and long bone fractures. Certain areas of Bangladesh vary this practice by not only having the abuser stand on the pole but also by repeatedly rolling the pole along the leg. Falanga is a method of torture where the soles of the feet are repeatedly beaten with sticks and other large objects. Victims often note persistent pain, difficulty with ambulation, and scarring of the plantar structures of the foot. This method is especially common in African nations. Generalized beatings and falanga can be administered with the

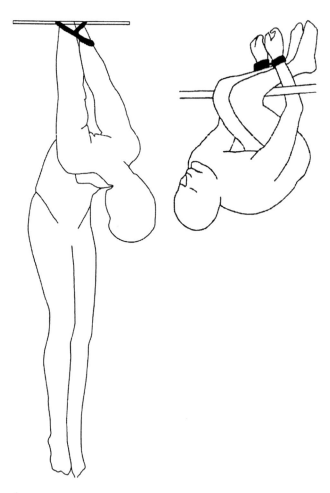

Figure 7.1   Types of Hanging

victim standing, sitting, or with the victim placed in a car tire to further contort the body and add an additional element of torture.

Evaluation of victims of torture

PT is a 21-year-old woman presenting to the urgent care section of the emergency department. Her chief complaint is intermittent headache and low-back pain over the past 18 months. She denies any medical history or surgical history. She is not taking any medications and has no known drug allergies. How should the examination proceed?

Caring for victims of torture is a challenging task. It is critical that all physicians, particularly those not practicing in refugee centers, consider that patients may be victims of torture. It has been estimated that 60 percent of all persons seeking

Table 7.1 Types of torture

Type	Examples	Country practiced
Direct	Kicking	
	Beating (fists, objects)	
	Binding	
	Hogtie	Turkey
Electric	Picana: Direct application of current	
	Parilla: Current through object	
Falanga		Africa
Ghonta		Bangladesh, India, Pakistan
Hanging	Kebab	Eastern Europe
	Palestinian	Middle East
	Traditional	
Psychological	Elephant	Former Soviet Union
	Mock execution	
	Near drowning	
	Threats (to self or family)	
Water	Deprivation	
	Nasal infusion	
	Submersion	

asylum in the United States have been tortured, as have many migrant workers and refugees.[14] It is particularly important for physicians to inquire about torture considering, as Yawar notes, that 'bogus asylum seekers report torture where none has happened; what tends to go unremarked is that those who have been tortured often underreport it.[18] Eisenmen administered the Detection of Torture Survivors Survey across a cross-sectional sample of foreign-born patients presenting to an urban primary care clinic to determine the prevalence of torture.[19] Eight of the 121 participants reported torture, none of whom had reported such during previous visits with the primary care providers at the clinic. Similarly, Crosby administered a self-designed questionnaire to foreign-born patients presenting to a different urban primary care clinic.[20] They found that one in nine patients met the UN definition of survivor of torture. They also found that only 39 percent of all subjects reported ever being asked about torture by a physician. These studies highlight the need for physicians to consider that a patient may be a survivor of torture. Silove notes that addressing physicians' anxiety about discussing the possibility of torture with patients may lead to more reporting of torture, particularly among victims not seen at designated centers.[21]

Table 7.2 Key screening questions

In which country were you born?
What is the current political situation there?
How were you treated in your country?
How did you escape from your country?
Did you live in other countries en route to living here?
Do you still have family members in your native country or here?

Although some may question the validity of the self-designed questionnaire, the work of Montgomery and Foldspang has shown that self-reporting is a reliable means of detecting torture.[22] Physicians should also note that survivors of torture may not immediately report a history of abuse, thus it is reasonable to repeatedly ask high-risk patients about a possible history of torture. Reasons for this delayed response include 'high emotional arousal with associated hyperbole or defensiveness for some individuals in reporting torture events, impaired memory secondary to psychiatric and neurological impairments, culturally prescribed sanctions that allow the trauma experience to be revealed only in highly confidential settings, and coping mechanisms that use denial and the avoidance of memories or situations associated with the trauma.'[23] This key component of a patient's medical history may do much to explain the etiology of somewhat vague, chronic symptoms.

Several key screening questions should be asked to all patients who may have survived torture. The first question to ask is to gather information about the patient's situation in his/her home country. Particular attention should be placed on the political situation and the family situation in the political context. It is also important to note the condition and location of family members as the psychosocial stresses of displacement can further complicate a victim's presentation. Questions relating to the actual escape from the home country should also be asked, particularly regarding all of the steps involved. Survivors are often exposed to less than ideal conditions while in refugee camps. The presence of family or other refugees in the new country is also important to note, as post-settlement stresses can play as significant a role in the victim's health as those stresses sustained in the home country.[23] If a survivor of torture was held in a detention facility in the home country, it is important to delineate the conditions in these facilities. A typical question would be 'while in captivity, did you ever experience physical or mental suffering, deliberately and systematically inflicted by an agent of a government or of an armed political group, or any person acting with the government's approval?'[14]

Now that PT has been identified as a survivor of torture, are there models to help guide her treatment?

Recovery over time is intrinsically linked to the 'reconstruction of social networks, achievement of economic independence, and making contact with appropriate cultural institutions against a background of respect for human rights and justice.'[17] Given the complexity of this undertaking, a multidisciplinary approach is believed to be the most effective means to serve this patient population. Feldman proposed a model for health care providers treating victims of torture.[24] He theorizes that a three-tiered system is needed to adequately address the varied needs of this patient population. The first component is the gateway to services where the role of outreach workers is emphasized. Core services provide the mainstay of evaluation and treatment, while ancillary services address the psychosocial needs of the patient population. This model is evident in the Rehabilitation and Research Center for Torture Victims (RCT) in Copenhagen, a model that has been copied worldwide. The RCT is staffed by physicians, psychologists, psychiatrists, nurses, social workers, physical therapists, and translators. All staff members are familiar with the signs and sequelae of torture and undergo training to maximize interactions with victims.[25] Miller interviewed 15 therapists and 15 interpreters to determine if the presence of an interpreter affected the patient–physician relationship.[26] Their self-designed survey revealed that therapists did not feel that the presence of the interpreter hindered the therapeutic relationship. In fact, most therapists felt the interpreter enhanced the therapeutic experience by filling key cultural gaps.

Are there any tips or strategies for assessing a patient's cultural situation that can be used in general medical practices, not just specialized refugee health centers?

Weine proposed a novel means of treating refugee populations. He recommends the integration of attitudes in an attempt to create a more cross-cultural atmosphere rather than a collection of seemingly random efforts to introduce the victims' culture into the therapeutic plan.[27] This method also attempts to break down perceived roles (such as interviewer and interviewee) and foster an environment of discussion. Hanscom proposes the mnemonic HEARTS to help physicians through the interview process:

> **H**istory
> **E**motions and reactions
> **A**sking questions about symptoms
> **R**easons for symptoms
> **T**eaching relaxation and coping skills
> **S**elf-change

She used this method in community settings and in refugee treatment centers and found that the method is easily applied by both trained professionals and local volunteers.[28]

Now that PT's cultural history has been elucidated, how should you follow-up this information?

A key element to working with victims of torture is the understanding of the political and cultural background of the victim's country of origin. The need for a culturally knowledgeable translator is also illustrated by cultural differences regarding health care. Some cultures consider asking questions of a health care provider to be a sign of disrespect. If the physician is unaware, key portions of the history may be missed. Similarly, some cultures do not want the patient to know details of his/her condition; rather, all information is given to family members. Not following this cultural belief could seriously jeopardize the patient–physician relationship.[29] These examples illustrate that knowledge of a patient's cultural background provides much needed insight that allows the victim to feel safe enough in a new environment to allow the evaluation to proceed. Ramaliu and Thurston emphasize the need to involve other immigrants resettled in the area as this helps to ameliorate the cultural differences that likely exist between patients and physicians.[30] Boersma notes that knowing the patient's country of origin may also help the physician identify the reason the victim was tortured.[31] She reviewed records of torture victims and found that those relocated from the Middle East, Europe, and Central America were more likely to have been tortured for religious reasons while those from Africa and South America were more likely to have suffered based on political or group affiliation.

How should I prepare for the examination in light of this information?

Another critical component to the examination of the survivor of torture is the need to conduct the examination in a manner that will not trigger memories of torture. Before the examination begins it is critical that the victim of torture not be left alone in a room. This seemingly benign act may actually trigger memories of isolation the victim may have experienced in captivity. Education as to possible triggers is crucial if the examination is to proceed. Electrocardiogram (ECG) leads may remind victims of previous electrocution/shock sessions and needles may remind victims of prodding during torture sessions. Particular care should be taken before performing a pelvic or rectal exam as many survivors of torture may view these procedures as being similar to abuses suffered during captivity.[23] The role of a translator, particularly one from the victim's home country, if possible, becomes evident during this educational process. Familiarity of the translator with the cultural norms of the victim's country of origin further facilitates the therapeutic relationship. The importance of the culturally appropriate translator is further magnified during the screening for psychological conditions as a significant stigma against mental illness exists in several countries.

While performing the physical examination it is important for the physician to carefully record any findings. This is particularly critical for patients who are

Table 7.3 Essentials of examination preparation

Consider the possibility of torture
Inquire about cultural beliefs
Use a culturally sensitive translator if it is possible
Incorporate cultural considerations into the examination area
Consider torture history when performing diagnostic tests

applying for asylum. Physicians should be familiar with state and national laws/ regulations regarding the use of digital cameras when attempting to document injuries. Also, the physician should be sure to obtain informed consent from the victim before taking any photographs or video of physical examination findings. Lastly, care of victims of torture is not without controversy. The ethics of performing invasive diagnostic procedures solely for the purpose of documentation of abuse with no definitive plans for treatment of discovered conditions is currently being debated.[16]

Medical sequelae of torture

Now that historical information has been gathered, how should the physical exam proceed and what findings should I expect?

Due to the nature of relocation and the time associated with such, most victims of torture come to the attention of a physician after a significant amount of time has elapsed since the last episode of torture. Although physicians are often aware of the need to proceed rapidly to physical examination in an attempt to document visible signs of abuse, many patients are wary of both the physician and the examination process, necessitating the physician to focus on building the patient–physician relationship before proceeding.

Moreno stresses the need for a formal intake session[32]

This may be difficult in a busy clinical area and may be deferred to an appropriate referral center if you are able to discuss the case with them, arrange a timely appointment, and determine that the patient has no emergent medical issues.

This time allows the physician to gather key historical data in an environment that is not intimidating for the victim of torture. Based on their experiences at the Boston Center for Refugee Health and Human Rights, his group's recommendations for intake are summarized in Table 7.4. This information should be gathered before beginning the physical examination. It is also important for the physician to consider the need for multiple interview/intake sessions before proceeding to the examination process.

Unfortunately for the physician, many of the physical signs of torture are not readily apparent as most obvious superficial lesions heal within six weeks of the

Table 7.4 Critical information

Background	Country of origin, marital status, family composition and location, date of arrival, current living conditions, education, occupation, language(s), religion
Trauma	Reason(s) for persecution, affected family members, age at first persecution, number of persecutions, conditions during capture, path taken to country of relocation
Medical history	Medications, surgery, current diagnoses, allergies, immunization status, dental history
Review of systems	
Screening test results	Laboratory and radiology results; psychological screening findings

Adapted from Moreno A, Piwowarczyk L, LaMorte WW, Grodin MA. Characteristics and utilization review of primary care services in a torture rehabilitation center. *Journal of Immigrant and Minority Health.* 2006b; 8(2): 163–71.[33]

occurrence, thus a thorough physical examination is necessary. However, physicians may occasionally be faced with treating the victim of torture in the days or weeks following the episode. Therefore, physicians should be familiar with the acute and subacute findings associated with torture as summarized in Table 7.5.

One of the most common presenting concerns of victims of torture, those seeking immediate and delayed treatment, is that of generalized pain. Olsen and colleagues surveyed 221 refugees at the Rehabilitation and Research Center for Torture Victims (RCT) to determine the prevalence of chronic pain and to identify pain trends in this patient population. They found a dose-related effect of trauma to the likelihood of the victim experiencing headaches. Of note, this trauma was generalized trauma, not specifically head trauma. Those who were suffocated as part of their torture were more likely to experience headache than those who did not. This finding is likely due to subacute hypoxia; however, the exact cellular mechanism has not yet

Table 7.5 Acute signs of torture

Body system	Findings
Skin	Lacerations, abrasions, ecchymosis, burns
Head and neck	Facial asymmetry, visual changes (diplopia), subconjunctival hemorrhage, proptosis, septal hematoma, tympanic membrane perforation, dental fractures/avulsions, trismus
Chest	Cardiac dysrhythmia, tenderness to palpation/crepitus (rib fractures)
Abdomen	Tenderness to palpation (splenic/liver laceration, ruptured viscus, ruptured diaphragm)
Extremities	Decreased range of motion, obvious deformity, inability to ambulate
Genitourinary	Males: testicular torsion, testicular rupture, hydrocoele, urethral rupture Females: Deformity, laceration, tear

been determined. Exposure to sexual trauma was a strong predictor for the survivor presenting with back pain (odds ratio 2.75). Physicians must consider the possibility that the survivor may have persistent peripheral nerve injury at the site of the direct torture, resulting in neuropathic-type pain. Lastly, Olsen and colleagues theorizes that it is possible that chronic pain is due to central sensitization or pain memory.[34]

Olsen and colleagues conducted a separate study of 97 refugees (69 of whom were included in the study) evaluated at the RCT to determine the presence of persistent pain. Subjects were interviewed at time zero (an average of 10.6 years from the last episode of torture), 9 months, and 23 months using a visual analog scale to assess pain. Initially, 81 percent reported head pain, 78 percent noted back pain, and 59 percent suffered from foot pain. At 23-month follow-up, 77 percent still had head pain, 81 percent still suffered from back pain, and 70 percent noted foot pain. The symptoms had not decreased in this time period despite multiple treatment modalities and significant time from injury. As in their previous study, Olsen and colleagues found that the number of generalized torture sessions did correlate to head pain. In addition to suffocation causing headaches as in the previous study, here they also note that low-back pain was significantly associated with a history of suffocation.[35]

Thomsen and colleagues sought to determine the nature of pain (nociceptive, visceral, or neuropathic) amongst survivors of torture.[36] The group defined nociceptive pain as that resulting from direct injury to bones, joints, and their associated structures. Direct trauma is usually responsible for nociceptive pain, making it relatively easy for the patient and the victim of torture to localize the site of the pain. Neuropathic pain is that resulting from disease or injury to a nerve(s). Given the long path most nerves travel, it may be difficult to pinpoint the original site of pain. Visceral pain results from injury or disease of internal organs; as there are fewer pain receptors in deep cavities. The classic example of visceral pain is the patient with appendicitis, who initially notes periumbilical pain that later localizes to the right lower quadrant. Eighteen randomly selected patients seeking treatment at the RCT, but not experiencing significant pain relief, were enrolled in this study. All subjects were male, and were an average of 14.9 years from the time of last torture. After history and physical examinations were repeated, the authors found that all subjects reported pain at multiple sites and 67 percent listed pain at greater than three areas. Additionally, all patients reported nociceptive and neuropathic pain symptoms but visceral pain was only found in four patients. Falanga was associated with peripheral neuropathy, blunt head trauma was linked to trigeminal neuralgia, and Palestinian hanging led to brachial plexopathy and shoulder dislocation. Thomsen and colleagues theorize that these findings are due to the likelihood that 'sensory cell somata in dorsal root ganglia are highly sensitive to mechanical distortion and the incidence of spontaneous and evoked dorsal root ganglion discharge is significantly augmented by chronic peripheral nerve injury' likely to have been induced by the original trauma.

Moisander and Edston conducted a study of 160 survivors of torture presenting to the Centre for Trauma Victims in Stockholm, Sweden. Victims hailed from Bangladesh, Iran, Peru, Syria, Turkey, and Uganda. Intake records were reviewed, showing the most common presenting concerns were chronic headache, low-back pain, and joint pain, consistent with the findings of other authors. Through this analysis, the authors were able to delineate the most common methods of torture in each of the countries of origin. Such background information may ultimately help establish a databank of torture methods that helps victims of torture obtain asylum in their countries of relocation.[13]

The skin examination may reveal a multitude of signs of abuse, including keloids, burn marks, fissuring from vitamin deficiency, and areas of hyper or hypo pigmentation from prolonged pressure. When examining the skin it is important to consider that certain culturally based methods of healing may have been attempted before the victim presented to a physician. Signs of such therapy, including cupping and coining, should not be mistaken for signs of abuse.[29]

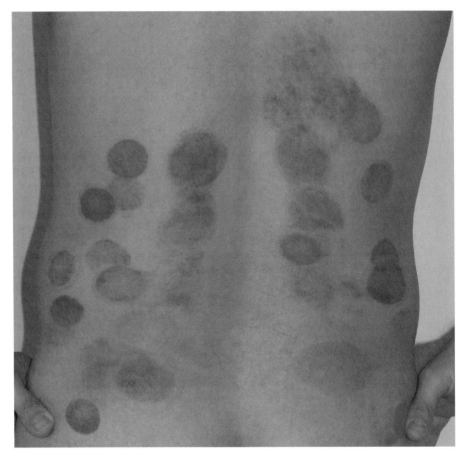

Figure 7.2   Example of Cupping

Examination of the head and neck may reveal evidence of torture. Subtle changes to the tympanic membrane may be evident, including scarring resulting from repeated blunt trauma directly to the ears (boxing of the ears). This scarring may result in decreased or complete loss of hearing. Scarring of the external auditory canal may also be noted in victims who sustained repeated foreign body insertion into the site. Victims who sustain considerable boxing of the ears or other forms of blunt head trauma also complain of tempormandibular. Attention should be paid to the victim's dentition; dental fractures and avulsions commonly follow trauma. Nasal fractures and septal deviation are commonly seen in torture victims. Unrepaired retinal detachments may be detected on physical examination, but would be accompanied by loss of vision. Cranial nerve deficits may also be apparent following head trauma and facial fractures. Lastly, survivors of water torture may experience chronic sinus infections; physicians should consider unusual etiologies of sinusitis based on the likelihood of contaminated water being used during the water torture.

Little published data exists regarding the effects of torture on the cardiovascular system. It is widely theorized that significant alterations in hemodynamic parameters would result from torture sessions; however, this has not been documented. Corovic and colleagues conducted a trial on 182 former Serbian prisoners of war and 182 age- and gender-matched controls. Subjects had been exposed to a variety of torture methods while in captivity, including 'hunger, extreme cold, lack of medication, beatings, forced to shower in cold water while outdoors in sub-zero weather, and other forms of abuse.' By report, none of the subjects (average age 35.8 years) had known cardiac disease or EKG changes before imprisonment. Survivors of torture had significantly higher rates of ST segment depression and arrhythmia (most commonly PVCs, incomplete left-bundle branch block, sinus bradycardia, and low QRS voltage) than the control groups. Study subjects also tended to have higher rates of post-infarction Q waves, negative T waves, and sinus tachycardia than the controls, however, these differences were not statistically significant. Although this study is small, it is impressive given the number of changes found in a young study population.[37]

Examination of the musculoskeletal system may reveal crepitus with joint movement or decreased range of motion at affected joints. Laxity is also a key feature of abuse, particularly at the shoulder of those subjected to Palestinian hanging. Winging of the scapula (due to injury to the long thoracic nerve) can be seen in these patients as well.[38] Pain over a particular area should trigger the use of x-rays to determine if there is an underlying fracture at the site of pain. Victims of torture may also be prone to malunion of fractures due to inappropriate immobilization and to non-union of fractures based on persistent abuse during captivity. These bony abnormalities can also have a significant effect on surrounding nerves and

Table 7.6 Chronic sequelae of torture: Skin and HEENT

Body system	Conditions
Skin	Keloids, burn scars (electrode, cigarettes), abrasions (may leave permanent marks if initial lesion contaminated with dirt/other objects), hair loss, nail loss/deformity
Facial bones	Facial asymmetry, crepitus, trismus, temporomandibular joint dysfunction
Facial structures	Lid lag, tympanic membrane scarring, collapsed nasal bridge, deviated septum
Oropharynx	Dental fractures/avulsions, gingival scarring, gingival disease, trismus
Neck	Hyoid crepitus, bruits, muscle spasm

muscles, resulting in neuropathy and weakness in many cases. Contractures may also be seen in those who sustained a significant neurologic or vascular injury that was not allowed to heal properly. Falanga can result in generalized tenderness of the plantar surface of the foot. Loss of arch function and posterior tibial tendinopathies are also commonly seen following this method of torture. Savnik published a case series of MRI studies of those who were subjected to falanga while in captivity. They examined 12 victims of falanga (undergoing treatment at the RCT) and 7 age- and gender-matched controls. All victims of torture had experienced their trauma from 5 to 15 years before the MRI. All 12 subjects noted pain with ambulation, ten noted sensory changes to the feet, and eight noted pain at rest. None of the controls had any history of foot injuries and none had active foot concerns at the time of the MRI. They found that all victims of falanga had significantly thicker plantar aponeuroses than controls. There was no difference between the area of the plantar muscles, the characteristics of the plantar muscles, the thickness of the plantar fat pad, or the amount of fibrous septae of the fat pad. It is postulated that this increased thickness of the aponeurosis contributes to the chronic pain via a combination of persistent plantar fasciitis and a chronic compartment syndrome. However, the exact cellular changes resulting in this finding are yet to be determined. This study, although small, provides the clinician and the forensic examiner with a readily available means of documenting prior torture.[39]

If MRI is not available, bone scanning can also be used to attempt to document a history of falanga. Altun and Durmus-Altun compared MRI to bone scanning in a victim of falanga. MRI showed aponeurotic thickening as previously described; bone scanning detected increased uptake in multiple areas of the foot on initial scan. The delayed scan also showed increased osteoblastic activity, another indication of recent trauma. The latter findings show the modality may be particularly useful when the falanga occurred relatively recently.[40]

The genitourinary system is particularly prone to trauma during abuse. The basic examination should include thorough inspection of the skin. Mutilation is common in both genders, with females subjected to circumcision in African nations. Hydroceoles commonly result after trauma to the male genitourinary (GU) system. Rectal trauma is also commonly seen in victims of sodomy. Rectal tears and a loss of the normal rugal patterns result.

Another sequelae of abuse to the GU system is the sexually transmitted disease. Gonorrhea, chlamydia, syphilis, and HIV should be considered in all victims of torture; however, routine screening of all refugees is not currently recommended by the World Health Organization. Those with signs of active infection should be treated immediately. When evaluating a victim of torture for signs of sexual abuse, it is important to remember that men tend to underreport sexual abuse considerably more often than females, presumably out of shame.[17]

Female genital mutilation has received considerable coverage in the press, as human rights groups work to ban this practice. The World Health Organization defines female genital mutilation as the 'complete or partial removal of female genital organs performed for cultural rather than therapeutic reasons.' This practice is classified into four types:

Type 1: excision of part or all of the clitoris
Type II: excision of all or part of the labia
Type III: type II with stitching/narrowing of the vaginal opening
Type IV: piercing/pricking the clitoris

It is difficult to determine how common these practices are, but estimates range varying on the region studied. The various types of mutilation are seen primarily in African nations, particularly those in the northern and central parts of the continent. However, as more people emigrate from this region, female genital mutilation is being seen around the world. Overall, approximately 100 to 140 million women are believed to be affected.[41]

In September 2001 the European Parliament passed a resolution banning female genital mutilation; however, this resolution is not legally binding. Since the passage of this measure, Austria, Belgium, Sweden, Switzerland, the UK, and Norway have all passed laws specifically banning female genital mutilation.[42] Although the spirit of the law is explicit, it has proven to be difficult to enforce such measures; further work is needed to determine how to best protect recent immigrants.

While the 'procedures' involved in female genital mutilation have significant morbidity associated, it is the conditions under which they occur that lead to significant mortality. Women subjected to such abuse are often forced to undergo the 'procedure' in less than sterile conditions and usually without anesthesia (either general or local). There are several reports of death from sepsis related to mutilation, but significantly more survivors of mutilation suffer from recurrent urinary tract infections, infertility, various fistulae, and sexual dysfunction.

Signs of torture are often particularly evident in the nervous system. The physician must be careful not to mistake language difficulties with changes in mental status. It is important to consider that the victim of torture may have sustained a traumatic brain injury, further complicating the evaluation process. Several of the sequelae of traumatic brain injury (TBI), including 'memory and attentional deficits, apathy, labile affect, impaired social judgment, distractibility, and impulsivity' overlap significantly with post traumatic stress disorder (PTSD)-associated symptoms. It is imperative that the clinician considers both diagnostic possibilities when evaluating survivors of torture. This is particularly important in regards to treatment, as those with TBI may not be able to fully participate in cognitive behavioral therapy, a mainstay of PTSD treatment.

Several studies of World War II prisoners of war and concentration camp survivors have linked excess weight loss ($<30\%$) while in captivity with significantly greater memory deficits than those who did not lose large amounts of body weight.[43] Adams and Duschen have theorized that hippocampal sensitivity to hypoxia may lead to higher rates of PTSD.[44] However, exact cellular mechanisms for PTSD have not yet been determined. These factors reinforce the need to obtain as much historical information as possible to best help the survivor of torture.

Post-traumatic seizures are another manifestation of torture. Rasmussen estimated that 73 percent of all torture victims sustained head trauma with 19 percent of these victims losing consciousness at some point during the torture.[45] Considering that Moreno and Peel state that the relative risk of seizure increases by 50 percent after head trauma involving a brief loss of consciousness, significant numbers of torture victims are at risk for seizures.[46]

When seizures do occur in victims of torture, they tend to follow the same pattern as in non-torture victims. There is some discussion as to whether victims of torture are susceptible to a particular type of seizure, the pilomotor seizure. In this subtype, patients experience symptoms resembling an anxiety attack; 'piloerection, anxiety, head tightness, nausea, difficulties sleeping, and cold sweats.'[46] As with all post-traumatic seizure patients, prophylaxis is controversial and is usually decided on a case-by-case basis.

These seizure patients differ from the non-tortured population in several key ways. Some survivors of torture are able to recall their initial seizure immediately after head trauma. The clinician must pay particular attention to these victims as recurrent seizures often trigger flares of PTSD or other psychiatric conditions. The ability to diagnose seizures is further complicated by the fact that the gold standard diagnostic test, the EEG, may also remind victims of previous torture. Formal diagnosis may be significantly delayed as the patient undergoes therapy to help

Table 7.7 Chronic sequelae of torture: Musculoskeletal, GU, CNS

Body system	Findings
Musculoskeletal	Deformity, decreased range of motion, contracture, distal neurovascular deficit
Genitourinary	Deformity, incontinence, STDs, discharge, diarrhea
Central Nervous System	Gait disturbance, cognitive/motor delays, sensory changes, posterior column changes, neuropathy/radiculopathy, seizure disorder

cope with this association. Lastly, the similarities between pilomotor seizures and exacerbations of psychiatric conditions further cloud the treatment and prophylaxis decisions the physician must make.

As mentioned previously, cranial nerve deficits may be seen after head trauma, particularly when facial fractures are involved. Particular attention should be paid to the oculomotor portion of the cranial nerve exam to detect subtle findings. Moreno and Grodin postulate two possible explanations for the prevalence of neuropathies that frequently follow trauma, particularly hanging. The first means of nerve damage is direct compression, which often occurs in the process of suspension. It is also likely that axonal damage results from the prolonged traction associated with certain types of suspension.[47] Changes in sensation (hypesthesia and hyposthesia) have been shown to occur in approximately 10 percent of torture survivors and tends to be more common in the upper extremities than in the lower extremities.[45] Lastly, changes in vibratory and positional sense should be considered, particularly in those who have sustained spinal trauma and in those with a possible history of sexually transmitted diseases. Gait abnormalities are commonly seen; it is important for the physician to consider the possible contribution of orthopedic trauma as well as neurologic etiologies when evaluating gait abnormalities.

Endemic illnesses

In addition to screening for signs of torture, the physician must consider the possibility that a victim of torture is suffering from a medical condition endemic to the individual's country of origin. Physicians examining victims of torture may consider consulting an infectious disease specialist as well as the Centers for Disease Control (CDC) website for further information regarding conditions endemic to a given country.

The CDC currently recommends screening all individuals from malaria endemic areas with hemoglobin values of less than 30 percent of age-recommended norms. However, they do not recommend a specific screening protocol. Stauffer attempted

Table 7.8 Infectious disease considerations

Region	Conditions
Africa	Dengue fever, HIV, Malaria, Marburg/Ebola virus, sickle cell disease, TB
Asia	Hepatitis B/C, HIV, malaria (South Pacific), TB
Central/South America	Chagas disease, HIV, malaria, typhoid
Middle East	G6PD deficiency, malaria, thalassemia

Adapted from the CDC at http://wwwn.cdc.gov/travel/destinationList.aspx.

to determine the efficacy of rapid antigen testing to detect asymptomatic parasitemia in this population. Using polymerase chain reaction (PCR) as the gold standard, they compared microscopy to the rapid antigen testing and they compared both to PCR. They found the sensitivity of combined blood smear and rapid antigen testing to be only 22 percent, thus leaving physicians without a convenient means of screening at-risk populations. Interestingly, they also note that low platelet counts (usually seen in cases of asymptomatic malaria) was not seen in any of the confirmed cases.[48] This, too, should serve to remind physicians to be particularly vigilant when treating this patient population.

Seybolt conducted a retrospective chart review of all refugees seen at an urban medical center to better determine the significance of asymptomatic eosinophilia. They found that 12 percent of asymptomatic patients from a variety of regions had an eosinophil count of greater than 450 cells per microliter. Of these patients, 29 percent had positive stool cultures and a significant number of patients had positive serologic studies for various parasites.[49] This study highlights the need for adequate follow-up of screening studies.

Pediatric considerations

In the course of PT's examination it is revealed that she has two young children. Should you consider the possibility that they were tortured, too?

Unfortunately, children are not immune to torture. While no specific data has been published documenting the actual number of children affected, it is believed that the number is easily on the scale of millions. Once in a new country, children who have survived torture may also go undetected based on the auspices under which they initially entered the new country. For example, children adopted by Western families may easily have been tortured in their homeland; unless a history of torture is explicitly sought, this group may easily be missed.

Screening guidelines for children entering the United States vary from those for adults. The CDC guidelines should be reviewed before treating such a child, as updates occur regularly. Currently, the initial evaluation focuses on screening for highly communicable diseases such as tuberculosis, HIV, syphilis, gonorrhea, and leprosy. These recommendations are similar to those for adults; however, unlike with adults, laboratory screening is not recommended in those younger than 15.[51] It is important to evaluate the immunization history of the immigrating child. Immunization practices of countries vary widely; it is likely that a child will need several vaccinations to 'catch up' to the recommended schedule. This is particularly evident with the newer vaccinations, such as hepatitis B, varicella, and pneumovax which are not readily available or used in many parts of the world. The American Academy of Pediatrics website (www.aap.org) is a useful resource for immunization-related questions.

Another key difference between adult and pediatric screening processes is that hearing and vision screening are recommended for all those under 15 years of age. Physicians may also want to consider screening for lead toxicity in immigrating children as several cultures still cook in clay pots with high lead levels. Thus, it is important for the physician to consider lead poisoning in patients well outside of the normally affected age range. Lastly, developmental assessments should be performed on all children as Johnson estimates that 'for every 4 months spent in an institution children will be delayed 1 month in all growth parameters.'[52]

As with adults, it is important to assess not only the pediatric patient's country of origin but also the path taken to the new country as the child may have been exposed to endemic diseases en route to the final destination.

Schwarzwald points out that dietary habits in the country of origin may pose health risks. For example, non-pasteurized dairy products are the norm in parts of Mexico, Central America, and India; this may be a source of infection.

Pickering estimates that 15 to 35 percent of internationally adopted children have a pathogen identified on screening.[54] Given that conditions in many international orphanages are not significantly different than those in refugee centers, it stands to reason that similar numbers of children surviving torture would be affected. Exposure to Hepatitis B and C should strongly be considered in children arriving from endemic areas (Asia and Africa). Similarly, a high index of suspicion should be maintained for malaria in those arriving from affected areas. Lastly, given varying immunization practices as mentioned, physicians examining refugee children should consider conditions not usually encountered in the United States (i.e., measles, rubella).

The dental health of pediatric survivors of torture should not be overlooked. Cote and colleagues performed dental screenings on 224 refugee children ranging in age from 6 months to 18 years (median age 10.7 years). Subjects were from Africa (53.6%), Eastern Europe (26.8%), and the Middle East (19.6%). They found significantly lower rates of caries in African children (38%) than in Eastern Europeans

Table 7.9 Adult vs. pediatric screening

Screening measure	Adult	Pediatric
Immunizations	Update as needed	Update as needed, start series based on CDC/AAP guidelines
Developmental milestones	Not required	Age-specific guidelines; delay may be due to growth delay
Growth delays	Not required	Gender-specific growth curves should be plotted
Dental screening	Should be performed	Should be performed, consider supplemental fluoride
Vision and hearing screening	Recommended based on patient concerns/ exam findings only	Recommended on all children <15 years of age

(79.7%); overall 51.3 percent experienced caries. This is comparable to rates seen in U.S. children (49.3%). Of all study groups, African children were the least likely to have seen a dentist in the country of origin. The authors postulate that the lower caries rate despite lack of dental care may be attributed to differences in natural fluoride content in water supplies and to dietary differences. This study highlights the need for clinicians to address dental health as well as overall health in the pediatric population.[55]

Psychiatric concerns must also be addressed in pediatric victims of torture. Ellis evaluated the UCLA PTSD for DSM-IV in Somali adolescents. This 22-question survey was administered to 41 males and 35 females ranging from 12 to 19 years of age. Subjects had been in the United States for a mean of 6.4 years and had experienced a mean of 7.6 traumas before resettlement. Responses on the UCLA scale were then compared to the War Trauma Screening Scale and the Depression Self-Rating Scale, both of which have been validated in this age group. The UCLA scale did prove to be reliable, sensitive, and specific in its ability to detect depression in adolescent refugees.[56] As this tool is shorter and easier to administer than the other collection devices, it may prove to be a useful adjunct in treating adolescents.

Halcon and colleagues conducted a cross-sectional study of Somali and Oromo youth (ages 18–25) living in Minnesota. Subjects sustained a mean of 17.3 episodes of torture in their homelands. Findings suggested that those who spoke English well were less likely to suffer PTSD as were those who came to the United States at a younger age and those who arrived with family members.[50] These results reinforce the notion of the resiliency of youth. Lastly, these findings emphasize the need for the clinician to obtain an adequate history when working with survivors of torture as such demographic information can help determine the likelihood of a survivor suffering from PTSD and can help better tailor therapy.

Sleep disturbance is one of the primary manifestations of depression and PTSD. Pediatric survivors of torture may be particularly vulnerable to this symptomology. Montgomery and Foldspang interviewed the parents of 311 children (range 3–15 years, mean 7.5) relocated to Denmark and seeking treatment at the RCT. Children experienced a mean of 8.7 episodes of torture/violence. The most important predictors for sleep disturbance were 'grandparent violent death before child's birth, mother tortured, and father scolds the child more' while the presence of both parents in Denmark decreased the risk of sleep symptoms.[57]

Psychological effects of torture

The physical examination portion of PT's evaluation is completed. Are there any other conditions to consider?

While the physical sequelae of torture can be devastating, the psychological consequences can also have a profound impact on the life of a survivor. Victims of torture often turn to coping mechanisms in an attempt to heal themselves. Commonly used methods include drug and alcohol abuse, high-risk sexual behavior, excessive behaviors (sleeping, eating), and self injury.[58] Anxiety, depression, and PTSD are extremely prevalent among survivors of torture. Interestingly, PTSD is more common in refugees than in those who remain in the country of origin, as the added stressors of relocation are thought to trigger exacerbations.[58]

Fazel and colleagues conducted a meta-analysis of refugee studies published from 1966 to 2002. They found a variety of different data collection devices used, but found that overall, 1 in 10 refugees suffered from PTSD, 1 in 20 met diagnostic criteria for major depression, and 1 in 25 were afflicted with anxiety disorder.[59]

Porter and Haslam also completed a meta-analysis of refugee studies to determine the role of sociopolitical factors on refugee mental health. They found that younger refugees tended to have better outcome than older ones and that males fared better than females. They also noted that European refugees tended to have worse outcomes than their African counterparts. They theorize that difference in the standards of living between the country of origin and the resettlement country is likely responsible for this discrepancy.[60]

Several studies have attempted to quantify the incidence of psychological disorders among survivors of torture. However, this is a difficult task given the large number of surveys available and in obtaining large, diverse sample sizes. This issue is further complicated by potential language subtleties that may result from translating the multitude of data collection devices available. While reviewing these efforts to determine the incidence of PTSD among victims of torture it is interesting to keep in mind that the rate of PTSD in the general U.S. population is 8 percent.[61]

Keller administered multiple questionnaires to 325 refugees from 60 countries. They found that 81 percent of patients had clinically significant anxiety, 84.5 percent had significant depression, and 45.7 percent had significant PTSD symptomatology. Furthermore, they found that women suffered from both depression and anxiety at significantly higher rates than did their male counterparts. The authors note that the findings are particularly striking given the length of time the subjects had been out of their home countries.[62]

Moreno conducted a similar study of 146 patients using the same screening tools. In this group, 70 percent of victims suffered from major depression and 58 percent met diagnostic criteria for PTSD. They also found that 77 percent of the study population had at least one somatic concern. Several other interesting trends were noted in this study. Moreno found that those with fewer than two visits to the Center were more likely to not be receiving psychological counseling.[32] Given the association of physical symptoms, somatic concerns, and psychological sequelae associated with torture, linking medical and psychiatric care of patients may significantly improve the overall health of these individuals. However, those referred for psychological counseling were more likely to also be receiving medical care than the converse group. This trend reinforces the need for medical providers to consider the impact of psychiatric illness on physical health. The Moreno group also noted that those without insurance were less likely to follow-up with any type of care, again highlighting the need for the team approach (particularly social workers) to treating victims of torture.[32]

Basoglu and colleagues went on to theorize that victims who felt that their torturers did not receive appropriate punishment were more likely to suffer from psychological sequelae than those who felt justice had been applied.[63]

Hollifield and colleagues compared eight different questionnaires in an attempt to validate the latter study device. Two hundred fifty two Vietnamese and Kurdish refugees relocated to the United States were included in the study. Multiple statistical analyses all revealed that all devices were both valid and reliable means of detecting torture and political violence among refugee populations.[64] This study should allow the clinician to feel comfortable using any of the data collection devices to assess this patient population.

de Jong and colleagues attempted to quantify the rates of PTSD and to identify risk factors for PTSD in post-conflict nations. They found rates of PTSD ranging from 15.8 percent to 37.4 percent among survivors from Algeria, Cambodia, Ethiopia, and Gaza. Exposure to torture, trauma after the age of 12, current illness (medical or psychiatric), and daily stressors were significant risk factors for the development of PTSD in all four populations. Of these, only exposure to trauma after the age of

12 was significant after regression analysis. The authors also highlight the different daily stressors encountered by refugees. Those still in conflict-ridden areas must worry about 'food, shelter, physical security, and human rights violations' while those resettled in Western nations are often concerned with 'asylum status and acculturation.'[65]

Eisenman and colleagues sought to determine the effect of exposure to political violence on immigrants from Mexico, Central America, and South America living in Los Angeles. They found that those exposed to political violence were significantly more likely to meet diagnostic criteria for PTSD, depression, and anxiety. Additionally, these patients were more likely to experience chronic pain and worse overall health than those that did not witness political upheaval in their home countries. Interestingly, only 3 percent of all study participants reported any history of violence to their physicians and no subjects reported being asked about such a history by their physicians.[66] This serves to reinforce the need of all physicians, not just those working in specialized centers, to inquire about possible exposure to violence and torture.

The effect of post-migratory stressors was further examined by Carlsson and colleagues. Working at the RCT in Copenhagen they attempted to identify predictors of mental health among male survivors of torture. Their findings, similar to de Jong and colleagues, were that previous torture and trauma, lower education, fewer social contacts, no occupation, and the presence of physical pain were significant predictors of emotional stress. Of these factors the lack of social contacts was the most significant predictor of poor health outcomes, again emphasizing the need for post-migratory social support. It was also found that emotional symptoms persisted years after relocation.[67]

Keller espouses the progression of torture victims through psychological recovery initially described by Dr. Judith Herman. Survivors progress from a sense of 'unpredictable danger to reliable safety, from dissociated trauma to acknowledged memory, and from stigmatized isolation to restored social connection.' Such a progression can be made through a variety of therapeutic interventions.[68]

Multiple psychiatric treatment modalities are available to help victims of torture. Medications are commonly used to treat the psychological sequelae of torture. Short term anxiolytic use may facilitate the initiation of therapy, however, long-term use of these agents is not recommended due to their addiction potential. Much PTSD treatment success has been achieved with selective serotonin reuptake inhibitors (SSRI); however, most studies recommend against use of medication only. A synergistic effect has been found when medication is combined with behavior modification and psychotherapy.

Cognitive behavioral therapy (CBT) is often used to treat PTSD and anxiety. This method is twofold. First, stimuli that trigger stress responses must be identified.

Table 7.10 Factors contributing to PTSD symptomatology

Genetic predisposition	Underlying psychiatric condition
Political situation in home country	Social situation in country of current residence
Dispersement of family members	Lack of income/meaningful employment
Language barriers	Methods of torture experienced
Country of origin	Suboptimal treatment modalities

Once these factors are known, the therapy consists of repeatedly exposing the victim to these stimuli in order to desensitize the individual. The ultimate goal of this method is to reach the point where previous triggers no longer elicit an emotional response in the survivor of torture.

Basoglu and colleagues presented the case of a 22-year-old victim of torture now living in Sweden. He was evaluated with the Structured Clinical Interview for DSM-IV and the Clinician Administered PTSD Scale at pre-treatment, weeks 6, 8, 12, and 16 of treatment and at 1-, 3-, and 6-month follow-up. During initial stages of treatment, scores on the stress indices did increase slightly, however, this has been shown to be a relatively common phenomenon as survivors begin to face their torture histories in depth.[70] Ultimately, scores on both scales improved in terms of social, work, family, and relationship parameters after CBT.

Given the wide range of therapeutic modalities available to victims of torture, the question of efficacy of treatment must be raised.

Carlsson and colleagues performed a longitudinal study of 69 patients enrolled at the RCT in Copenhagen. Patients were evaluated by three screening devices at enrollment and at nine months. Despite receiving treatment during the study period, follow-up questionnaires did not reveal a decrease in psychological symptoms or an improvement in quality of life.[71] Findings in this study were reinforced by a second Carlsson study which looked at patients a minimum of ten years (mean 15 years) after the initial presentation to the RCT. Again, three screening devices were administered to all participants with a randomly selected subgroup given a

Table 7.11 Key PTSD treatment modalities

Modality	Example
Medication	
	SSRI
	Short-term benzodiazepines
Cognitive-behavioral therapy	
	Trigger identification
	Trigger desensitization

general health screening questionnaire as well. Again, scores on both psychological scales remained high and the scores on the general health survey remained low at follow-up.[72] These studies reinforce that the length of time psychological treatment is needed for this group is still to be determined and that there is a need for continued therapy in this vulnerable population.

Several studies have attempted to determine the incidence of PTSD and other psychiatric conditions among different ethnicities and nationalities. Al-Safar administered the Self-rating Inventory for Posttraumatic Stress Disorder (SIP) to Iranian, Arab, and Turk refugees relocated to Sweden. They found PTSD rates of 69 percent for Iranians, 59 percent for Arabs, 53 percent for Turks, and 29 percent for Swedes. Repeated trauma to relatives was a stronger predictor than trauma to the victim among all ethnic groups; no gender differences were detected either among or between groups.[73] This effort should remind the physician of the importance of inquiring about the status and location of family members when interviewing a survivor of torture.

Jaranson and colleagues administered the PTSD Checklist to a group of 1,134 Somali and Oromo (Ethiopian) refugees resettled in Minnesota. Forty-four percent of study subjects had been tortured. PTSD incidence was 25 percent in those that were tortured and 4 percent in those who were not. These rates did not vary significantly between ethnic groups or between genders. However, females, Somalis, and those who decreased their religious practices since immigrating to the United States tended to be more susceptible to PTSD.[74]

Special considerations

Physicians, particularly military physicians, may find themselves treating a subset of survivors of torture, the prisoner of war (POW). Basic treatment guidelines for this patient population are put forth by the Geneva Conventions. There are four tenets of the Conventions which should be understood by the medical practitioner.

> Geneva I: Address the care of the sick and wounded (Geneva I),
> Geneva II: Care for the shipwrecked wounded and sick (Geneva II),
> Geneva III: Care for POWs (Geneva III), and
> Geneva IV: Care for civilian populations (Geneva IV).

Geneva I states that medical personnel can not be made POWs but could be retained only if the health status and numbers of existing POWs made it necessary. Thus, the military physician may be treating POWs captured by his/her own army or those from his/her army captured by the enemy. Such battlefield conditions are likely to be less than ideal, forcing the physician to use available resources in sometimes creative ways. Rather than adhere to the standard of care at which the physician is used to practicing, it is recommended that the standard be that of the local community before the conflict developed.

Howe raises two interesting ethical questions faced by physicians working at battle-side field hospitals: how should triage principles by applied? Should all U.S. soldiers be triaged and then all enemy soldiers triaged or should all injuries be triaged based on severity instead of on country of origin? Once triage is complete, should all U.S. soldiers with similarly severe injuries be treated before all detained soldiers with comparable injuries or should care be administered in an alternating fashion? These questions are further clouded by the role of military triage which espouses that soldiers who can quickly return to the battle should be treated first to 'allow the war effort to continue' even though treating these relatively minor injuries may result in the death of more severely injured soldiers.[76]

Another controversy centers on whether detainees should be given medications/vaccines to prevent against biological/chemical warfare or if such resources should be reserved for allied forces. These questions are further complicated by the fact that in some cases care rendered by military physicians may exceed the local standard of care, particularly in regards to chronic disease, leading some to give lower priority to these individuals. The U.S. military, in conjunction with ethicists and legal experts, is currently trying to come up with ways to answer these questions and better handle their implications.

The role of the camp physician is multifold. Every prisoner of war brought to a holding facility should undergo a thorough screening. This process is similar to that experienced by the survivor of torture upon arrival to a new country. History, physical examination, dental examination, and screening for tuberculosis (either chest x-ray or PPD testing) occur after the POW is screened for weapons. Prisoners with any condition requiring treatment are put into the 'infirmary' while those without significant findings are placed in the general holding area. The physician is responsible for the daily management of those in the infirmary as well as for addressing acute issues that may arise in those in the general population. Triage becomes an issue for the camp physician, both in terms of determining which prisoners are treated first and in some cases in terms of which prisoners get available supplies. This is particularly an issue for those physicians stationed at camps closer to the actual battle, where supplies are more limited without clear restocking abilities.

As with stateside health care providers, translation is a concern for the military physician. While locals are occasionally used as interpreters, Place recommends against using natives to translate for security reasons. If local people do participate in the care of POWs, their identities must be protected as retribution may be borne against these individuals if the POW is released from camp. He also notes that it has been found that 'simulation of mental illness by captured persons is a potential technique for evading interrogation, especially when they are paired with a captured interpreter.'[75] Although it is preferable to have a live interpreter, the U.S. Department of Defense does have medical phrasebooks available in several languages.

Recent controversies at Abu Ghraib and Guantanamo Bay have raised the possibility of physician participation in torture. These cases once again highlight the need for the military physician to practice medicine only and not participate in the interrogation of POWs. Behavioral scientists have reportedly been involved in the interrogation process at Guantanamo Bay. Various reports from the detainment center report mistreatment of prisoners, including denying dental care (to the point where detainees were no longer able to eat solid food due to deterioration of oral health), destruction of religious icons in front of prisoners, and using information from the patient's medical record as the basis for interrogation (i.e., capitalizing on known phobias to heighten psychological torture).

Many of the techniques used today are the converse of those developed by a group of military 'behavioral psychologists and psychiatrists,' also known as the Behavioral Science Consult Team (BSCT). This group is essential in 'developing integrated interrogation strategies and assessing interrogation intelligence production' as well as for working with U.S. soldiers to prepare them for possible capture and interrogation.[77] This program for U.S. soldiers, known as Survival, Evasion, Resistance, and Escape (SERE), was started by the U.S. Air Force at the end of the Korean conflict and was subsequently expanded to the U.S. Army and U.S. Navy after Vietnam. Mayer goes on to discuss the current SERE training parameters, which focus on 'creating an environment of radical uncertainty: trainees are hooded, their sleep patterns are disrupted, they are starved for extended periods, they are stripped of their clothes, they are exposed to extreme temperatures, and they are subjected to harsh interrogations by officials impersonating enemy captors.' She goes on to report that several 'graduates' of SERE also report destruction of the Bible as part of the training program and note that 'it was a crushing blow, even though this was just a school.' Perhaps the most compelling evidence that SERE training has significant psychological impact is the fact that, as of 2004, graduates of the program are required to 'sign a statement promising not to apply the program's counter resistance methods to U.S.-held detainees.'[77]

It stands to reason that if U.S. military/intelligence officials expect this treatment for captured U.S. soldiers, they expect to handle enemy detainees in a similar fashion. However, this list of training methods contains several modalities that are clearly considered torture by the standards of the Geneva Conventions. Given that the Geneva Conventions explicitly state that any physician participating in the torture of a POW loses the protections afforded by the Conventions, physicians implicated in the torture of prisoners of war are not only compromising the health and well-being of prisoners but are also placing themselves at significant risk of significant physical and legal harm. Lastly, it is also important to note that a physician can be held responsible for torturing a prisoner directly but can also be found in violation of the Geneva Conventions by not reporting witnessed abuse.

Events at Guantanamo Bay have also raised the issue of physician involvement in hunger strikes. The formal definition of a hunger strike, according to the International Red Cross, requires 'fasting, voluntariness, and a stated purpose.' The World Medical Association goes on to state that physicians 'should not participate in the force-feeding of prisoners.'[78] A key aspect of this debate centers on the voluntary nature of a hunger strike as opposed to decreased intake in response to a certain condition. Although some argue that as a hunger strike continues, the prisoner may become incapable of making informed decisions; military ethics tenets state that the physician must follow the known wishes of the patient and not participate in force-feedings. This thought process was challenged by the Bush administration but was ultimately upheld (along with the Geneva Conventions applying to those at Guantanamo Bay) by the U.S. Supreme Court.

The debate over how to treat detainees in Guantanamo Bay has focused on the U.S. Department of Defense, which favors the more aggressive techniques of SERE, and the U.S. Federal Bureau of Investigation (FBI), which favors 'slowly establishing a dynamic of friendly rapport.'[77] FBI officials argue that intelligence obtained under duress is not reliable and not able to be used in court, be it a U.S. court or a military tribunal. The role of physicians in torture was further expanded by former Secretary of Defense Donald Rumsfeld, who required that prisoners have 'medical clearance before combination techniques were applied,' further implicating medical personnel by clearing individuals prematurely with the sole intent of beginning the interrogation process as quickly as possible.[7] The debate is currently under investigation by the Department of Justice (DOJ). However, several legal experts question the value of the DOJ work given previous comments on torture made by former legal counsel to the President and current U.S. Attorney General Alberto Gonzales.

Professional considerations

It is clear from the data presented that health care providers can reasonably expect to treat a victim of torture at some point in one's medical career. The first step to effectively treating victims of torture, and those from various cultures in general, is to develop physicians with a sense of cultural competence. A recent meta-analysis by Beach and colleagues showed that cultural competency did improve physician knowledge, but to date has not improved health outcomes for patients seen by these physicians. The authors theorize that this may be due to the relatively small number of physicians who have actually undergone formal training in this area.[79] Small gains made by trained physicians are easily negated by other specialists lacking this educational focus. Traditional culture-based curricula tend to focus on physician interaction with only one culture. Given the multinational nature of immigration today, this model is likely outdated. The curriculum issue is further clouded by the lack of consensus as to exactly what the curriculum should cover, creating an additional educational barrier.

Koehn and Swick propose that transcultural competence is more applicable to the immigration situation today. This approach emphasizes that the physician first gathers and analyzes information about the culture of interest instead of relying on previously held beliefs.[80] It is thus critical that the physician inquires about a history of torture as well as conditions in the patient's country of origin. It is also imperative that practitioners of western medicine realize that many other cultures rely heavily on emotional aspects of healing. By incorporating the patient's cultural beliefs into the treatment plan the physician not only strengthens the patient–physician relationship but also significantly involves the patient in his/her own care, which may ultimately improve compliance. A creative approach encourages physicians to not only recognize the various components of the survivor's experience, but to tie these events together in a cause–effect relationship. By linking cultural experiences with psychological and physical symptoms, the physician is more likely to develop a treatment plan that addresses not only these needs, but the patient's social needs as well.

Communication is perhaps the most difficult aspect of treating this patient population, as it is not practical for the physician to learn the multitude of languages that survivors speak. It is estimated that over 150 languages are spoken in New York City, further illustrating the need for translators, preferably those from the victim's home country.[81] Physician familiarity with local resources available to the survivor population may also facilitate treatment. Depending on the geographical area there may be traditional healers and other ex-patriots that may further enhance the patient's emotional connection to treatment.

The UNHCR also attempted to provide a means for effectively treating victims of torture. The Istanbul Protocol, released in 2000, is a step-by-step guideline for the evaluation and documentation practices involved with treating victims of torture. However, the document wasn't widely used by medical professionals. Pincock reports of the European Union's efforts to implement the guidelines. The RCT and the World Medical Association (WMA) were awarded a $1.2 million dollar grant to implement a pilot program in Mexico, Morocco, Uganda, Sri Lanka, and Georgia aiming to train 250 physicians and 125 legal experts in the document's use. Pincock, along with WMA officials, feels that that for the Protocol to be effective it must be adapted to regional cultures and practices. The grant aims to use demographic data from mentioned studies to create 'torture practice databanks' and use this information to make the Protocol more broadly applicable.[82]

Evans touches on the risk of transformative reactions in those examining survivors of torture. He questions whether it is possible for the examiner to truly remain neutral in the face of significant human suffering. This case report serves as a reminder of the importance of debriefing of the clinicians involved to maintain some semblance of neutrality throughout the asylum process and to prevent emotional exhaustion in health care providers working with this patient population.[83] Similarly, Miller and colleagues examined the risk of interpreters experiencing transformative reactions. This group is particularly at risk considering that the majority of translators used in Western nations are refugees themselves. This study showed that while interpreters occasionally had some emotional response to the therapy session, these reactions were not disruptive to the therapy session or to the overall well-being of the interpreter. The authors do recommend paying particular attention to the well-being of the interpreter as well as assuring that the interpreter continues any therapy he or she was receiving.[26]

Physicians working with victims of torture may also face persecution themselves. Wenzel and colleagues report the case of two Turkish physicians persecuted by the Turkish government.[84] While the two physicians in this example were ultimately cleared of all charges, the case highlights the potential risks associated with treating victims of torture, particularly in countries where torture is still extensively practiced.

References

1. Vinar MN. The specificity of torture as trauma: the human wilderness when words fail. *International Journal of Psychoanalysis*. 2005; 86: 311–33.

2. Norredam M, Mygind A, Krasnik A. Access to health care for asylum seekers in the European Union – a comparative study of country policies. *European Journal of Public Health*. 2005; 16(3): 285–9.

3. Amnesty International., Facts and Figures Report 2006. http://news.amnesty.org/index/ENGPOL100232006.

4. United Nations High Commission for Refugees. Legal and Protection Policy Research Series: Protection Mechanisms Outside of the 1951 Convention ("Complementary Protection"). Available at http://www.unhcr.org/protect/PROTECTION/435df0aa2.pdf.

5. United Nations General Assembly. March 12, 2001. Resolution adapted by the General Assembly. Available at http://www.un.org/documents/ga/docs/56/a566s23.pdf.

6. McAdam J. Part III – Rights and remedies: the convention against torture. Alternative asylum mechanisms: the convention against torture and other cruel, inhuman or degrading treatment or punishment. *International Journal of Law and Psychiatry*. 2004; 27: 627–43.

7. Annas GJ. Unspeakably cruel – torture, medical ethics, and the law. *New England Journal of Medicine*. 2005; 352(20): 2127–32.

8. Moreno A, Piwowarczyk L, Grodin MA. Human rights violations and refugee health. *Journal of the American Medical Association*. 2001; 285(9): 1215.

9. European Council. January 27, 2003. European Council Directive 2003/9/EC – laying down minimum standards for the reception of asylum seekers. Available at http://eur-lex.europa. eu/LexUriServ/site/en/oj/2003/l_031/l_03120030206en00180025.pdf.

10. Steel Z, Frommer N, Silove D. Part I – The mental health impacts of migration: the law and its effects. Failing to understand: refugee determination and the traumatized application. *International Journal of Law and Psychiatry*. 2004; 27: 511–28.

11. Crock M. Part II – Movement and stasis: Re-reading refugee and migration laws. Immigration mindsets – how our thinking has shaped migration law in Australia. *International Journal of Law and Psychiatry*. 2004; 27: 571–85.

12. Worth H. Unconditional hospitality: HIV, ethics and the refugee 'problem.' *Bioethics*. 2006; 20(5): 223–32.

13. Moisander PA, Edston E. Torture and its sequel – a comparison between victims from six countries. *Forensic Science International*. 2003; 137: 133–40.

14. Mollica RF. Global health: Surviving torture. *New England Journal of Medicine*. 2004; 351(1): 5–7.

15. Asirdizer M, Yavuz MS, Sari H, Canturk G, Yorulmaz C. Unusual torture methods and mass murders applied by a terror organization. *American Journal of Forensic Medicine and Pathology*. 2004; 25(4): 314–20.

16. Leth PM, Banner J. Forensic medical examination of refugees who claim to have been tortured. *American Journal of Forensic Medicine and Pathology*. 2005; 26(2): 125–30.

17. Burnett A, Peel M. The health of survivors of torture and organised violence. *British Medical Journal*. 2001; 322: 606–09.

18. Yawar A. Healing in survivors of torture. *Journal of the Royal Society of Medicine*. 2004; 97: 366–70.

19. Eisenman DP, Keller AS, Kim G. Survivors of torture in a general medical setting: how often have patients been tortured, and how often is it missed? *Western Journal of Medicine*. 2000; 172(5): 301–04.

20. Crosby SS, Norredam M, Paasche-Orlow MK, Piwowarczyk L, Heeren T, Grodin MA. Prevalence of torture survivors among foreign-born patients presenting to an urban ambulatory care practice. *Journal of General Internal Medicine*. 2006; 21: 764–8.

21. Silove D. Overcoming obstacles in confronting torture. *Lancet*. 2003; 361: 1555.

22. Montgomery E, Foldspang A. Criterion-related validity of screening for exposure to torture. *Danish Medical Bulletin*. 1994; 41: 588–91.

23. Piwowarczyk L, Moreno A, Grodin MA. Health care of torture survivors. *Journal of the American Medical Association*. 2000; 284(5): 539–41.

24. Feldman R. Primary health care for refugees and asylum seekers: A review of the literature and a framework for services. *Journal of the Royal Institute of Public Health*. 2006; 120: 809–16.

25. Bohannon J. Laying abominable ghosts to rest. *Science*. 2004; 304(5678): 1735–6.

26. Miller KE, Martell ZL, Pazdirek L, Caruth M, Lopez D. The role of interpreter in psychotherapy with refugees: An exploratory study. *American Journal of Orthopsychiatry*. 2005; 75(1): 27–39.

27. Weine S. From war zone to contact zone: culture and refugee mental health services. *Journal of the American Medical Association*. 2001; 285(9): 1214.

28. Hanscom KL. Treating survivors of war trauma and torture. *American Psychologist*. 2001; 56(11): 1032–9.

29. Goodridge E. Meeting the health needs of refugees and immigrants. *Journal of the American Association of Physician Assistants*. 2002; 15: 20–32.

30. Ramaliu A, Thurston WE. Identifying best practices of community participation in providing services to refugee survivors of torture: A case description. *Journal of Immigrant Health*. 2003; 5(4): 165–72.

31. Boersma R. Forensic nursing practice with asylum seekers in the USA – advocacy and international human rights: a pilot study. *Journal of Psychiatric and Mental Health*. 2003; 10: 526–33.

32. Moreno A, Piwowarczyk L, LoMorte WW, Grodin MA. Characteristics and utilization of primary care services in a torture rehabilitation center. *Journal of Immigrant and Minority Health*. 2006a; 8(2): 163–71.

33. Moreno A, Piwowarczyk L, LaMorte WW, Grodin MA. Characteristics and utilization review of primary care services in a torture rehabilitation center. *Journal of Immigrant and Minority Health*. 2006b; 8(2): 163–71.

34. Olsen DR, Montgomery E, Bojholm S, Foldspang A. Prevalent musculoskeletal pain as a correlate of previous exposure to torture. *Scandinavian Journal of Public Health*. 2006; 34: 496–503.

35. Olsen DR, Montgomery E, Carlsson J, Foldspang A. Prevalent pain and pain level among torture survivors. *Danish Medical Bulletin*. 2006; 53(2): 210–14.

36. Thomsen AB, Eriksen J, Smidt-Nielsen K. Chronic pain in torture survivors. *Forensic Science International*. 2000; 108: 155–63.

37. Corovic N, Durakovic Z, Zavalic M, Zrinscak J. Electrocardiographic changes in ex-prisoners of war released from detention camps. *International Journal of Legal Medicine*. 2000; 113: 197–200.

38. Hargreaves S. A body of evidence: torture among asylum seekers to the West. *Lancet*. 2002; 359: 793–4.

39. Savnik A, Amris K, Rogind H, Prip K, Danneskiold-Samsoe B, Bojsen-Moller F, et al. MRI of the plantar structures of the foot after falanga torture. *European Radiology*. 2000; 10: 1655–9.

40. Altun G, Durmus-Altun G. Confirmation of alleged falanga torture by bone scintigraphy – case report. *International Journal of Legal Medicine*. 2003; 117: 365–6.

41. World Health Organization, 2007. Available at http://www.who.int/hhr/Convention_torture.pdf.

42. Powell RA, Leye E, Jayakody A, Mwangi-Powell FN, Morison L. Female genital mutilation, asylum seekers and refugees: the need for an integrated European Union agenda. *Health Policy*. 2004; 70: 151–62.

43. Weinstein CS, Fucteola R, Mollica RF. Neuropsychological issues in the assessment of refugees and victims of mass violence. *Neuropsychology Review*. 2001; 11(3): 131–41.

44. Adams JH, Duschen LW. (1992). *Greenfield's Neuropathology. 5th edition*. New York: Oxford University Press.

45. Rasmussen O. Medical aspects of torture. *Danish Med Bull*. 1990; 37(Supp 1): 1–88.

46. Moreno A, Peel M. Posttraumatic seizures in survivors of torture: manifestations, diagnosis and treatment. *Journal of Immigrant Health*. 2004; 6(4): 179–86.

47. Moreno A, Grodin MA. Torture and its neurological sequelae. *Spinal Cord*. 2002; 40: 213–23.

48. Stauffer WM, Newberry AM, Cartwright CP, Rosenblatt JE, Hanson KL, Sloan L, et al. Evaluation of malaria screening in newly arrived refugees to the united states by microscopy and rapid antigen capture enzyme assay. *Pediatric Infectious Disease Journal*. 2006; 25(10): 948–50.

49. Seybolt LM, Christiansen D, Barnett ED. Diagnostic evaluation of newly arrived asymptomatic refugees with eosinophilia. *Clinical Infectious Diseases*. 2006; 42: 363–7.

50. Halcon LL, Robertson CL, Savik K, Johnson DR, Spring MA, Butcher JN, et al. Trauma and coping in somali and oromo refugee youth. *Journal of Adolescent Health*. 2004; 35: 17–25.

51. CDC. Available at http://www.cdc.gov/ncidod/dq/health.htm. Accessed January 17, 2007.

52. Johnson D. Long-term medical issues in international adoptees. *Pediatr Ann*. 2000; 29: 234–41.

53. Schwarzwald H. Illnesses among recently immigrated children. *Seminars in Pediatric Infectious Diseases*. 2005; 16: 78–83.

54. Pickering L. (2000). *Medical Evaluation in Internationally Adopted Children*. 2000 Red Book: Report of the Committee on Infectious Diseases, 25th Edition.

55. Cote S, Geltman P, Nunn M, Lituri K, Henshaw M, Garcia RI. Dental Caries of Refugee Children Compared With U.S. Children. *Pediatrics*. 2004; 114(6): 733–40.

56. Ellis BH, Lhewa D, Charney M, Cabral H. Screening for PTSD Among among Somali adolescent refugees: psychometric properties of the UCLA PTSD Index. *Journal of Traumatic Stress*. 2006; 19(4): 547–51.

57. Montgomery E, Foldspang A. Traumatic experience and sleep disturbance in refugee children from the Middle East. *European Journal of Public Health*. 2001; 11(1): 18–22.

58. McCullough-Zander K, Larson S. The fear is still in me: caring for survivors of torture. *American Journal of Nursing*. 2004; 104(10): 54–64.

59. Fazel M, Wheeler J, Danesh J. Prevalence of serious mental disorder in 7000 refugees resettled in western countries: a systemic review. *Lancet*. 2005; 365: 1309–14.

60. Porter M, Haslam N. Predisplacement and postdisplacement factors associated with mental health of refugees and internally displaced persons. *Journal of the American Medical Association*. 2005; 294(5): 602–12.

61. Kessler RC, Sonnega A, Bromet E, Hughes M, Nelson CB. Posttraumatic stress disorder in the National Comorbidity Survey. *Arch Gen Psychiatry*. 1995; 52: 1048–60.

62. Keller A, Lhewa D, Rosenfeld B, Sachs E, Aladjem A, Cohen I, et al. Traumatic experiences and psychological distress in an urban refugee population seeking treatment services. *Journal of Nervous and Mental Disease*. 2006; 194(3): 188–94.

63. Basoglu M, Livanou M, Crnobaric C, Franciskovic T, Suljic E, Duric D, et al. Psychiatric and cognitive effects of war in former Yugoslavia. *JAMA*. 2005; 294: 580–90.

64. Hollifield M, Warner TD, Jenkins J, Sinclair-Lian N, Krakow B, Eckert V, et al. Assessing war trauma in refugees: properties of the Comprehensive Trauma Inventory-104. *Journal of Traumatic Stress*. 2006; 19(4): 527–40.

65. de Jong JT, Komroe IH, Van Ommeren M, El Masri M, Araya M, Khaled N, et al. Lifetime events and posttraumatic stress disorder in 4 post-conflict settings. *Journal of the American Medical Association*. 2001; 286(5): 555–62.

66. Eisenman DP, Gelberg L, Liu H, Shapiro MF. Mental health and health-related quality of life among adult latino primary care patients living in the United States with previous exposure to political violence. *Journal of the American Medical Association*. 2003; 290(5): 627–34.

67. Carlsson J, Mortensen EL, Kastrup M. Predictors of mental health and quality of life in male tortured refugees. *Nordic Journal of Psychiatry*. 2006; 60(1): 51–7.

68. Keller AS, Saul JM, Eisenman DP. Caring for survivors of torture in an urban, municipal hospital. *Journal of Ambulatory Care Management*. 1998; 21(2): 20–9.

69. Basoglu M, Ekblad S, Baarnhielm S, Livanou M. Cognitive-behavioral treatment of tortured asylum seekers: a case study. *Anxiety Disorders*. 2004; 18: 357–69.

70. Basoglu M, Aker T. Cognitive-behavioral treatment of torture survivors: a case study. *Torture*. 1996; 3: 61–5.

71. Carlsson J, Mortensen EL, Kastrup M. A Follow-up study of mental health and health-related quality of life in tortured refugees in multidisciplinary Treatment. *Journal of Nervous and Mental Disease*. 2005; 193(10): 651–7.

72. Carlsson JM, Olsen DR, Mortensen EL, Kastrup M. Mental health and health-related quality of life. A 10 year follow-up of tortured refugees. *Journal of Nervous and Mental Disease*. 2006; 194(10): 725–31.

73. Al-Saffar S, Borga P, Edman G, Hallstrom T. The aetiology of posttraumatic stress disorder in four ethnic groups in outpatient psychiatry. *Social Psychiatry Psychiatric Epidemiology*. 2003; 38: 456–62.

74. Jaranson J, Butcher J, Halcon L, Johnson DR, Robertson C, Savik K, et al. Somali and Oromo refugees: correlates of torture and trauma history. *American Journal of Public Health*. 2004; 94(4): 591–8.

75. Place RJ. Caring for non-combatants, refugees, and detainees. *Surgical Clinics of North America*. 2006; 86: 765–77.

76. Howe EG. Dilemmas in military medical ethics since 9/11. *Kennedy Institute of Ethics Journal*. 2003; 13(2): 175–88.

77. Mayer J. The experiment. *The New Yorker*. July 11–18, 2005; pp. 60–71.

78. Annas GJ. Hunger strikes at Guantanamo – medical ethics and human rights in a "Legal Black Hole." *New England Journal of Medicine*. 2006; 355(13): 1377–82.

79. Beach M, Price E, Gary T. Cultural competence: a systemic review of health care provider educational interventions. *Med Care*. 2005; 43: 356–73.

80. Koehn PH, Swick HM. Medical education for a changing world: moving beyond cultural competence into transnational competence. *Academic Medicine*. 2006; 81(6): 548–56.

81. Zweifler J, Gonzalez A. Teaching residents to care for culturally diverse populations. *Acad Med*. 1998; 73: 1056–61.

82. Pincock S. Exposing the horror of torture. *Lancet*. 2003; 362: 1462–3.

83. Evans FB III. Trauma, torture, and transformation in the forensic assessor. *Journal of Personality Assessment*. 2005; 84(1): 25–8.

84. Wenzel T, Jaranson J, Sibitz I, Kastrup M. Torture and the scientific community. *Lancet*. 2000; 355: 1550.

85. Nadeau L, Measham T. Caring for migrant and refugee children: challenges associated with mental health care in pediatrics. *Developmental and Behavioral Pediatrics*. 2006; 27(2): 145–54.

86. Wenzel T, Griengl H, Stompe T, Mirzaei S, Kieffer W. Psychological disorders in survivors of torture: exhaustion, impairment and depression. *Psychopathology*. 2000; 33: 292–6.

Quick Reference Pages

I. Screening questions for a possible survivor of torture

In which country were you born?
What is the current political situation there?
How were you treated in your country?
How did you escape from your country?
Did you live in other countries en route to living here?
Do you still have family members in your native country or here?

II. Examining a possible survivor of torture

Consider the possibility of torture
Inquire about cultural beliefs
Use a culturally sensitive translator if it is possible
Incorporate cultural considerations into the examination area
Consider torture history when performing diagnostic tests

III. Information to gather on a survivor of torture

Background	Country of origin
	Marital status
	Family composition and location
	Date of arrival
	Current living conditions
	Education
	Occupation
	Language(s)
	Religion
Trauma	Reason(s) for persecution
	Affected family members
	Age at first persecution
	Number of persecutions
	Conditions during capture
	Path taken to country of relocation
Medical	Medications
History	Surgery
	Current diagnoses
	Allergies
	Immunization status
	Dental history
Review of systems	
Screening test results	Laboratory results
	Radiology results
	Psychological screening findings

IV. Acute signs of torture

Body system	Findings
Skin	Lacerations, abrasions, ecchymosis, burns
Head and neck	Facial asymmetry, visual changes (diplopia), subconjunctival hemorrhage, proptosis, septal hematoma, tympanic membrane perforation, dental fractures/avulsions, trismus
Chest	Cardiac dysrhythmia, tenderness to palpation/crepitus (rib fractures)
Abdomen	Tenderness to palpation (splenic/liver laceration, ruptured viscus, ruptured diaphragm)
Extremities	Decreased range of motion, obvious deformity, inability to ambulate
Genitourinary	Males: testicular torsion, testicular rupture, hydrocoele, urethral rupture
	Females: Deformity, laceration, tear

V. Chronic sequelae of torture

Body system	Conditions
Skin	Keloids, burn scars (electrode, cigarettes), abrasions (may leave permanent marks if initial lesion contaminated with dirt/other objects), hair loss, nail loss/deformity
Facial bones	Facial asymmetry, crepitus, trismus, temporomandibular joint dysfunction
Facial structures	Lid lag, tympanic membrane scarring, collapsed nasal bridge, deviated septum
Oropharynx	Dental fractures/avulsions, gingival scarring, gingival disease, trismus
Neck	Hyoid crepitus, bruits, muscle spasm
Musculoskeletal	Deformity, decreased range of motion, contracture, distal neurovascular deficit
Genitourinary	Deformity, incontinence, STDs, discharge, diarrhea
Central Nervous System	Gait disturbance, cognitive/motor delays, sensory changes, posterior column changes, neuropathy/radiculopathy, seizure disorder

VI. Infectious disease considerations

Region	Conditions
Africa	Dengue fever, HIV, Malaria, Marburg/Ebola virus, sickle cell disease, TB
Asia	Hepatitis B/C, HIV, malaria (South Pacific), TB
Central/South America	Chagas disease, HIV, malaria, typhoid
Middle East	G6PD deficiency, malaria, thalassemia

VII. Adult vs. pediatric screening

Screening measure	Adult	Pediatric
Immunizations	Update as needed	Update as needed, start series based on CDC/AAP guidelines
Developmental milestones	Not required	Age-specific guidelines; delay may be due to growth delay
Growth delays	Not required	Gender-specific growth curves should be plotted
Dental screening	Should be performed	Should be performed, consider supplemental fluoride
Vision and hearing screening	Recommended based on patient concerns/exam findings only	Recommended on all children <15 years of age

VIII. Key PTSD treatment modalities

Modality	Example
Medication	SSRI Short term benzodiazepines
Cognitive-behavioral therapy	Trigger identification Trigger desensitization

IX. Some potential resources to consider for a survivor of torture

1. Social work:
   a. To assist in locating a specialty referral center for torture survivors
   b. To assist patient in qualifying for Medicaid or medical insurance
2. Psychiatry
   a. To assist in screening patient for PTSD or other psychiatric sequelae
   b. To treat and follow patients suffering from PTSD
3. Neurology
   a. To assist in managing chronic headaches or seizures in torture survivors
   b. To assist in evaluation of neurovascular deficits in survivors of torture
4. Infectious Disease
   a. If patient may be suffering from endemic illness
5. Primary Care (Adult or Pediatrics)

8

Trafficking victims

Fiona Gallahue, M.D., F.A.C.E.P

Goals and objectives

1. To understand what trafficking in human beings entails, the scope of the problem and how victims are trafficked
2. To learn how to screen a potentially trafficked patient and interview a trafficked patient
3. To learn how to appropriately medically manage and refer a trafficked patient

Human trafficking

A 13-year-old Guatemalan native presents to an emergency department, pregnant and in premature labor. Her medical issues are managed routinely but what the emergency attending and staff do not recognize is that this patient is a victim of human trafficking. As a result, she is not rescued until several months later. This girl was sold by her parents for sex and domestic servitude. One of her brutal beatings by her trafficker stimulated her premature labor. This is the true story of one of thousands of trafficking victims living in the United States.[1]

Trafficking in human beings is a form of modern slavery, which expressly forces, defrauds, or coerces people for the purpose of forced labor or commercial sexual exploitation. There is no nation immune to the threat of having residents trafficked or harboring trafficked workers.[2] Human trafficking is the world's fastest growing criminal enterprise, with profits rivaling that of the drugs and arms trades. Because of the lucrative nature of human trafficking and low risk to the traffickers, the problem continues despite the growing awareness of this issue.

While true numbers are obscured by the clandestine and illegal nature of trafficking, commonly cited sources include the following:

- The ILO (International Labour Organization) estimates that 12.3 million people are enslaved in forced labor of which at least 2.4 million are victims of trafficking operations.[3]

- The U.S. Department of State approximates 600,000 to 800,000 people are trafficked across international borders each year, approximately 80 percent are women and girls, and up to 50 percent are minors. The majority of transnational victims were trafficked into commercial sexual exploitation.[4]
- The annual revenue from trafficking in persons has been estimated to be about 31 billion dollars.[3]

Trafficking: Definitions

Human trafficking is one of the greatest human rights challenges of our generation. As such, the United Nations, the United States Department of State, and the Council of Europe have all created legal definitions of trafficking, strengthened laws to convict traffickers, and enhanced the resources to protect victims of trafficking. If you as a practitioner believe your patient is a victim of trafficking, it can be helpful to understand the different forms trafficking can take and the legal terms for them.

The United Nations

The United Nations Protocol to Prevent, Suppress and Punish Trafficking in Persons, Especially Women and Children (Trafficking in Persons Protocol) defines trafficking as the action of recruitment, transportation, transfer, harboring, or receipt of persons by means of the threat or use of force, coercion, abduction, fraud, deception, abuse of power or vulnerability, or payments or benefits to achieve the consent of a person for the purpose of exploitation.[5]

United States

The Federal Government has recently developed federal laws to aggressively address the problem of trafficking, prosecute traffickers, and assist victims of trafficking. Washington and Texas are two states that have their own state anti-trafficking laws, who can pursue prosecution of traffickers on a state level.

U.S. Federal anti-trafficking law is defined by the *Trafficking Victims Protection Act of 2000 (TVPA)* and reaffirmed by the *Trafficking Victims Protection Reauthorization Act (TVPRA) of 2005*. The TVPA enacts criminal penalties against traffickers and provides services for victims of "severe forms of trafficking in persons."

Definitions

"*Severe forms of trafficking in persons*" is defined as (A) sex trafficking in which a commercial sex act is induced by force, fraud, or coercion, or in which the person induced to perform such act has not attained 18 years of age; or (B) the recruitment, harboring, transportation, provision, or obtaining of a person for labor or services, through the use of force, fraud, or coercion for the purpose of subjection to involuntary servitude, peonage, debt bondage, or slavery.

"Commercial sex act" means any sex act on account of which anything of value is given to or received by any person.

"Coercion" means (A) threats of serious harm to or physical restraint against any person; (B) any scheme, plan, or pattern intended to cause a person to believe that failure to perform an act would result in serious harm to or physical restraint against any person, or (C) the abuse or threatened abuse of the legal process.

"Debt bondage" means the status or condition of a debtor arising from a pledge by the debtor of his or her personal services or of those of a person under his or her control as a security for debt, if the value of those services as reasonably assessed is not applied toward the liquidation of the debt or the length and nature of those services are not respectively limited and defined.

"Involuntary servitude" includes a condition of servitude induced by means of (A) any scheme, plan, or pattern intended to cause a person to believe that, if the person did not enter into or continue in such condition, that person or another person would suffer serious harm or physical restraint; or (B) the abuse or threatened abuse of the legal process.

"Peonage" means holding someone against his or her will to pay off a debt.[6]

Human trafficking versus smuggling

The term "human trafficking" is differentiated from "smuggling of migrants" in three distinct ways.

First is the issue of consent: A victim of trafficking has not consented to the treatment he/she receive or, if he/she initially consented, this consent is considered meaningless because of the coercive, fraudulent, abusive, or deceptive actions by the traffickers. Additionally, children under the age of 18 cannot give valid consent, so any recruitment, transportation, transfer, harboring, or receipt of children for the purpose of exploitation is a form of trafficking regardless of the means used. Custodians of minors also cannot give consent to the human trafficking act for the purpose of exploitation.

Second is the duration of time that a person is subjected to degrading and/or dangerous conditions. A trafficked person continues to be exploited once he/she has reached his/her destination in order to generate profits for the traffickers. Smuggling ends once the migrant has reached his/her destination.

Third is the fact that smuggling always requires the migrant to cross national borders whereas trafficking victims may or may not ever leave their country of origin.[5]

Human trafficking is a process, not a single offence

The process of trafficking in persons generally includes the following steps:

1. RECRUITMENT: The process of human trafficking begins with the abduction or recruitment of a person.
2. TRANSPORTATION: It continues with the transportation from the place of origin to the place of destination. In case of transnational trafficking in persons, the process includes the entry of the individual into another country.
3. EXPLOITATION: This is followed by the exploitation phase during which the victim is forced into sexual or labor servitude. This often includes violence against the victim.
4. PROFIT LAUNDERING: The criminal organization may find it necessary to launder the criminal proceeds. There may be further links to other criminal offences such as the smuggling of migrants, weapons, or drugs.[5]

The role of organized crime in trafficking

Because of the highly organized requirements of human trafficking, nearly all operations are conducted by organized crime groups. This greatly complicates the process of rescuing victims.

An "organized crime group" as defined by The United Nations Convention against Transnational Organized Crime is "a structured group of three or more persons existing for a period of time and acting in concert with the aim of committing one or more serious crimes or offences established in accordance with the Convention, in order to obtain, directly, or indirectly, a financial or other material benefit."[5]

Two distinct patterns dominate the diverse structures of organized crime groups, either a hierarchy with a clear leadership or a core group with a limited number of individuals forming a tight core surrounded by a loose network of associates. In all the criminal groups engaging in the trafficking of persons, the groups involved had cooperation with other organized crime groups.

Because these operations are conducted by organized crime groups, the victim of trafficking is at high risk if he/she escapes their traffickers. The traffickers usually retaliate with violence and the victim may be murdered if found or his/her immediate family killed or injured if he/she is not. Rescued victims also face significant danger of being retrafficked if adequate resources and assistance are not set up for them. Many times, a victim of trafficking has been sent back to the area from which he/she was trafficked immediately after being rescued, identified by his/her traffickers and retrafficked into the same or worse situation from which he/she was "rescued."

Currently, many countries are now aware of this problem and increasing efforts to assist victims through social services, legal assistance, and issuing visas to allow the victims to remain in the country where they were found. Unfortunately, even with the increased awareness, the legal process for protecting these victims can be daunting and the social services may be inadequate in many places to prevent the retrafficking of rescued victims.[2]

Who are the recruiters?

In many cases, recruiters share predetermined characteristics to appeal to potential victims. Most suspected traffickers are over 30 years old, reinforcing their credibility and authority. Many of the traffickers are the same nationality as the victims. Although a majority of traffickers are male, there is some evidence that women as recruiters give more credibility to the job offers used as bait to lure victims who were inexperienced in the sex market.[7,8]

Interestingly enough, it has been demonstrated that the gender of the trafficker influences the gender of the victims. Male traffickers or male/female teams have victims who are men; female-only traffickers generally have victims who are women or girls.

Traffickers often manage to win their victim's trust without revealing information about themselves. Interviews with victims from Romania demonstrated that in a large number of cases, the recruiter was acquainted with the victim or the victim's family, yet, often, no detailed information about the recruiter, including his/her occupation, place of residence, or family status was known by the victim.

In Nepal, cases commonly involving families, neighbors, and friends play an active role in trafficking by creating fictitious marriage and job offers, contacting recruiters and brokers, or by luring girls away from home on outings or errands, and then kidnapping and selling them.[8]

In some cases, the recruiter may have also been a victim of trafficking. In a report by Human Rights Watch on the trafficking of Nepali girls and women to India, some Nepali trafficking victims working as prostitutes procure their release by the brothel keeper if they furnish a substitute. These women may travel to their own villages and attempt to lure a female relative, friend, or a village woman to accompany them to India to be the next victim of human trafficking for commercial sexual exploitation.[8]

Trafficked forced laborers and annual profits generated by them[7]

Region of destination	Trafficked people	% of regional total of forced laborers	Profits generated by traffickers (millions)
Asia and Pacific	1,360,000	14%	9,704
Industrialized Countries	270,000	75%	15,513
Latin America & Caribbean	250,000	19%	1,348
Mid-East & North Africa	230,000	88%	1,508
Transition Countries	200,000	95%	3,422
Sub-Saharan Africa	130,000	20%	159
TOTAL	**2,440,000**	**20%**	**31,654**

Trafficking rates continue to rise, spurred on by the large profits generated and minimal legal deterrents. Traffickers receive steady profits from forced labor or sexual exploitation for prolonged periods of time. Furthermore, human victims can be sold repeatedly, creating huge profit margins. In many countries, traffickers enjoy "virtually no risk of prosecution." Even when prosecuted, the criminal penalties are light and harmless compared to sentences given to dealers in drugs or weapons.

Additionally, global and economic conditions are creating more vulnerable victims: weak economies, unemployment, and scarce job opportunities in foreign countries. Although legal protections are now being instituted, these protections are unlikely to stem the growing tide of trafficking.[2]

Where do victims come from? Where do they work?

The horrifying accounts from survivors range widely in the types of servitude and their countries of origin but not in the basic fact that they were not given the rights of personhood to be allowed to leave these situations.

Generally, trafficked victims come from any country where poverty is high; they may be moved to more affluent areas to make money for their traffickers, as is often the case in prostitution, or fall into involuntary servitude within their own countries. A lack of educational and training opportunities, a financial need to support their families, cultural attitudes toward children and women, and inadequate laws and protections make these victims vulnerable to trafficking. Victims also come from families displaced from a war-torn area or area that has been ravaged by a natural disaster. Shortly after the Indian Ocean tsunami in 2005, numerous cases of rape, kidnapping, and trafficking of children orphaned by the tsunami were reported.[9]

Within the United States, 300,000 children are estimated to be at risk of becoming victims of trafficking, many of these start out running away from homes where they

All Trafficking Prosecutions[6]	2001	2002	2003	2004	2005
Investigations – Total	63	65	82	129	139
Cases Filed					
Labor	6	3	6	6	8
Sex	4	7	8	23	26
Total	**10**	**10**	**11**	**26**	**34**
Defendants Charged					
Labor	9	17	6	7	20
Sex	26	27	21	40	75
Total	**35**	**41**	**27**	**47**	**95**
Convictions					
Labor	8	5	5	3	10
Sex	15	23	16	30	25
Total	**23**	**28**	**21**	**33**	**35**

Figure 8.1 All trafficking prosecutions. *Note*: From United States Department of Justice. (2006, September). *Assessment of U.S. Government Efforts to Combat Trafficking in Persons in Fiscal Year 2005*. (14/37) Retrieved December 1, 2006, from http://www.usdoj.gov/ag/annualreports/tr2006/assessment_of_efforts_to_combat_tip.pdf. *Some cases include both labor and sexual elements, making it difficult to categorize.*

were already physically or sexually abused. These children are usually exploited within the borders of the United States.[10]

The greatest number of documented trafficking victims come from Asia (approximately 250,000 per year), the former Soviet Union (about 100,000 per year), and from central and eastern Europe (about 175,000 per year). An estimated 100,000 trafficked women come from Latin America and the Caribbean annually, and more than 50,000 from Africa.[11]

Most victims of trafficking are children or young men and women. Their youth makes them more likely to trust an older, mature trafficker and less likely to ask questions that will protect them or raise red flags that might otherwise give them pause.

In fieldwork investigating the trafficking of women from Romania to Germany, the average age was just over 21 years of age with the youngest victim being 14 years old. Most of the victims came from rural areas, from families with more than four children and few income sources, and had a low level of education. The Human Rights Watch report on Nepali girls and women trafficked to India found the average age of victims to be between 14 and 16 in the 1980s, dropping to between 10 and 14 years of age in 1991. The increasing demand by brothels and customers for younger, virginal girls who are thought to be less likely to harbor the HIV virus is assumed to account for this shift.[8] Unfortunately, these younger victims have more long-term medical complications related to their abuse than older teens and women. In fact, these younger girls have a higher rate of HIV/AIDS than prostituted women (27.7% vs. 8.4%).[12]

The overwhelming majority of transnational victims are trafficked into commercial sexual exploitation. Some victims are subject to more than one form of exploitation.

People trafficked within their own national borders outnumber those trafficked transnationally per estimate of the U.S. Department of State. These victims are enslaved as domestic servants, factory workers, sold as brides, beggars, camel jockeys, stone-quarry workers, soldiers, field laborers, and used for commercial sexual exploitation. The number of victims trafficked intranationally are believed to be overwhelmingly underreported as compared to transnational victims because there are fewer legal authorities to intercept the victim and traffickers.

Victims of trafficking are at risk for being re-trafficked after being rescued. Often, these victims are especially vulnerable because they lack the resources of citizenship in the destination county, are unable to speak the language, and are often young and inexperienced. Stories of victims being rescued and sent back immediately to their country of origin only to be picked up at the airport by their traffickers are common. The traffickers sometimes bribe the authorities entrusted to protect these victims and the rescued victim is victimized again.

Many countries have inadequate protection for victims. One such example is Russia where the only adult trafficking-specific shelters are run by NGOs with no government funding or assistance; these NGOs are expected to provide legal, medical, and psychological support for these victims. At least three Russian trafficking victims were re-trafficked in 2005, due in part to the lack of a trafficking shelter in Moscow. The victims returned to Moscow, were identified by their traffickers, and quickly re-trafficked.[12]

Victims may also be re-trafficked by being vulnerable to further exploitation in attempts to get out of a terrible environment. Girls trafficked into sweatshop factory environments are ripe for traffickers looking for brothel workers, lured by promises that they are going into domestic service and a better environment than the one they are currently in.

Some children are trafficked in order to be human sacrifices. Children trafficked for ritual sacrifice first emerged into the public eye in September 2001 when a child's torso was found in the Thames River in London. The child was not identified though he was named Adam by the police, but his background was traced to Nigeria. In London, it has been reported that boys "unblemished" by circumcision are being sacrificed in some African churches in the United Kingdom because this type of human sacrifice is required for powerful spells. There are approximately 300 of these churches currently in the United Kingdom though the majority of them are not believed to be involved. The children are trafficked from Africa for as little as ten British pounds (approximately $22). In one three-month period in 2005, Scotland Yard revealed that 280 black boys between the ages of four to seven were reported missing from London schools with no trace. There is concern in the United Kingdom that the true number of missing boys and girls may be several thousand a year.[13]

The role of globalization and cultural values on trafficking

Globalization has provided opportunity to both those who wish to migrate and those who traffic the unwilling. In 2000, the United Nations estimated that almost 13 million people or 2 percent of the world population, are on the move at any given time.[14]

Emigrating youth are especially vulnerable to traffickers. Since 2004, 120 Chinese children have disappeared from Swedish immigration centers. In all of these cases, the children arrived in Sweden on a plane from Beijing or Moscow requesting immediate political asylum. Within days, they disappeared while cases were pending. Swedish law enforcement authorities believe a network of traffickers is behind the disappearances.[12]

In some cases, the country of origin is complicit with the trafficking that occurs either overtly or covertly. In some countries, such as Burma, slavery is state sponsored with children as young as 11 being forced into the military. Covertly, many countries such as India have laws against trafficking but the policing of these crimes are minimal by many accounts. In 2005, 13 suspected sex traffickers were arrested in Mumbai, India's largest city with the highest concentration of victims of commercial sexual exploitation, but no prosecutions or convictions were pursued. Between June and September of 2005, 16,000 children were reported rescued from forced labor workshops in Mumbai and 694 children rescued in Delhi in November but there were no documented arrests or prosecutions of the factory owners exploiting these children despite strict laws that subject employers to imprisonment and fines for forced child labor.[12]

The unequal status of women and children in most countries contributes to the lack of attention to this problem, making them more vulnerable as victims of both forced labor and sexual exploitation (80% of transnational trafficking victims are women, 40–50% are children).[12]

It is clear that cultural attitudes toward gender affect the trafficking victim's gender. In most countries, many more girls are exploited into commercial sex than boys. However, in Sri Lanka where girls receive a greater proportion of protection in the family, the majority of children exploited are boys.[14]

Lack of individual and societal protective mechanisms makes children especially vulnerable. Effective child protection projects only receive 60 percent of the United Nations Consolidated Appeals (CAP) requested funding while other projects receive 73 percent of requested funding.

Children are especially targeted in conflict areas. Close to ten thousand children were deliberately maimed in Sierra Leone making them more vulnerable to later physical or sexual abuse. At any time, more than 300,000 children are fighting as soldiers worldwide. In the Democratic Republic of Congo, where over 2.3 million people have been displaced, displaced children suffer the most. A study by Save the Children found that one in five children will die before reaching the age of five, 38 percent of children under five have stunted growth due to hunger and malnutrition, only 50 percent of children aged 6 to 11 attend school, girls as young as 13 were regularly subjected to exploitative sexual relations by peacekeepers in exchange for food or money.[15] Refugee adolescents are the most underserved groups, only 3 percent of the 1.5 million refugee children between the ages of 12 and 17 worldwide have access to education.[15] Without education, these children are especially at risk to be trafficked. In Cambodia, children as young as four years old are trafficked as beggars, some with "unnatural deformities," likely mutilated by their traffickers because handicapped children bring in more money.[16]

The unequal status of women is especially demonstrated in some countries such as China, Taiwan, South Korea, India, Pakistan, and some sub-Saharan African countries where the ratio of men to women is higher than would be expected from the typical sex ratio at birth and typical differential mortality. High female mortality rates resulting from sex-selected abortion, female infanticide, and the systematic and often fatal neglect of the health and nutritional needs of girls cause this demographic inequality.

Worldwide, it is estimated that between 60 and 100 million girls and women are "missing." This is reflected in the 1991 Indian census. After adjustment for expected differences in fertility and life-expectancy, the 1991 figures suggests that between 22 and 37 million Indian girls and women are "missing" with the greatest excess mortality in girls younger than four years.[11]

The trafficking of girls and women by their families can be understood in context as accepted practice in these communities given the low societal value placed on their well-being and the often desperate circumstances surrounding the family.

Role of law enforcement in trafficking

In almost all countries, the official role of law enforcement is to enforce the international laws against human trafficking. Unfortunately, in many countries the official role and actual role of law enforcement are very different.

Anecdotal stories of the police accepting bribes from traffickers and being complicit in the enslavement of women in the commercial sex industry are common. This includes raping victims who have escaped their traffickers or having sex with the enslaved victims at the brothels as a benefit of complicity with the traffickers and/or brothel keepers. Violence toward women in the sex industry by police is common in many areas. In a survey of 540 female prostitutes in Bangladesh, 49 percent had been raped and 59 percent had been beaten by police in the past year.[11]

In some countries, the law officer may arrest these women for violating their "contracts." Women who escape their traffickers may face litigation for working as prostitutes or for not fulfilling the "terms of their employment" to their traffickers if they signed contracts initially for what they believed to be legitimate employment.

Even when law officers are not corrupt, they may hold negative views of women especially those who have been working in the commercial sex industry. Prostitutes are often vilified and even if trafficked, are assumed complicit in their own exploitation. This is a pervasive societal belief in many cultures and it may override the officer's understanding that the victim be treated with respect and accepted as a victim. Rescued trafficking victims have been arrested for their work in the sex industry, held in jails as prostitutes, and even shackled while in jail like common prisoners, their captive state reinforcing feelings of vulnerability and negative emotional states.

In many cases, victims are also threatened with deportation to their countries of origin by the legal authorities, where they face the risk of being trafficked again or may have no support system if they were orphaned, trafficked by their families, or had lost contact with their families who may have relocated.

As a health care practitioner, you may find yourself needing to advocate for your patient to the law enforcement officials who are supposed to protect them.

Victims of trafficking may be wary of law enforcement given their prior experiences. Additionally, law enforcement and legal authorities who do work with trafficking victims may not always be aware of the new laws and protections for victims since most of these protections are new or recent. However, many countries are now aware of this limitation and have hotline numbers to assist anyone in contact with a potential trafficking victim. These numbers are listed in the "Resources" section at the end of this chapter.

The federal response in the United States

The Victims of Trafficking and Violence Protection Act (TVPA) was passed by the U.S. Congress and signed into law on October 28, 2000 and reauthorized on January 10, 2006. The TVPA endeavors to protect victims of trafficking by providing stiffer penalties for trafficking, to create new standards of eligibility for governmental assistance regardless of legal immigration status, and to grant victims a T visa that gives them temporary residency status in the United States. Although the TVPA is a positive step toward addressing trafficking victims, the criteria to meet the T visa's eligibility is strict and requires the victim to assist with the investigation and prosecution of their traffickers. Additionally, even if the victims comply with all of the requirements there is often a lag time before they can receive the benefits they are entitled to with no interim provisions.[2]

Assisting the trafficked patient

Because a majority of trafficking victims are women and girls, the feminine pronoun is used throughout this section, it should be remembered however, that trafficking victims may be men or boys.

Groups that assist labor trafficking victims report that the most commonly required services are advocacy (97%) and medical services (97%). The greatest needs reported for sex trafficking victims are legal/paralegal services (99%), medical services (98%), and information/referral services (97%).[2]

Differences between trafficking victims and victims of other crimes

Although trafficking victims may seem similar to victims of sexual assault or domestic violence, there are significant differences between these groups.

- Trafficking victims may be running from an entire network of organized crime in contrast to the domestic violence victims who are running from a single perpetrator.
- Trafficking victims may have been sexually assaulted multiple times over a long time period by multiple perpetrators leaving them with more physical and mental health damage in comparison to sexual assault victims usually assaulted by a single person over a discrete time period.
- Trafficking victims are less stable overall because they often have no home, no job, no U.S. citizenship, no savings, and no family in the area.
- Trafficking victims have more extreme trauma and mental health needs than the average domestic violence or sexual assault victim.
- Trafficking victims are more socially isolated than the average domestic violence victim.
- Trafficking victims may have less understanding of the criminal justice system.
- Trafficking victims are often young adults and minors without family support or guidance.

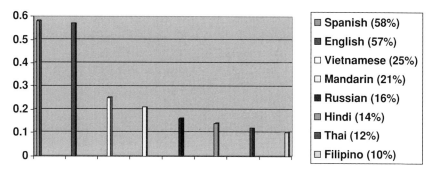

Figure 8.2   From Clawson et al., *Needs Assessment for Service Providers and Trafficking Victims*. U.S. Department of Justice, National Institute of Justice. October 2003. Available online at http://www.ncjrs.gov/pdffiles1/nij/grants/202469.pdf.

Language barriers

A survey of American groups working with trafficking victims reported that English is not the primary language of a large proportion of their clients.[2] Professional translation services are recommended in assisting any person not fluent in English.

A victim-centered approach to trafficking: The three R's

The three R's of the victim-centered approach are rescue, rehabilitation, and reintegration.[12]

Clues to suspect a patient may be a trafficking victim[17]

1) Evidence of being controlled
2) Evidence of inability to move or leave a job
3) Bruises or other signs of physical abuse
4) Fear or depression
5) Not speaking on one's own behalf and/or non-English speaking
6) No passport or other forms of identification or documentation

Screening questions to help determine if your patient is a trafficking victim

(From the "Rescue and Restore Campaign" by the Department of Health and Human Services' Administration for Children and Families)

1) What type of work do you do?
2) Are you being paid?

3) Can you leave your job if you want to?

4) Can you come and go as you please?

5) Have you or your family been threatened?

6) What are your working and living conditions like?

7) Where do you sleep and eat?

8) Do you have to ask permission to eat/sleep/go to the bathroom?

9) Are there locks on your door/windows so you cannot get out?

10) Has your identification or documentation been taken from you?

The World Health Organization's set of recommendations for service providers who are unfamiliar with the situation of trafficked victims (modified here for the health care practitioner).

Ten guiding principles in interviewing a person who has been trafficked

1) ***Do no harm:*** Assume that the potential for harm is extreme for your patient until there is evidence to the contrary. Do not undertake any interview that will make a patient's situation worse in the short or long term. Ensure confidentiality of all consultants working with this patient. Your patient's trafficker may be nearby, and your patient may not be in a position to answer your questions freely. Be very careful about putting your patient at risk and minimize risk to your patient as much as possible. Your patient's children, spouse, or other family may all have been threatened and targeted as a means of coercion by the trafficker. Your patient may be unwilling to speak with you and risk placing loved ones in harm's way. Understand that these are credible threats that may be acted on by the traffickers.

2) ***Know your subject and assess the risks:*** This is a difficult task in a busy clinical area but if you are unable to take the time to learn the risks associated with trafficking and the specific risks to your patient, limit the interview as much as possible and focus your efforts on getting someone who will be able to devote the time with your patient (i.e., social work, agencies who specialize in trafficking, etc.)

3) ***Prepare referral information. Do not make promises you cannot fulfill:*** Be prepared to provide information in your patient's native language and the local language about appropriate legal, health, shelter, social support, and security services. Be prepared to hold your patient until such referrals can be made. Victims who are referred inadequately are at significant risk for being retrafficked or found by their trafficker.

4) ***Adequately select and prepare interpreters and co-workers:*** Assume that your patient's traffickers may be nearby, limit conversation about the patient in

public areas, work on getting an appropriate translator (not family members, etc.) and preparing the translator for the interview. Be sure that your co-workers limit any public conversation about the patient.

5) ***Ensure anonymity and confidentiality:*** Protect your patient's confidentiality as much as possible. If your patient is in the hospital or emergency department, involve administration, and consider registering the patient under an alias so that hospital operators can not confirm that your patient is in the hospital to traffickers who may be searching for them.

6) ***Get informed consent:*** Make sure that your patient is aware that the interview can be terminated at any time, that she can decide what services she would like to access, and that she has the right not to answer any questions.

7) ***Listen to and respect the victim's assessment of the situation and safety risks:*** Each victim has different concerns and the way she views her concerns may be different from how others might assess them.

8) ***Do not re-traumatize the patient:*** Do not ask questions intended to provoke an emotionally charged response. Be prepared to respond to your patient's distress. Be careful not to place judgment on the patient's situation, the patient's family who may have been involved in their trafficking, or how they became trafficked.

9) ***Be prepared for emergency intervention:*** Be prepared to respond if your patient reports being in imminent danger. Believe your patient if she states that she is in danger.

10) ***Put information collected to good use:*** Use information in a way that benefits the individual victim. Limit your questions to those that will help assess safety and how you can best assist your patient medically and emotionally.[18]

Interview with a trafficked patient

Ideally, this should occur in a quiet, private place with no distractions. While this may be difficult, if not impossible, in a busy clinical area such as an emergency department, it may be possible to limit distractions or delegate one member of the health care team to dedicate to this patient.

Find a translator if the patient is not fluent in English, even if you can communicate non-fluently. The details that you record may be used in litigation and getting any recorded details correct is imperative. Additionally, a translator may be aware of certain cultural details that are important to understand during your history and physical. The translator who understands the cultural background of the patient may be able to prepare you for certain taboos in touching, feeding, and questioning your patient. Do not underestimate the value of being culturally sensitive. Confirm that the translator does not know the trafficker so that there is no conflict of interest.

Patients generally do not identify themselves as victims of trafficking. These victims may not appear to need social services because they have a place to live, food to eat, medical care, and what they think is a paying job. Children especially may not be aware that they are victims of trafficking believing that they are paying off a "debt" to their trafficker by working for them.[17]

Ask your patient if she prefers to speak with a practitioner of a specific gender. Culturally, some patients may not be comfortable with a practitioner of the opposite gender examining them. Additionally, many victims of trafficking have been sexually assaulted, even if they were not working in the sex industry and will be less open speaking with a member of a specific gender. Women who have been trafficked into the sex industry may be especially distrustful of speaking with a male practitioner. Since the victim has had very little opportunity to assert her own opinions or preferences while in captivity, it is imperative to respect the wishes of your patient now. Ensuring your patient's emotional comfort during the history and physical exam reiterates her value as an individual and survivor.

Develop trust in the interview, being careful not to make assumptions or judgments. This may be difficult to do, especially if you find out that her own family may have sold her to traffickers or if she does not want to leave her traffickers.

Assess your patient's general physical condition, is there any pressing medical intervention required that should pre-empt your interview?

Assess your patient's safety. Is she currently being abused by her employer or anyone else? Is she in danger?

Find out what your patient's expectations are – what does she want or need from you?

Learn as much as you can about your patient's background and her current situation. Explain to your patient why you are asking this information and understand if your patient withholds information or lies to you.

Assess your patient's emotional state especially regarding whether she is considering suicide. Some patients do consider killing themselves out of the shame of what they have endured.

With child victims, be careful to ask only open-ended questions and limit your interview until a trained interviewer can assist you. Children may be more suggestible and also may be less capable of answering multiple interviewers with consistent answers. Any inconsistency will weaken later prosecution.

Because children may not know their birth date and may have been told that they are older than they are, a trafficked patient may actually be under 18 and eligible for more protection under the current laws. If you suspect this is the case, you are required to inform the state-appropriate child protection agency and you may need to hold the patient in protective custody at your institution as a suspected child abuse victim.

Unless the patient has an emergency medical condition and needs emergent stabilization, it is best for trafficked children to be transferred to a specialized center, if available, for a forensic examination, especially if sexual abuse is involved.

Things to keep in mind during your interview with a trafficking victim

1. Your patient may not tell you the entire story or be entirely truthful with you. She may be embarrassed, she may be afraid of reprisal by her trafficker, or be afraid of being turned over to law authorities. Your patient may have been misled by people they cared about and trusted; she may be unlikely to trust anyone who offers to assist them. She may be afraid to speak the truth or be trying to protect herself. Your patient may be using drugs or alcohol as a coping mechanism.

2. Your patient may not know the truth about everything. Often, traffickers deceive victims in order to enforce their power over them. Some victims are drugged during their captivity, which may interfere with their ability to recall details.

3. Don't assume that your patient hates the trafficker, brothel owner, husband (in an arranged marriage), or employer. Because your patient has been depending on these people for survival, she may not want to risk the relationship with them. To the contrary, your patient may have feelings of love for these people or have other complicated relationships with them.

4. Don't assume that the patient wants to change the situation. She may choose to stay in the current situation. Allow her to make her own choices and be careful to be as non-judgmental as you can.

5. Don't assume that your patient can read or write.

6. Don't assume your patient is uneducated.

7. Don't assume that your patient wants to contact the authorities or wants you to take action.

8. Do not assume that your patient has not been sexually assaulted if she was not trafficked into the sex industry.

9. Your patient may be shut down emotionally or express a wide variety of emotions (hostility, joy, guilt) if she was severely abused. Understand that her experiences may be beyond your ability to comprehend and that her emotional state does not reflect upon the validity of her experience. Be careful not to get defensive if your patient is hostile but do ask if she is responding to something you said or did. Apologize if you were insensitive.

10. Ask about drugs or alcohol use. Your patient may have been encouraged to use drugs and alcohol but may not be forthcoming about this information.

11. Ask about suicidality and depression.

12. Be careful to ask for permission prior to touching your patient at any time. Even the most benign touching may feel threatening to a victim of trafficking.

13. Be especially careful about releasing children to anyone's care, as traffickers will often claim to be the parents. Strongly consider holding children in protective custody until the family situation can be carefully investigated.
14. Limit your interviews with children who have been trafficked since they are more impressionable and leading questions may interfere with an in-depth interview with authorities later.
15. If a victim is unsure of her age or appears younger than her stated age, assume that she are under the age of 18. It is common practice for victims to be told to report an age over 18 to protect the traffickers from laws against exploiting minors.

Health concerns for trafficking victims

Specific health concerns for victims trafficked expressly for sexual exploitation will be discussed later. However, do not to assume that because your patient was not trafficked into sexual exploitation that she has not been sexually assaulted.

Although your patient may not tell you her age or the age she was when she was first enslaved, be aware that child victims are especially vulnerable medically and psychologically. Many of these children have no family to return to if they have been separated from them for a significant period of time. Malnourishment and dental problems are prevalent in these child victims due to a poor diet which does not meet their physiologic needs. As a result they may suffer from growth retardation, poorly formed or rotted teeth, and nutritional deficiencies such as scurvy or rickets.

Many victims of trafficking suffer from chronic conditions that have not been treated such as hypertension or diabetes. One case of a woman in domestic servitude for many years was taken to an emergency department by a neighbor for the evaluation of a large tumor. The doctor treating her recognized her as a trafficking victim and assisted her in escaping her situation and getting the medical care she needed.[17]

Health concerns that are commonly seen in trafficking victims may be specific to the type of work they were trafficked into.

Sweatshop workers often suffer from chronic back, hearing, cardiovascular, or respiratory problems due to dangerous work environments. Weak eyes and eye problems due to strain from dim light are also common.

Agricultural workers are at high risk for chronic back problems, and musculoskeletal complaints. Respiratory, skin, or other constitutional symptoms may arise from exposure to pesticides and other environmental toxins. Tuberculosis and parasites such as lice may spread rapidly in cramped environments without medical care.

Trafficking victims are closely guarded, but may be brought for emergency medical treatment for injuries sustained by a brutal beating or a workplace accident, or for an untreated medical condition that has reached a critical stage, or for complications from inept medical care by an unqualified person working with the traffickers, such as a botched abortion. This may be the only opportunity to rescue them from their enslavement.

Trafficking for sexual exploitation

The demand from sex industries and their customers for sex industry workers along with limited employment opportunities for women, the feminization of poverty globally, the increasing economic marginalization of women, and the globalization of organized crime networks have made trafficking in women and girls for sexual exploitation a growing problem internationally.

The trafficking of women and girls for sexual exploitation is an issue that involves every country, whether they are the source, transit, or destination country for these women and girls.

According to the Human Rights Watch, more than a million women and children are employed in Indian brothels. Many are the victims of trafficking across international borders, often from Nepal, held in slavery and subjected to serious physical abuse. Trafficked Nepali girls and women make up about half of Bombay's estimated 100,000 brothel workers. Many of these girls and women are brought to India as virgins, and if they survive, many return to Nepal with HIV or AIDS. The average age of a trafficking victim in this area is about thirteen. Twenty percent of these workers are under 18 and up to 50 percent may be infected with HIV.[8]

According to research by the Home Office, it is estimated that 50 percent of London's sex industry workers are migrant women and that 5 percent have been trafficked. In another prostitution investigation, a majority of the women were found to be migrants, mostly from the Balkans. Although it cannot be presumed that all of the women were trafficked, it is likely that a proportion of them were.

The UK has also been identified as a transit country for women from West Africa into the Italian sex industry. All of the known cases involved girls under 18 years old from West Africa, primarily Nigeria.[19]

Women from Russia and the CIS (the Commonwealth of Independent States, consisting of eleven former Soviet Republics: Armenia, Azerbaijan, Belarus, Georgia, Kazakhstan, Kyrgyzstan, Moldova, Russia, Tajikistan, Ukraine, and Uzbekistan) are trafficked for the global sex trade to over 50 countries around the world. In some countries, such as Israel and Turkey, women from Russia and the CIS are so prevalent, that prostitutes are called "Natashas."

Russia is not only a major source country but also a receiving country for the international trafficking in women and children, child prostitution, child sex tourism, and child pornography. Although the sexual exploitation of minors occurs in all regions of Russia, it manifests most acutely in Moscow. More than 70,000 victims of trafficking for prostitution are currently in Moscow, ninety percent of them are women and girls, and eighty percent are under 18 years of age. There is no system of rescue or rehabilitation for these victims, no specific shelters for these victims, and if they do escape to a shelter, may be easily found by their traffickers and re-exploited.[20]

Often, the trafficker exploits their own cultural community knowing that they are not likely to be reported if there are financial or other incentives to be gained by other influential people in the same community. In Berkeley, California, a man originally from India, was discovered using fraudulent visas, sham marriages, and fake identities to bring men, women, and children to the United States. Additionally, he brought dalit (the lowest caste in India) girls to the United States for his own sexual use. These activities continued for years before being discovered by the U.S. authorities.[6]

Public health impacts of sex trafficking

The impacts of sex trafficking have significant health consequences for the victim. The physical and psychological trauma is impossible to quantify. Even if rescued, the long-term consequences of a victim's experiences may be devastating. Victims suffer from physical and emotional damage from violent sexual activity, forced substance abuse, exposure to sexually transmitted diseases including HIV/AIDS, food deprivation, and psychological torture. Some victims have permanent damage to their reproductive organs. Many victims die as a result of being trafficked, and when the victim is trafficked to an area where she does not speak or understand the language, the psychological damage caused by isolation and domination of the traffickers is compounded.[12] Victims may not be able to locate their families if they have been enslaved for a significant period of time and this loss may be even more devastating.

In some communities, victims of commercial sex trafficking are shunned by their families and communities because of the stigma associated with loss of virginity, prostitution, or HIV/AIDS if they have contracted the disease. Some victims were originally sold to traffickers by their own families. This loss of support and/or betrayal also negatively impacts the victim's sense of identity and value, and may lead to feelings of hopelessness and even suicide. Post traumatic stress disorder (PTSD) is common and 68 percent of female sexual trafficking victims meet criteria.[21]

In a survey of survivors/victims of prostitution in Portland, Oregon, looking at injuries suffered from clients while in prostitution, 78 percent reported being raped, on average, 49 times per year. Eighty-four percent had been physically assaulted requiring emergency department treatment, 53 percent had been sexually abused and tortured, and 23 percent had been mutilated. Another study investigating injuries sustained by victims who had been prostituted demonstrated the following: 71 percent reported being bruised, 41 percent had mouth and teeth injuries, 59 percent had vaginal bleeding, 41 percent had "other" bleeding, 65 percent reported internal pain, 24 percent had head injuries, and 12 percent had broken bones.[21]

Victims of sex trafficking in East Africa reported widespread rape, physical abuse, sexually transmitted diseases (STDs), and tuberculosis (TB). In Nepal, 38 percent of rescued victims suffered from HIV/AIDS as well as STDs and TB. According to one study, 65 percent of female victims of sex trafficking sustain serious physical internal injuries, 24 percent experience head injuries, and 12 percent report broken bones.[22] Women trafficked to the European Union had health problems ranging from broken bones to loss of consciousness and gang rape. Also reported were complications related to abortions, gastrointestinal problems, unhealthy weight loss, lice, suicidal depression, and drug and/or alcohol addiction. One study of women trafficked to the European Union found that 95 percent of victims had been violently assaulted or coerced into a sexual act and over 60 percent of victims reported fatigue, neurological symptoms, gastrointestinal problems, back pain, vaginal discharges, and gynecological infections. Later health consequences may include cervical cancer caused by the human papilloma virus, a sexually transmitted disease.

The history and physical exam

Any patient suspected of being trafficked should be separated from anyone accompanying her without arousing suspicion and interviewed in a private space with a translator. Take care that any potential trafficker will not overhear the interview.

Be certain to spend some time gaining the trust of your patient and explain clearly that she may refuse any part of the medical exam if she so chooses. Explain that if she chooses to refuse part of the exam, that you will still do everything you can to assist her.

Remember that all documents may be used for legal prosecution of the traffickers. If you have little time to see this patient and there will be someone else documenting the patient's entire history (i.e., social worker), limit your history, focus on the physical examination and treatment, and keep all documentation simple and clear so that there will be no conflicting statements that could jeopardize your patient's case later on.

Due to the comprehensive nature of this type of crime and the large number of needs that the patient will have, enlist as much assistance as you are able to. Social workers and government agencies are excellent places to start. In the United States, there is a hotline available 24 hours a day, 7 days a week to assist. The Trafficking Information and Referral Hotline (1-888-3737-888) is set up to assist in identifying local resources available, coordinate with local social service agencies to help protect and serve victims, and to start the process of connecting victims to the services they need to rebuild their lives.[17] Other countries may have similar hotlines (see resources section).

Up to 71 percent of trafficked children exhibit suicidal tendencies and 68 percent of female sex trafficking victims meet criteria for post traumatic stress disorder, so a psychiatric screening for depression and suicide should be a part of the history.[10,21]

In the case of young victims and sexual abuse, if there is an outside agency or specialized clinic that is well established to do forensic examinations in this population and will perform this exam in a timely manner, it is appropriate to transfer your patient to this agency to avoid further trauma to the patient and to allow for the most specialized care available. You can refer to the chapter on the Care of the Sexual Assault Victim for more detailed instructions.

The physical exam should be as comprehensive as your clinical area and the patient allow. Be certain to do a full head to toe physical exam and document any scars, bruises, or injuries even if they seem insignificant. Even examining areas such as the ears to look for perforated tympanic membranes from trauma or the teeth to look for dental caries (due to poor nutrition) may be helpful to your patient's case. If you are able to photograph any injuries, obtain consent from the patient and take photographic evidence of any visible injuries. If your clinical area has charts that contain a pictorial image of the entire body and genitalia, such as for sexual assault, you should use them since they have a larger area to document every visible physical injury. If you do not have access to this type of pictogram, please refer to the sexual assault section in this book for a copy which may be utilized.

Almost a quarter of female victims will experience head trauma, so a thorough head and neurological examination is warranted. Back injuries are common in both labor and sexual trafficking victims. A full genital exam should be completed in any patient reporting a history of sexual abuse, if your patient permits, due to the high probability of sexually transmitted diseases and physical injuries.

Tests requested should be appropriate to the type of exploitation and abuse that the patient was exposed to. If your patient has been recently sexually abused, offer post-exposure prophylaxis for HIV, hepatitis, gonorrhea, chlamydia, and trichomonas. Many hospitals have specific forensic examiners available for cases of sexual assault, if this is the case at your institution, make use of this service. The most experienced clinician available should do the forensic examination. If there is any history of sexual abuse, HIV screening or referral should be offered along with testing for hepatitis, syphilis, gonorrhea, and chlamydia.

Orthopedic injuries are common in both labor and sexual trafficking victims so x-rays of currently or previously injured areas may be appropriate to document old or new fractures.

Tuberculosis is a common illness for trafficking victims who have been exposed to crowded living quarters and a screening chest x-ray should be considered.

Getting assistance

There are often multiple sources that may be able to assist you in evaluating, treating, and providing referrals for this patient. Given the myriad needs these patients have, consider the following sources for assistance.

1) The Trafficking Information and Referral Hotline (1-888-3737-888)
2) Social Work
3) Sexual Assault Forensic Examiner
4) Child Advocacy and Rape Crisis Centers
5) Psychiatry
6) Translation Services

Referrals and follow-up

Identifying and treating the victim of trafficking is only the first step in a long process. These patients often have no resources of their own and are at high risk for being re-trafficked if they are not provided for immediately. You may find yourself in a position of holding your patient in a busy emergency department or clinic until appropriate shelter placement can be met. If this is the case, try to secure your patient in as safe a location as possible to ensure that her trafficker will have difficulty finding her. Additionally, try to identify and make the appropriate referrals prior to her departure from the medical area.

Resources for assisting the trafficking victim

United States

1) The Trafficking Information and Referral Hotline **1-888-3737-888** through the U.S. Department of Health and Human Services, more information available at http://www.acf.hhs.gov/trafficking/index.html. This toll-free hotline operates 24 hours a day, 7 days a week; it provides information and supportive services for victims of trafficking. Interpreters are available at this number. This hotline may be able to identify local resources for victims of trafficking such as medical assistance, shelter, legal services, and non-governmental organizations (NGOs) who will assist the patient.[17]
2) The Angel Coalition Trafficking Victims Assistance Center Hotline: For Russian Trafficking Victims, 24 hours a day, 7 days a week, operators are Russian speaking only. Toll free call from USA (to Russia): **+1-866-800-0270**.[20,23]

Canada

Web site resource: http://www.humantrafficking.ca.

A resource for non-governmental agencies and victims of human trafficking in Canada. The Web site will offer information and a database of shelters, community organizations, translators, legal aid providers, and government agencies concerned with human trafficking.

Anti-Trafficking Hotline, **1-866-227-2124**.[24]

Europe

The Angel Coalition Trafficking Victims Assistance Center Hotline: For Russian trafficking victims, 24 hours a day, 7 days a week: operators are Russian speaking only. Toll free call from Netherlands, Belgium, Germany (to Russia): **0080045505555**.[23]

Italy

(800) 290–290. This is a toll-free number, which functions throughout Italy. Directed through Rome and then transferred to regional centers. The service provides help, information, and advice to victims.

Australia

The Child Wise Support and Information Service is a free advisory service available to all.

Free phone (inside Australia) – **1800 99 10 99**

Outside Australia – **61 3 9645 8911**

Child Wise specializes in child protection strategies to prevent child sexual abuse in organizations, child pornography, child prostitution, and child sexual abuse outside the family. Available by phone 9:00 AM – 5:00 PM, Monday to Friday.

Ukraine

527: National toll-free hotline established to assist victims of trafficking.[25]

Russia

The Angel Coalition Trafficking Victim Assistance Center: Russian speaking operators only, toll free number calls from anywhere in Russia (to the Angel Coalition/TVAC in Moscow): **88002002400**.

Israel

Hotline for migrant workers: **972 3 5602530**, Web site: http://www.hotline.org.il/.

Web sites to learn more about trafficking

1) http://www.acf.hhs.gov/trafficking/index.html

   The U.S. Government's Health and Human Services Web site on trafficking and assisting victims.

2) www.ecpat.net

   A non-profit group, ECPAT stands for End Child Prostitution, Child Pornography and Trafficking of Children for Sexual Purposes. Their work is both in the United States and International.

3) www.childtrafficking.org

   The UNICEF Innocenti Research Centre is the independent research arm of the United Nations agency dedicated to the protection of children and the promotion of child rights. The Centre has a specific global mandate to fill knowledge gaps in current issues, address sensitive or controversial issues, and flag new and emerging issues.

4) www.childtrafficking.net

   The International Labour Organization (ILO) works to identify issues of child trafficking. The ILO creates programs to assist children at risk and rescue children in exploitive work environments.

5) www.childtrafficking.com

   The Swiss Foundation of Terre des hommes (Tdh) with headquarters in Lausanne, Switzerland, is the largest Swiss children's aid organization operating outside Switzerland. Since 1960, the movement has been active wherever children are in need.

6) www.antislavery.org

   Anti-Slavery International, founded in 1839, is the world's oldest international human rights organization and the only charity in the United Kingdom to work exclusively against slavery and related abuses.

7) www.iom.int

   An intergovernmental organization established in 1951, The International Organization for Migration (the IOM) is committed to the principle that humane and orderly migration benefits migrants and society.

8) www.humantrafficking.org

The purpose of this Web site is to bring Government and NGOs in the East Asia and Pacific together to cooperate and learn from each other's experiences in their efforts to combat human trafficking. This Web site has country-specific information such as national laws and action plans and contact information on useful governmental agencies. It also has a description of NGO activities in different countries and their contact information.

9) www.interpol.int

INTERPOL is the world's largest international police organization, with 186 member countries. Created in 1923, it facilitates cross-border police co-operation, and supports and assists all organizations, authorities, and services whose mission is to prevent or combat international crime.

10) www.childcentre.info

The Child Centre is the web support of a regional cooperation to raise the level of knowledge and to coordinate the activities targeting children at risk in the Baltic Sea Region.

References

1. Garza V. Modern-day slavery: human trafficking. *On The Edge*. Summer 2007; 13(2). Available from http://www.forensicnurse.org/publication/ote/oteSummer2007.cfm.
2. Clawson HJ, Small KM, Go ES, Myles BW. Needs Assessment for Service Providers and Trafficking Victims. U.S. Department of Justice, National Institute of Justice, editor. October 2003. Available from http://www.ncjrs.gov/pdffiles1/nij/grants/202469.pdf.
3. Loyn D. Forced Labour – Global Problem. BBC, Editor. May 11, 2005. Available from http://news.bbc.co.uk/1/hi/world/europe/4521921.stm.
4. United Nations Office on Drugs and Crime, Global Programme Against Trafficking in Human Beings, Toolkit to Combat Trafficking in Persons. United Nations, Editor. New York, 2006. Available from http://www.unodc.org/pdf/Trafficking_toolkit_Oct06.pdf.
5. United Nations Office on Drugs and Crime, Global Programme Against Trafficking in Human Beings, Trafficking in Persons: Global Patterns. United Nations, Editor. April 2006. Available from http://www.unodc.org/pdf/traffickinginpersons_report_2006ver2.pdf.
6. Hughes DM. Hiding in Plain Sight: A Practical Guide to Identifying Victims of Trafficking in the United States. October 2003. Available from http://www.acf.hhs.gov/trafficking/resources/plain_site.html.
7. BBC News Online. Forced Labour: Global Problem. Facts and Figures. [cited 2007 April 15]; Available from: http://news.bbc.co.uk/1/shared/spl/hi/world/05/slavery/html/4.stm.

8. Staff, Human Rights Watch. Rape for Profit: Trafficking of Nepali Girls and Women to India's Brothels. Human Rights Watch, Vol. 12 (5A), October, 1995. Available from http://www.hrw.org/reports/1995/India.htm.

9. The U.S. State Department, "U.S. "Horrified" at Child Trafficking in Tsunami Aftermath," January 5, 2005. Available from http://usinfo.state.gov/xarchives/display.html?p=washfile-english&y=2005&m=January&x=20050105172231cmretrop0.4135248.

10. Kain EJ. Prostitution of Children and Child-Sex Tourism: An Analysis of Domestic and International Responses. National Center for Missing and Exploited Children. April 1999. Available from http://www.missingkids.com/enˉUS/publications/NC73.pdf.

11. Watts C, Zimmerman C. Violence against women: global scope and magnitude. *The Lancet*. April 6, 2002; 359: 1232–7.

12. U.S. Department of State. 2006 Trafficking in Persons Report. Office to Monitor and Combat Trafficking in Persons, June 5, 2006. Available from http://www.state.gov/g/tip/rls/tiprpt/2006/.

13. Edwards R. "Child Sacrifices in London," thisislondon.co.uk. Evening Standard. June 16, 2005: London. Available from http://www.thisislondon.co.uk/news/article-19328071-details/'Child+sacrifices+in+London'/article.do;jsessionid=CxrtGQTF1lHhxf0Y4rpDthMmpTn1zlB46QlThLbkV2m8dRlK9hJL.

14. International Labour Office, International Programme on the Elimination of Child Labour. Unbearable to the human heart: Trafficking in children and action to combat it. ILO, 2002. Available from http://www.no-trafficking.org/content/web/05reading‗rooms/unbearable‗to‗the‗human‗heart.pdf.

15. Save the Children. Protecting Children in Emergencies: Escalating Threats to Children Must Be Addressed. Policy Brief. Vol. 1(1), Spring 2005. Available from http://www.essex.ac.uk/armedcon/story‗id/000259.pdf.

16. International Labour Office. A new kind of trafficking: child beggars in Asia. *The World of Work*. 1998; 26: 17–9.

17. The U.S. Department of Health and Human Services, Administration for Children and Families. The Campaign to Rescue and Restore Victims of Human Trafficking. Available from http://www.acf.hhs.gov/trafficking/.

18. United Nations Office on Drugs and Crime, Global Programme Against Trafficking in Human Beings. Toolkit to Combat Trafficking in Persons. United Nations, New York, 2006. Available from: http://www.unodc.org/pdf/Trafficking‗toolkit‗Oct06.pdf.

19. Kelly L, Regan L. Police Research Series, Paper 125. Stopping Traffic: Exploring the extent of, and responses to, trafficking in women for sexual exploitation in the UK. Home Office, 2000. Available from: http://www.homeoffice.gov.uk/rds/prgpdfs/fprs125.pdf.

20. The Angel Coalition. Combatting and Prevention of Human Trafficking. Available from: http://www.angelcoalition.org/epjs/e‗history.html. Accessed April 12, 2007.

21. U.S. Department of State. 2005 Trafficking in Persons Report. Office to Monitor and Combat Trafficking in Persons, June 3, 2005. Available from http://www.state.gov/g/tip/rls/tiprpt/2005/.

22. Hynes HP, Raymond JG. Chapter 8: *Put in Harm's Way: The Neglected Health Consequences of Sex Trafficking in the United States from Policing the National Body: Sex, Race, and*

Criminalization, eds. Silliman, J. and Bhattacharjee. South End Press, Cambridge, 2002. Available from http://action.web.ca/home/catw/readingroom.shtml?x=21563.

23. Staff, Human Rights Watch. Available from: http://www.humantrafficking.org/links/79. Accessed September 14, 2007.

24. Cabral GV, Marengo F. *Assisting Victims of Trafficking in Human Beings.* January 2003. Available from http://www.esclavagemoderne.org/img_doc/traite_etres_humains_uk.pdf.

25. The United Nations. "Victim of Trafficking Helped Through "527" Hotline." July 9, 2007. Available from http://www.un.org.ua/en/news/2007-09-07/.

Quick Reference Pages

Clues to suspect a patient may be a trafficking victim*

1) Evidence of being controlled
2) Evidence of inability to move or leave job
3) Bruises or other signs of physical abuse
4) Fear or depression
5) Not speaking on own behalf and/or non-English speaking
6) No passport or other forms of identification or documentation

Screening questions to help determine if your patient is a trafficking victim*

1) What type of work do you do?
2) Are you being paid?
3) Can you leave your job if you want to?
4) Can you come and go as you please?
5) Have you or your family been threatened?
6) What are your working and living conditions like?
7) Where do you sleep and eat?
8) Do you have to ask permission to eat/sleep/go to the bathroom?
9) Are there locks on your door/windows so you cannot get out?
10) Has your identification or documentation been taken from you?

---

* From The U.S. Department of Health and Human Services, Administration for Children and Families. The Campaign to Rescue and Restore Victims of Human Trafficking. Available from http://www.acf.hhs.gov/trafficking/.

Screening questions to help determine if your patient is a trafficking victim: Spanish*

1) What type of work do you do?

    1. ¿A qué se dedica usted?

2) Are you being paid?

    1. ¿Le pagan?

3) Can you leave your job if you want to?

    1. ¿Puede dejar su empleo si quisiera?

4) Can you come and go as you please?

    1. ¿Puede ir y venir a su gusto?

5) Have you or your family been threatened?

    1. ¿Ha sido usted o algún miembro de su familia amenazado?

6) What are your working and living conditions like?

    1. ¿Cómo son sus condiciones de trabajo y de domicilio?

7) Where do you sleep and eat?

    1. ¿Dónde duerme y come usted?

8) Do you have to ask permission to eat/sleep/go to the bathroom?

    1. ¿Tiene que pedir permiso para comer/dormir/ir al baño?

9) Are there locks on your door/windows so you cannot get out?

    1. ¿Hay candados o cerraduras en sus puertas/ventanas para que no pueda salir?

10) Has your identification or documentation been taken from you?

    1. ¿Le han quitado su identificación o documentación?

Translation courtesy of Sabrina Abreu.

Screening questions for a potentially trafficked patient: Mandarin Chinese*

1. What type of work do you do?
   你是作什麻工作的?
2. Are you being paid?
   他們付你錢嗎?
3. Can you leave your job if you want to?
   你要的話可以不繼續去作工嗎?
4. Can you come and go as you please?
   你能隨心所欲的來來去去嗎?
5. Have you or your family been threatened?
   有人恐嚇過你或你的家人嗎?
6. What are your working and living conditions like?
   你的工作條件和居住環境怎麻樣?
7. Where do you sleep and eat?
   你在那兒睡覺?在那兒吃飯?
8. Do you have to ask permission to eat/sleep/go to the bathroom?
   你吃飯,睡覺或上洗手間都得有人批准嗎?
9. Are there locks on your door/windows so you cannot get out?
   你的門,窗有沒有被鎖住而不能出去?
10. Has your identification or documentation been taken from you?
    你的身份證明和文件有人拿去嗎?

Translation courtesy of Dr. Christine Yang Kauh.

Screening questions to help determine if your patient is a trafficking victim: Russian*

1) What type of work do you do?
2) Are you being paid?
3) Can you leave your job if you want to?
4) Can you come and go as you please?
5) Have you or your family been threatened?
6) What are your working and living conditions like?
7) Where do you sleep and eat?
8) Do you have to ask permission to eat/sleep/go to the bathroom?
9) Are there locks on your door/windows so you cannot get out?
10) Has your identification or documentation been taken from you?

1. какая у вас работа?
2. вы получаете плату за эту работу?
3. смогли-бы вы оставить работу если захотели?
4. вы свободны передвигатся по желанию?

5. были ли вы или баша семья запуганы кем-либо?

6. каковы обстая тельства вашей работы и домаш него жилья?

7. где бы спите и питаетесь?

8. приходтся ли вам просить разрешения чтобы есть/спать/ходить в туалет?

9. бывает ле такое что вы замкнуты дома и не можете выйти?

10. не забрал кто-либо ваши документы или пасспорт?

Translation courtesy of Dr. Ilya Saltykov.

Forensic photography

Mary Ryan, M.D.

Introduction

Recognition and documentation of injuries is an essential step in the evaluation of victims of sexual assault, domestic violence, or other forms of abuse in which injuries are incurred. Although many of these injuries are medically "insignificant," they can still have significant forensic value if adequately documented. Physicians and nurses who examine these patients may find themselves with the additional role of forensic photographer. While most providers will not have the benefit of formal training in photography, it is important to understand some basic principles of forensic photography. This chapter is intended to outline these principles to allow you to maximize the use of photography in the care of assault victims. Many photographs referred to are included in the color insert.

Injury documentation

When an injury is identified, it is important to record the findings. Ideally, injuries should be recorded in three ways: a written description, complemented by diagrams and finally by photography.

a) Written description

The written description of the injury should be simple and accurate. It should include the location of the injury and describe the type of injury (e.g., contusion / burn / stab wound). Both the width and length of the injury should be noted. If the injury has a specific shape or pattern, describe it (circular, curvilinear, linear, triangular, etc.).

Even in experienced hands, some injuries can be difficult to describe and often words alone fail to describe the injuries adequately. For this reason, supplementing the written description with body diagrams and photographs is essential.

b) Body diagrams

These serve as an adjunct and not as an alternative to the written record. Record the patients name and date of exam on the body diagram. Remember to sign and date the diagram for future reference.

c) Photography

Photography is important for recording any notable injuries on the body, including genital injuries. Vaginal and cervical injuries will require use of a colposcope with photographic capabilities.

Importance of photography in the acute care setting

Cameras are commonly found in the emergency department (ED) and often used for educational as well as forensic purposes. When a health care provider records injuries, which may be later used in legal proceedings, the term medical forensic photography applies. Reasons to undertake photography in the ED include the following:

1) Written descriptions, even in the best hands, are often inadequate to describe injuries.
2) Photographs serve as an aid to memory. At a later date, the examiner may be called to testify in court. The medical record, including the photographs, will be available for review and can be very helpful when preparing to testify.
3) Much physical evidence is short lived and if not recorded early may be lost permanently. Injuries heal faster than the legal system operates. The appearance of injuries can change significantly in a short time. Most injuries will quickly heal completely, leaving little evidence that they existed.
4) Photos can often say more than victims. Photographs create a permanent record of the acute injury and reduce subjectivity. They permit the court and jurors to "see the evidence" as it was.
5) Photography can assist in demonstrating malice or criminal intent.

Physics of photography: the basics

A basic understanding of the physics and principles behind photography can be helpful. For those interested in a more in-depth understanding, please refer to the "Recommended Reading" section.

Lens, aperture, shutter speed, film

When the camera shutter opens, light is allowed to enter. The light passes through the lens, which focuses it onto light-sensitive film. Lenses are available in different focal lengths. In practical terms, the larger the focal length, the greater the magnification produced. "Macrolenses" are specifically designed for close-up work. "Zoom" lenses have adjustable focal length allowing for variable magnification. The amount of light allowed to enter depends on the aperture size and the shutter speed, both of which can be adjusted. The aperture size refers to the size of the opening allowing the light through. It is expressed as f/-. Shutter speed is expressed as a fraction of a second, a shutter speed of "60" for example, allows the shutter to open for 1/60 of a second. The higher (faster) the shutter speed setting, the less time allowed for light to expose the film. Thirty-five (35) mm film is available in different ratings as described by the International Standards Organization (ISO). The higher the ISO number, the more sensitive it is to light. ISO 200 film is generally adequate for ED forensic purposes. Heat and humidity can damage film and ideally, film should be refrigerated until ready for use. It should be allowed to reach room temperature immediately prior to use.

Adequate lighting is essential to expose the film properly. The addition of a flash provides more light, and is often necessary in the forensic setting. Many cameras have a built-in flash and the flash function is activated automatically when lighting levels are low. Other cameras allow for a separate top-mounted flash to be attached in order to enhance lighting further. "Ring" flashes encircle the lens and illuminate the finding from all sides and are specifically designed for close-up work, for example, a bite mark.

In reality, the equipment available to most practitioners is of the basic "point and shoot" variety and requires little in the way of annual adjustment. As technology advances, even these fully automated units are quite sophisticated and are adequate for most purposes.

Photography in court

Admissibility

Once a photograph is taken, it will remain part of the medical record and may be used at a later date as evidence in court proceedings. When a case goes to trial, some evidence, photographs included, may be "admitted into evidence" in the case. The decision of whether photographs are admitted rests with the Judge – this is the concept of admissibility. Many factors influence this decision and include the following:

1) The photo must first be "substantiated" – that is, a person must verify that it "is a true and accurate representation" of the injuries at the time the photo was taken. The person who took the photo or someone who was present when it was taken can verify this. Signing and dating the back of the picture and recording

in the chart who took the image will make this task much easier at a future date in court.

2) The photo may not be introduced into evidence if it is deemed to be "inflammatory." In legal terms this means that the photo may "inflame the passions of the jury making it difficult for them to render a dispassionate verdict. The image should not be 'overly prejudicial'." While images of injured victims may by their very nature be unpleasant, they should not be "unduly gruesome or inflammatory."

3) Unnecessary distractions such as blood-stained gauze should be removed before the picture is taken. These may deem the photo "objectionable" and the photographic evidence may be inadmissible.

4) The photos taken by an "occupational photographer" will not be judged against professional photography standards, but they must meet certain minimum criteria. The image should be in focus, the injury of interest should be clearly visible, and the photograph should not be over exposed distorting colors and giving a "washed-out" appearance to the picture.

Chain of custody

The concept of chain of custody applies to forensic photographs as it does to other evidence in court. A record should be kept of who took the photographs and to whom they were given. Although the photographs become part of the medical record of the patient, hospitals may differ on their policy and practice of whether the photographs stay with the medical records or are archived separately. You should be familiar with the policy at the institution in which you practice. The policy should address issues relating to processing and storage of images.

Consent

States vary on their laws governing consent for medical photography. In many states, general consent for medical treatment is not adequate for medical or forensic photography and separate consent is needed. The same concept of "informed" consent applies here as it does to any "procedure" being undertaken during the care of the patient. The patient should be informed of what is involved in the procedure. The potential advantages and disadvantages should be outlined as well as the alternatives. The patient should be allowed to ask any questions and have their concerns addressed before proceeding. No attempt should be made to coerce the patient and if a patient declines to have photographs taken, their decision should be respected.

The potential advantage is of preserving a record of the injury as it was on the day of presentation. The potential disadvantage is that some patients feel intimidated and self-conscious and may find the added step of taking photographs unpleasant. This is especially true when photographs are being taken of the face. Patients should be reassured that the rules governing confidentiality of medical records extend to photographs also. Patients should also be informed that if photos are admitted into evidence in court, questions may arise about any findings in the photographs, e.g., for example, old injuries recorded incidentally.

The alternatives include a written description along with drawings and trauma diagrams but even in experienced hands, narrative descriptions and drawings on trauma diagrams often fail to capture the injury as well as a photo can.

Exceptions to informed consent

Two exceptions exist to the requirement for obtaining informed consent. The first is when a patient is unable to consent, in which case the concept of implied consent may be invoked in the best interest of the patient. The second is when a court order is issued for photographs to be taken.

Implied consent

In cases where informed consent cannot be obtained at the time but "a reasonably prudent person" would consent in the given situation, the concept of "implied" consent can be employed. An example would be an assault that rendered the person unconscious and unable to give informed consent at that moment. The examiner could proceed to take the photographs in the belief that the person would consent if he/she was able to consent. The photographs would then be preserved and at a later date, when the patient (or proxy) is able, his/her consent should be obtained. It is important to remember that while the concept of implied consent can be used initially, true, informed consent must be obtained later.

Court order

Although uncommon, a written order may be signed by a judge to proceed with photography regardless of the patient's wishes. It would be highly unusual for a court order to be issued for photography of a victim against his/her wishes and is more likely to be the case for photographs of a potential suspect who may also have injuries, for example, a bite mark. In cases of suspected child abuse, a court order may be issued as the victim is a minor. When faced with a Court Order, verify that the order is valid and signed. A verbal court order is not acceptable. A copy of the written court order should be placed in the medical record and a note made in the chart that it was issued. If any doubt exists, involvement of the Risk Management department at the institution should be sought before proceeding.

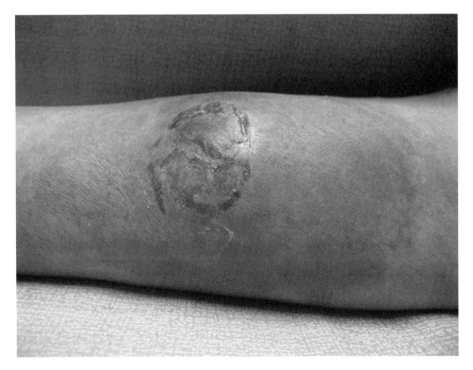

Figure 9.1   Neutral background.

Technique – how best to take good images

Once you identify an injury and decide to undertake photography, give some thought to how best to proceed. The following are suggestions on how to maximize the usefulness of the photo.

Background

Start by setting the stage for the photo. Unnecessary distractions should be removed from the field, for example, bloodied gauze. Metallic objects that may reflect the flash should be covered or removed if possible. Disposable surgical drapes in a neutral color are ideal (see Figure 9.1).

Scales/measuring device

A tape measure or other measuring device should be at hand. Without a reference of measure, the size of the injury will be unclear, especially in close-up views. Take the same image with and without the tape measure to confirm that the device was not covering anything of significance.

A variety of measuring devices exist. A traditional ruler or tape measure is acceptable as long as the numbers are easy to read and the surface is not too reflective.

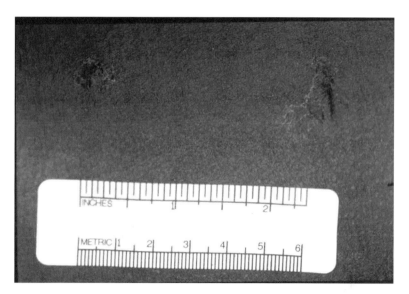

Figure 9.2   Using a tape measure.

Commercially available adhesive paper scales are also available (see Figure 9.2). They have the advantage of also serving as labels allowing the date and medical record or case number to be written on them. They are cheap, easy to apply, and are disposable.

An AFBO No. 2 device allows both dimensions of the injury to be measured on one image (see Figure 9.3). This scale also displays circles, which serve as a reference to check for possible distortion. This is particularly helpful for recording bite mark injuries.

If you have no standard scale available, improvise by placing a coin or other object of standard size in the photograph. While not ideal, it will serve the same function, giving an objective measure of size. Remember to use the same units of measurement in written description as displayed on the scale to avoid unnecessary confusion.

Next check that your equipment is ready. Ideally this should be done before entering the room! Check that the batteries are charged. If you are using 35 mm film, check the expiration date. If you are using digital technology, confirm that the flashcard or compact flash is in place, is functioning, and has enough space to accommodate the number of images you anticipate you will need.

Optimize lighting in the room. Ideally there should be adequate light to provide good exposure and avoid unwanted shadows. Most cameras used by the examiner will have built-in flash capabilities, which can be useful but may provide excessive lighting in some settings. The artificial lighting used in many Emergency

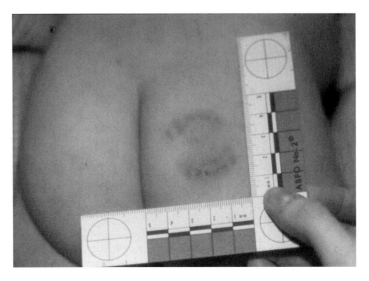

Figure 9.3   Bite mark, using an ABFO.

Departments may provide enough lighting to work without a flash though flu-
orescent lighting may give a washed-out appearance to the image. A red-eye
reduction function is available in most cameras and can be helpful for the I.D.
photograph.

   Obtain informed consent and explain the procedure to the patient. You are now
ready to begin.

- First obtain an identification picture ("ID Shot") of the patient. This should be a
  frontal view of the victim and should clearly show the victim's face. This photo
  is important as it serves to identify the victim with the subsequent photographs
  of the injuries. Use the "red-eye" reduction function if available.
- Next take an "orientation" photograph of the injury. This photograph is an
  overview of the injury and serves primarily to show the location of the injury.
- Next take a photograph of the injury itself. The injury should occupy the center
  portion of the photograph and be in focus (see Figure 9.4). If the injury is very
  small, a macro lens may be required. A minimum of two views of each injury
  should be taken to show the length and width of the injury. Photos should be taken
  at 90 degrees to the surface to avoid distortion of the shape and size. Remember
  the same photo should be taken with and without the tape measure to confirm
  that no part of the injury was hidden under the tape or scale. This series of
  photographs aims to objectively show the characteristics of the injury.
- If an injury requires specific treatment (e.g., suturing), if possible, take a photograph of the injury before and after repair.

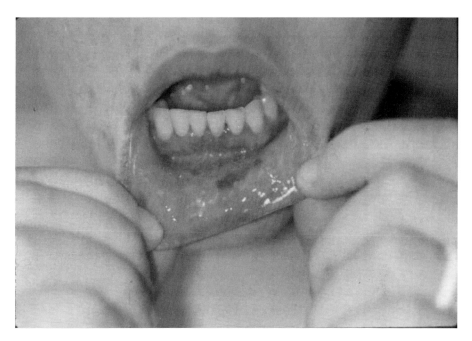

Figure 9.4   This image is well centered and in focus.

What injury to photograph?

In general this will be a straightforward decision but at times, injuries may be in hidden areas and can be easily overlooked. It is also easy to be distracted by larger injuries and overlook minor ones (Figure 9.5). A thorough search should be made for all injuries and efforts to document them equally well no matter how trivial.

Medically significant versus forensically significant injuries

It is important to remember that the majority of injuries sustained in victims of assaults seen in the ED are not medically significant – but even minor injuries can have tremendous forensic significance and should not be dismissed as trivial (Figure 9.6). Remember to look in key areas where injuries may be hidden or concealed from the casual observer, for example, behind the ears, under the chin, the axillae. These findings may be the only objective evidence that a struggle took place and may be important factors to corroborate (or dispute) the story offered.

Bite mark photography

Bite mark injuries deserve special mention. While evidence collection from bite marks can be useful for DNA evidence and perpetrator identification, in selected

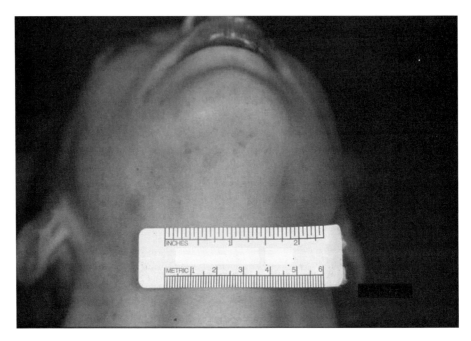

Figure 9.5   Hidden submental injury.

cases, bite mark photography can also play a role. The first step is to recognize the injury as a bite mark. A classic bite mark consists of two opposing arches, which are patterned abraded contusions. In many instances the bite mark is "incomplete" and the pattern is not so obvious. If a patient reports that an injury is a bite mark, the injury should be treated as such regardless of its appearance.

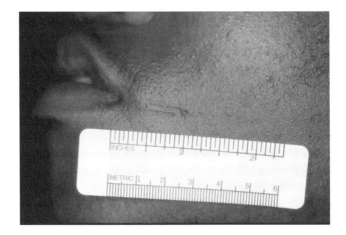

Figure 9.6   Forensically significant versus medically significant.

In selected cases, a forensic odontologist may be involved in review of bite mark photographs. Adequate photographic documentation is essential for it to be of value for review and interpretation.

• Photograph the bite mark before any manipulation if possible (e.g., swabbing or cleaning).
• Photograph the injury at 90 degrees to the surface to avoid distortion of its size and shape.
• Take several photos of the injury.
• It is important to include a reference. A measuring scale is essential and measurements of both the horizontal and vertical dimensions of the injury should be made. The ABFO #2 scale is ideal as it incorporates both a circular and linear scale.
• As with all forensic photographs, label the photo with the victim's name, and the date and time the photo was taken. Sign the back of the photo and indicate in the medical records the number of photographs taken.

Equipment

The selection of available cameras is extensive and continues to grow, especially with the ongoing evolution of digital technology. Although the choice is large, most fall into one of three categories – conventional 35mm, instant, and digital – each with its own set of advantages and disadvantages.

Conventional 35mm single lens reflex (SLR) camera

Conventional 35mm cameras remain the gold standard and are the system preferred for legal work. When used properly, they produce very high quality images. The main disadvantage is that the images cannot be viewed until later when the film is developed. If on review, the image quality is poor, the opportunity is lost forever. Another disadvantage is that many centers do not have access to police or other secure photo labs and patient confidentiality and chain of custody often preclude commercial photo shops from handling such material. Film and development costs also can be significant and should be taken into consideration when planning and implementing a forensic program.

Thirty-five mm film (ISO rating 200 or above) is available for negatives and slides. Film quality and storage is important. Film can degrade with heat and humidity. Always remember to check expiration date before starting!

Polaroid "instant" cameras

"Instant" cameras are commonly found in emergency departments and clinics where victims are examined. The main advantages to this system include that it allows viewing of the image immediately and eliminates concerns about developing images outside the facility. Additional copies can be produced at the push of a button. The cost of the film is offset by the fact that there are no additional processing costs to develop the film. The main disadvantage is that the image quality and color reproduction tends to be less reliable than conventional cameras. Older models have limited zoom capability making close-up work difficult. The development of newer "forensic grade" models have attempted to address these shortcomings and models such as the Macro5 are widely used for forensic purposes.

Digital cameras

Digital technology continues to expand and the use of digital cameras for forensic purposes is becoming increasingly popular. As technology advances, images approaching "film quality" are both available and affordable. The advantages are numerous. The images can be viewed immediately and large numbers can be stored easily. With the availability of high quality photo-printers, prints can be made without the involvement of outside facilities thus avoiding the confidentiality issues for developing images and copies can be made with ease.

Digital systems are not without their problems however. Although their use is gaining acceptance in the Courts, they are not yet the Gold Standard for forensic use in many judicial districts. Concerns continue to be raised about the potential for image "manipulation." Even with high-resolution cameras and high quality printers, the images are still not 35mm film quality. Maintaining chain of custody can be difficult when files are stored on computers where multiple users may have access. Concerns have been raised also about the ease with which files / images can be copied and sent electronically over the Internet.

Adjuncts to injury detection and documentation in sexual assault

Gross visualization of the genital area post-sexual assault identifies some but not all injuries. To assist further in the identification and documentation of micro injuries, the use of toluidine blue dye and colposcopy are often employed.

Toluidine blue

Toluidine blue is a stain that is preferentially taken up by nucleated cells. It is used primarily for detecting superficial injuries to the anogenital region. Following injury, disruption of the normal skin allows dye to bind nuclei in the exposed deeper layers. The uptake is seen as thin blue lines, which represent linear areas of micro lacerations. Lauber and Souma studied the use of toluidine blue for micro injury identification following sexual assault in 1982 and found 40 percent of victims displayed micro injury.[1] Subsequently, McCauley and colleagues report an increased detection of injury from 4 percent on gross examination alone to 58 percent following the use of toluidine blue.[2]

The dye is used in a 1 percent aqueous solution and is applied to the anogenital region using cotton gauze. Particular attention should be paid to the posterior fourchette. It is intended for application to skin, not to mucosal surfaces. The dye should be allowed to remain for a few minutes and then wiped away with lubricating jelly. Close inspection is then made of the area for dye uptake, which is considered a "positive finding." Photography should be undertaken before and after application of the dye.

Note: Some centers advise application of toluidine blue before insertion of the speculum to exclude the possibility of trauma from the insertion of the speculum itself.[3]

Colposcopy

History

The colposcope was designed and developed in the 1920s in Germany by Hinselmann. He recognized that examination of the cervix with the naked eye alone was inadequate and developed a "magnifying instrument," the colposcope, to assist in his study of leukoplakias of the cervix.[4] It was not until the 1950s that colposcopy was introduced into the United States by Bolten. By the late 1970s its importance was accepted and its practice was widespread. Today it plays a central role along with Papanicolaou smears in the detection and management of early cervical cancer.

Forensic versus medical uses

Although developed primarily for evaluation of cervical abnormalities in routine gynecological care, the potential for its use in evaluation of victims of sexual assault was soon recognized. Colposcopy provided an important tool to assist in the evaluation of victims of sexual assault by improving detection and documentation of injuries not otherwise visible to the naked eye. In a study by Slaughter and colleagues in 1992,[5] colposcopic magnification increased injury identification from approximately 10 to 30 percent to 87 percent. Lenehan and colleagues found an increase in injury detection from 6 percent on gross exam alone to 53 percent when a colposcope was used.[6]

The most common sites of injury were the posterior fourchette, fossa navicularis, hymen, and labia minora.[7]

Equipment/physics

The modern colposcope essentially consists of a portable binocular operating microscope that has been adapted for examination of the cervix and lower genital

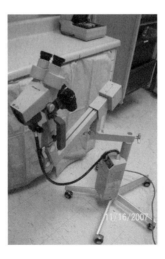

Figure 9.7   Colposcope with 35mm camera.

tract (see Figures 9.7, 9.8, and 9.9). It allows for variable magnification, binocular vision, and is equipped with a high intensity light source (e.g., halogen). The main objective lens allows light to converge on the image ensuring excellent illumination. Colposcopes used for forensic purposes require the additional ability to take high resolution photographs (35 mm or digital) or video clips to document the findings.

Colposcopy allows direct visualization of the entire genital tract and the binocular system provides a clear stereoscopic image. Although most systems allow for magnification ranging from 5 to 30, a magnification of 15 is the most commonly used. The higher the magnification used, the smaller the field of vision. Coarse focus can be achieved by simply moving the entire unit forward or backward. In addition, most units are also equipped with a fine-focus knob.

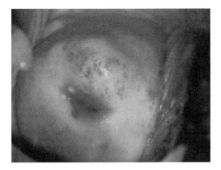

Figure 9.8   Cervix with petechiae and contusions. Colopscopic photograph courtesy of Bronx SART.

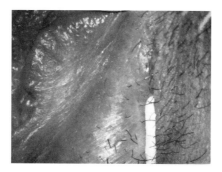

Figure 9.9   Labia minora abrasion and superficial laceration. Colposcopic photograph courtesy of Bronx SART.

Filter selection

Most medical colposcopes are equipped with a green or blue filter. The filter reduces the amount of long wavelength light and enhances the detail of the vascular pattern of the epithelium. The vessels appear blacker, which sharpens the contrast with the surrounding tissue. In general, for forensic purposes the filter function should be disengaged before photo documentation.

Procedure

Consideration should be given in advance to the exam room in which the exam is to be preformed – additional space may be needed for the equipment involved. An assistant should be available as coordination of the speculum, colposcope, and camera is important and difficult at times. The cervix and vaginal vault should be initially examined with the aid of a speculum and then with the colposcope. In cases where metallic speculums are used, the reflective surface may interfere with photography. Disposable plastic units are generally adequate. A systematic approach to the exam is essential and the lower genital tract should be evaluated in its entirety. When an area of interest is identified, it should be brought into focus and photo documented.

The same principles apply to images taken using a colposcope as apply to photography for non-genital injuries (consent, chain of custody, recording in the medical record, and signing and dating the images). The same checklist should be employed before and after each case. Make a note of the magnification setting used for colpophotography.

When possible, a follow-up colposcopy is ideal to establish that the findings have gone, that is, genital injuries heal quickly and other genital findings, for example, congenital or acquired will persist.

Although primarily used for female genital examination, the colposcope can be used for non-genital injuries also, for example, oropharyngeal, where the magnification and illumination provided can help identify and record injuries better than direct visualization alone. Some investigators have used colposcopy combined with anoscopy in male victims of sexual assault and found that the combined exam improved detection of ano-rectal injuries when compared to either modality alone.[8]

Colposcopy references

1. Lauber A, Souma M. Use of toluidine blue for documentation of traumatic intercourse. *Obstet Gynecol*. 1982; 60(5): 648.
2. McCauley J, Guzinski G, Welch R, et al. Toluidine blue in the corroboration of rape in the adult victim. *Am J Emerg Med*. 1987; 5(2): 105–8.
3. Jones JS, Dunnuck C, Rossman L, et al. Significance of toluidine blue positive findings after speculum examination for sexual assault. *Am J Emerg Med*. 2004 May; 22(3): 201–3.
4. Hinselmann H. Verbesserung der Inspekionsmoglchkeiten von vulva, vagina and portio. *Munchen Mrd Wchuschr*. 1925; 72: 1733.
5. Slaughter L, Brown C. Colposcopy to establish findings in rape victims. *Am J OB Gyn*. 1992; 166: 83.
6. Lenahan LC, Ernst A, Johnson B. Colposcopy in evaluation of the adult sexual assault victim. *Am J Emerg Med*. 1998 Mar; 16(2): 183–4.
7. Slaughter L, Brown C, Crowley S, et al. Pattern of genital injury in female sexual assault victims. *Am J Obstet Gynecol*. 1997; 176: 609–16.
8. Ernst AA, Green E, Ferguson MT, et al. The utility of anoscopy and colposcopy in the evaluation of male sexual assault victims. *Ann Emerg Med*. 2000 Nov; 36(5): 432–7.

Suggested reading

Forensic photography

Bell K. Identification and documentation of bite marks. *J Emerg Nursing*. 2000 Dec; 26(6): 628–30.

Olshaker JS, Jackson MC, Smock W. Forensic Emergency Medicine. Lippencott Williams and Wilkins, 2001.

Henham AP, Lee KA. Photography in forensic medicine. *J Audiov Media Med*. 1994 Jan; 17(1): 15–20.

Pasqualone GA. Forensic RN's as photographers. Documentation in the ED. *J Psychosoc Nurs Ment Health Serv*. 1996 Oct; 34(10): 47–51.

Pasqualone GA. The importance of forensic photography in the emergency department. *J Emerg Nursing*. 1995 Dec; 21(6): 566–7.

Sheridan DJ. Forensic documentation in battered pregnant women. *J Nurse Midwifery*. 1996 Nov–Dec; 41(6): 467–72.

Smith J. Digital imaging: a viable alternative to conventional medico-legal photography. *J Audiov Media Med.* 2001 Sept; 24(3): 129–31.

Wright FD. Photography in bite mark and patterned injury documentation – Part 1. *J Forensic Sci.* 1998 Jul; 43(4): 877–80.

Wright FD. Photography in bite mark and patterned injury documentation – Part 2: A case. *J Forensic Sci.* 1998 Jul; 43(4): 881–7.

Colposcopy

Obstetrics and Gynecology Clinics of North America. Wright, CV. Contemporary Colposcopy. W. B. Saunders Company. March 1993. Volume 20, Number 1.

Adams JA, Girardin B, Faugno D. Adolescent sexual assault: documentation of acute injuries using photocolposcopy. *J Pediatr Adolesc Gynecol.* 2001 Nov; 14(4): 175–80.

Mears CJ, Helfin AH, Finkel MA, et al. Adolescent response to sexual abuse evaluation including the use of video colposcopy. *J Adolesc Health.* 2003 Jul; 33(1): 18–24.

Muram D, Arheart KL, Jennings SG. Diagnostic accuracy of colposcopic photographs in child sexual abuse evaluations. *J Pediatr Adolesc Gynecol.* 1999 May; 12(2): 58–61.

Palusci VJ, Cyris TA. Reaction to videocolposcopy in the assessment of child sexual abuse. *Child Abuse Negl.* 2001 Nov; 25(11): 1535–46.

Sommers MS, Fisher BS, Karjane HM. Using colposcopy in the rape exam: healthcare, forensic and criminal justice issues. *J Forensic Nurs.* 2005 Spring; 1(1): 28–34.

Quick Reference Pages

Forensic photography

- A separate consent is required for medical or forensic photography in most states.
- Choose a neutral, non-reflective background for the image.
- Check that the batteries are charged and that the film is not expired (if applicable).
- Have a measuring device at hand, preferably an AFBO no. 2.
- Use the same unit of measurement in your written description as are displayed in the image.
- Remember to take an I.D. photo of the patient.
- Remember to sign and date the images.
- Document in the medical record that photographs were taken and to whom they were given.
- Photographs should not to be placed into the evidence collection kit (SAECK). They should be placed in an envelope, stapled to the chart where they become part of the medical record.
- Colposcopy can be a very powerful tool, but some degree of training is advisable before undertaking its use with patients who have been assaulted.

Remember, the objective of a photograph is to provide clarification, not add confusion!

Regardless of the exact type of camera in use, it is important to be very familiar with the equipment at the facility where you work. You should also be familiar with the policies and procedures at your institution and the laws in your state as practice and requirements will vary from place to place.

Index

abandonment, 139

abdominal injuries, 19–20

ABFO. *See* American Board of Forensic
    Odontology

ABFO No. 2 device, 271, 272, 275

abrasion, 8, 196, 279

Abu Ghraib, 192, 221

abuse. *See also* child abuse; elder abuse; ethnic
    minorities, abuse of; intellectually
    disabled people, abuse of; intimate
    partner violence; mentally ill people,
    abuse of; neglect; sexual abuse
    cultural definitions of, 174–176, 178, 190
    economic, 76–77, 138, 151
    emotional, 75, 76, 139
    peer, 151
    as public health issue, 150
    religion influencing, 176, 180

acupuncture, 175–177

adaptive device, constraint of, 151

adolescents
    PEP assessment of, 58, 71
    pregnancy test for, 58
    sexually active, 54
    STDs and, 55

adult protective service (APS), 139,
    141–143

agricultural workers, 250

AIDS. *See* HIV/AIDS

alcohol, in DFSA, 52

alternative medicine, 174–177

American Board of Forensic Odontology
    (ABFO), 10, 271, 272, 275

American Professional Society of the Abuse of
    Children (APSAC), 42

anal/rectal examination, 44–45

anal swabs and smears, 120

aperture, 266–267

APS. *See* adult protective service

APSAC. *See* American Professional Society of
    the Abuse of Children

asphyxia, research regarding, 26

assault. *See* sexual assault

asylum seekers, 194–196

asymptomatic eosinophilia, 212

Australia, 195, 256

ayurvedic medicine, 177

azithromycin (Zithromax), 56–57, 72–73, 123

back injuries, 205, 254

bacterial vaginosis (BV), 50, 56–57, 72–73

beds, falls from, 22–24

Behavioral Science Consult Team (BSCT), 221

belt mark

benzodiazepines, 103

bite marks
    documentation of, 9, 272–275
    evidence collection of, 119
    as physical abuse, 9–10, 119, 272–275

blood-letting, 174

blood sample, 122

body diagrams, 116, 266

body injury map, 84, 85

bone scanning, 208

bone scintigraphy, 20–21

brain injury, 18, 210